THE ROLL MODEL

A Step-by-Step Guide to Erase Pain, Improve Mobility, and Live Better in Your Body

by Jill Miller

Victory Belt Publishing Inc.

Las Vegas

With deepest gratitude for my husband, Robert, who saw me as a "Roll Model" for my students, encouraged me to bring my work to the world, and helped me create a business that empowers people.

I wrote this book while pregnant with my first child, Lilah Iris Faust. She was my muse, she filled my dreams, and she is now a loved and loving manifestation of my commitment to self-care healthcare.

May you live peacefully and playfully in your body forever and ever.

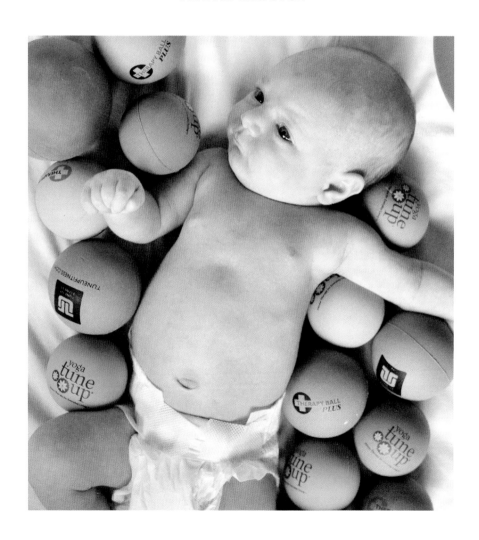

Everyone has a doctor in him or her; we just have to help it in its work. The natural healing force within each one of us is the greatest force in getting well.

–Hippocrates

The doctor of the future will give no medicines, but will interest his patients in the care of the human frame, in diet, and in the causes and prevention of disease.

–Thomas Edison

Movement is life. Life is a process. Improve the quality of the process and you improve the quality of life itself.

–Moshe Feldenkrais

Table of Contents

ROLL MODEL SUCCESS STORIES

Foreword

by Dr. Kelly Starrett

When you finally get to meet Jill Miller in person, you begin to understand what people mean when they say someone's eyes shine. To be more exact, her eyes burn brightly as if lit by a great and wondrous fire. And they do. For Jill has discovered a great secret about us all: that we all have the innate capacity to heal ourselves. She knows that each of us has the right and real ability to rid ourselves of pain and the terrible, self-made shackles of our own immobility.

Have you ever read the fantastic novel *Narcissus and Goldmund*? What? When you are searching for an appropriate metaphor to describe Jill as the brilliant teacher she so clearly is, you don't reach for an esoteric Hermann Hesse novel? Indulge me for a moment and I'll elaborate. You see, *Narcissus and Goldmund* is about two young best friends who take radically different life paths toward enlightenment and ultimately self-knowledge and understanding. One chooses a seemingly ideal, straightforward, formal, and literally cloistered path. Narcissus (whose name is not to be confused with a narcissistic personality) clearly knows his life path and purpose. His contemporary, however, lives a more ragged and uneven life as an adventurer gypsy-poet. He is slower to self-awareness and is filled with terrible self-doubt and the need to discover his own compass, which he does, beautifully. They end up in the same place at the end of their lives, of course, having taken radically different paths. This is one of my favorite points of the novel and serves as a backbone of my Jill Miller/Hermann Hesse metaphor.

When you encounter Jill and her work for the first time, you are struck by the profound feeling that she has always known how to do what it is she does—that from the moment she opened her eyes, she was on a Narcissus-like mission to change the lives of the people she met with her teachings. And yet that carefully crafted, step-wise grooming of skill fails to account for her incredible Goldmund-like commitment to self-discovery, self-improvement, experience, and humility. Let's be honest: Jill is just about the oldest soul you or I are ever likely to encounter. Jill is empathy and experience meets hard-fought clinical expertise and ability. She is the embodiment of Hesse's two heroes.

One of Jill's favorite sayings is "We have to seek out our bodies' blind spots." This could sound like a throwaway quote in a book about self-healing and self-treatment. But when you realize that it is delivered by a powerful teacher with the life experience and mad skill to back it up, you'd better listen well and believe it. And it was under these circumstances that I first met Jill Miller. A mutual coaching friend set us up and claimed the encounter would be like two long-lost siblings reuniting after being separated at birth. True fact. And when she highlighted areas for me that were being neglected in our care in the highest domains of sport, like down-regulation, diaphragm and breathing efficiency, and pelvic floor dysfunction, I realized immediately the truth of what she was saying. Common practice and base knowledge to her was literal gold to the thousands of athletes, soldiers, and average moms and dads we work with.

One of the things I regularly write about and say in interviews is that as modern humans, we are not the first people to have taken a crack at both improving and solving the problems of the human condition. On the contrary, I'm sure that for as long as there have been people, we have been taking our best swing at fixing ourselves. For example, my wife and I were traveling for work in Korea recently (Juliet, also my business partner, is the co-founder and CEO of San Francisco CrossFit and MobilityWOD.com) when we found ourselves in a small, very traditional neighborhood in the old part of Seoul. On a sidestreet vendor's table was a pile of horns and bones. In two seconds I knew what they were for.

When I called Juliet over to see, even she recognized that pile on the table for what it was. It was a pile of homemade hand-scraping tools to treat fascia, junky tissue, and adhesions. When we picked them up and starting scraping ourselves, the elderly Korean woman was delighted that we knew what was up. People have always known what is up. We just don't always connect the dots, revamp old concepts, or innovate based on what we have already learned.

Whenever I find myself addressing initiate clinician providers or fledgling physicians, I always ask them if they have a movement practice. Usually everyone in a room full of healthcare providers nods that of course they "exercise." But when I probe, it turns out that very few of them actually have a regular movement practice that has participants express all of the positions and physiology of which their bodies are capable. What do I mean? Running is exercise, and Pilates is a movement practice. Biking is exercise, and CrossFit is a movement practice. Swimming is exercise, and yoga is a movement practice. We believe that much of the orthopedic dysfunction we encounter in our physiotherapy and human performance coaching practice results from people either not having a movement practice or exercising like fiends in poor positions and in narrow ranges of motion.

These points are crucial to understanding both Jill Miller and the impact of this book. Jill is a yoga expert. Even if you don't understand the impact of the previous sentence, know that her master-level knowledge of yoga means that she understands how the body actually moves and functions. And here is the second point to be made. Jill has been able to translate and innovate upon very tried and very effective practices that are as old as yoga itself. **That means this book is full of function-oriented self-treatment practices based on solid movement foundations, and very real and actionable solutions to physiological problems.** This book isn't about "press and guess." This incredible work is a virtual medicine cabinet for self-treatment. You'll untack common pain ailments of the low back, neck, and ankle, and you'll also improve complex

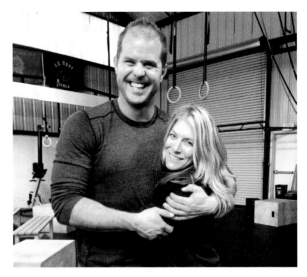

Kelly and Jill, known to one another as Kibbles and Bits.

functional disorders like asthma and pelvic floor dysfunction.

You are pretty brilliant at your normal life. You are a machine when it comes to your career, family, and hobbies. The problem is, most people have no idea how the body works or how to fix it when it breaks, or is about to break. Don't underestimate the significance of this book. **Jill has put forth one of the great works of public health of our time.** And here's the rub. As a modern human forced to sit, who's mostly inactive except when you try to exercise, you can't afford not to understand the basics when it comes to addressing your pain and dysfunction. You are Narcissus in your life, but you have to be a little Goldmund when it comes to understanding how you have the power to begin healing yourself.

If you are already familiar with Jill's work, then you are finally holding the textbook that explains the models and methods that enable her to teach so many people to effectively solve pain and dysfunction. If you are an athlete, you will discover performance blind spots that will unlock hidden athletic potential. And if you are holding this book and reading about Jill Miller for the first time, then you are holding a literal guidebook about how to reclaim your full, pain-free, and extraordinary humanity. Roll on!

Introduction

The US has 4.6 percent of the world's population and consumes 80 percent of the globe's painkilling opiate supply.*

As the daughter of a doctor, I was brought up to believe that pills and specialists could fix whatever hurt you. I now understand that this is a lie. And I'm on a mission to change the way you think about pain "management."

Collectively, we have come to rely on some*one* or some*thing* outside of ourselves to solve our physical ailments. Yes, in certain severe cases, your only chance for survival is an outside intervention, but a majority of our pain issues are self-treatable and, more important, preventable. Why is medicine the first resort? How did our consciousness shift from self-reliance to dependency? When did we, as a society, give our power over to the medical community?

I am here to tell you that *you* have the power to self-heal many of the aches that you might otherwise pay someone else to manage. The power is yours; it always has been and always will be. The work you're about to discover in these pages has helped people get off pain meds, avoid costly surgeries, relieve anxiety, and bring life back into body parts that had lain dormant for years.

You are designed to be a self-healing organism; you just need some basic knowledge of how your body is put together and a few tools to help keep it well oiled. This book provides both: some easily digestible education on the miracle that is the human body and an outline of how to use some simple tools to keep that miracle in tune. You'll learn to treat your own aches and pains with a new medicine cabinet that contains no prescriptions and comes with no side effects and no loss of dignity. Inside your new medicine cabinet is your own empowerment and (forgive my pun) *a new pair of balls.*

My childhood medicine cabinet was quickly and easily filled with prescription drugs for every fever, infection, or flu. In fact, I took so much penicillin for chronic strep throat that I developed an allergy to the drug. (I'll save that journey for another book!) Thankfully, my illnesses were never life-threatening, and I was one of those lucky kids who managed to escape childhood without breaking a bone or doing significant physical harm to myself (but keep reading and you'll learn how I chose to damage myself in other ways). The last time I had stitches, I was 2 years old. As the years roll on, I can rejoice in the fact that I have never been hospitalized for an injury** and rarely spend a day of downtime due to aches, pain, cold, or flu–quite an accomplishment considering that I travel to teach nearly two weeks out of every month.

You may be thinking that I live in a protective bubble, but I don't. I am simply the queen of self-care. This doesn't mean that I carry hand sanitizer in my purse at all times, nor do I spend thirty minutes every Saturday with a face mask and cucumber slices on my eyes. It doesn't mean that I avoid certain situations, people, or activities. It just means that I place a high priority on tending to the stresses that accumulate in my body before they take root and manifest as pain, "accidents," or illness.

You could say that I'm pain averse. While it's not always easy to avoid certain catastrophes that happen to everyone at one point or another, so much of our pain is preventable. And my mission is to provide you with the information and tools you need to keep pain at bay and let your body thrive and perform at its optimal level.

I am here to teach you a new standard for day-to-day living that's even simpler and less messy

* L. Manchikanti and A. Singh, "Therapeutic opioids: a ten-year perspective on the complexities and complications of the escalating use, abuse, and nonmedical use of opioids," www.ncbi.nlm.nih.gov/pubmed/18443641

** I have, however, been hospitalized for another devastating issue; find that story on page 386.

than flossing your teeth. You don't have to let the nagging pain in your neck remain there. You don't need to continue getting cortisone shots for your funked-up shoulder. You don't need to spend five days in bed each month because your back "went out." You don't need to let plantar fasciitis persist for eleven months. You don't need to depend on drugs to manage your fibromyalgia or your sciatic pain.

You are about to get your power back. You are about to stop chasing after doctors and thera-pists to diagnose and fix you. You are about to stop reaching into your wallet to pay for the next "quick fix" that will take your pain away. You are about to keep your money in the bank. You will learn how to live comfortably in your own body. And you'll be doing it yourself, with no need for a middleman. You have the ability to fix yourself and interrupt the downward spiral of pain, dys-function, and loss of pleasure in your life. You are about to become a "roll model" to yourself and to others living with pain.

If you've picked up this book, you are hungry for change. Nothing has eradicated your pain. Aches and pains cycle through you like injury whack-a-mole. Just when you've tamped down one twinge, another one pops up, and then another.

If you've picked up this book, you are no longer progressing in your workouts or your athletic endeavors, and you're looking to take it to the next level.

If you've picked up this book, you've tried other self-treatment methods, but they haven't fully addressed the foundational issues that imprison your pain or dysfunction in your body and mind.

If you've picked up this book, you know the emotional devastation that pain brings into your life. You feel a total loss of control, hopelessness, and the prospect of aging quickly in your broken-down body.

If you've picked up this book, you've attended or seen one of my Yoga Tune Up classes, videos, seminars, or webinars or worked with an instructor, coach, trainer, or therapist who introduced you to the famously effective Therapy Balls, and you want to know more.

If you've picked up this book, you've seen a friend, colleague, or relative transform his or her life with two grippy, pliable balls, and you want to know how to do it yourself.

Congratulations! You've picked up the right book. In just a few pages, you'll be on your way to pressing the reset button on your life and becoming a Roll Model.

What you'll find in these pages is not just a how-to for using the Roll Model Method and the Therapy Balls, but also information about why they are so helpful. You'll read real stories from real people who have changed the course of their lives by using these tools. Some of them have worked directly with me, others have worked with our worldwide team of teachers, and others have simply used our products or YouTube videos and gleaned a few basics. The stories are inspir-ing beyond imagination—these folks have liter-ally *taken life by the balls* and conducted their own healing in the privacy of their own homes, on their own time, completely self-directed and empowered. You'll read stories of people who have reversed chronic pain and disease, dumped medications, sidestepped surgeries, healed from emotional trauma and violence, broken national sports records, and triumphed in spite of odds and obstacles.

Who I Am and How I Can Help

I was an inactive child. I played with dolls, read books, and stayed indoors. I skipped first grade and was a year younger than all the other kids in my class, so I constantly used my intellect to prove myself. I was a studious smarty-pants, wore thick glasses, and aspired to be a microbiologist. Because of my completely sedentary junk food-filled childhood, I weighed 100 pounds by the time I was 11 years old. At 4'9", I was chubby and got teased all the time. I never could have predicted that my life's mission would be to teach you how to "Live Better in Your Body," or that my mantra would be "Movement Is Medicine."

My father's specialty is infectious diseases, and some of my earliest memories are of leafing through his anatomy and medical books, looking at pictures of diseased bodies and decayed anomalies of the human form. They have fascinated me for as long as I can remember. Some of my other early memories are of my mother, gasping for breath when severe asthma attacks took hold of her. She was frequently rushed to the hospital, unable to breathe. There was nothing scarier than being with my mother while she struggled to inhale. I also remember massaging her to help her relax. She would "tip" me, and I loved making the extra money as much as I liked knowing that I was helping her breathe better. My father's work in medicine and my mother's helplessness set the stage for my primal drive to help others live better.

At age 11, I found fitness and yoga. At the time, we lived off the grid in Santa Fe, New Mexico. We didn't have TV and instead relied on Betamax videos to entertain us. My mom brought home the latest fad: the *Jane Fonda Workout* and Raquel Welch's yoga videos. We practiced them together for a few weeks. She gave up, but I became obsessed. The videos were the perfect stimulus at the perfect time for me. They became my best friend and babysitter, and they changed the course of my life. I dropped 35 pounds by the time I turned 12 and was clearly no longer chubby. Instead, I swung to the other end of the spectrum and soon became anorexic. For the rest of my teen years, I struggled with weight, self-worth, body dysmorphia, and bulimia.

Every teen goes through a rebellious phase. Some do drugs, others run away. I took it out on my body through exercise and food.

Even though I was studying yoga, eating a vegetarian diet, and becoming fanatical about every calorie I put in my mouth, I knew that I was not okay mentally. I surged ahead with my eating disorder even though I knew that I was acting weird with food. I was so aware of my issue, in fact, that I studied it while hiding it from my parents; my bedside books included texts about anorexia and bulimia. I was fascinated by these eating disorders while I hid my shame from the world. By the time I went to college, bulimia was a weekend ritual for me. How I managed to hide it in the dorms at Northwestern University I'll never know.

During my freshman year of college, I happened upon an open house at a local shiatsu school. This ancient form of Japanese pressure-point massage was certainly not on my to-do list as a busy coed, but when the teacher touched me during a demonstration for the group, I felt completely at peace for the first time ever. It soothed my racing mind, halted the progression of time and space, and gave me a reprieve from worrying about my body. I promptly enrolled as a work/study student. I needed to chase that feeling of bliss. Nothing in my life had touched me so deeply, and I needed to learn this art inside and out. I felt the potential for real healing, but it was still not quite within my reach.

My shiatsu studies complemented the dance training I was doing at school. It also seemed to swirl into a greater body dialogue with the yoga, Pilates, and Feldenkrais studies I was engaged in as part of my quest to overcome my eating disorder. And yet even with all this conscious movement, I still struggled with bulimia.

I studied theater in London during my junior year. My bulimia was out of control. Looking back, I don't even recognize myself. A friend and I spent a free weekend in Paris. I hadn't thrown up the entire weekend, but on the train ride back toward the English Channel, I binged on a bag of pastries and then tried to throw up in the bathroom of that moving train. I was on my hands and knees on a dirty floor, over a disgusting commode, and nothing would come out of my pastry-filled stomach. I thought that if I ate some more, I might be able to make it happen. So I went back to my seat with blood-red eyes, ate some more, and then tried again. Nothing worked. I was stuffed and broken. It was on that grimy bathroom floor in the middle of France that I knew I had hit rock bottom. I could go no lower. The only way out was up, and I would have to confront my demons if I wanted to heal.

Meeting My Mentor and Finding My Path

While I found little comfort in being back at college, my next and most definitive step toward healing my inner wounds occurred through my shiatsu school. They connected me to my turning point: a job at the Omega Institute for Holistic Studies.

The summer between my junior and senior years of college, I worked at the Omega Institute in Rhinebeck, New York. Omega is a holistic playground for adults that offers continuing education in everything from human potential to alternative medicine, art, yoga, and bodywork. The campus is an idyllic paradise nestled in the woods, adjacent to a lake. I lived in a tent all summer and worked in the sundries store, selling to participants and faculty: flashlights to Deepak Chopra, alarm clocks to Ram Dass, shampoo to Rosanne Cash, breath mints to Iyanla Vanzant, and sunscreen to Phil Jackson and Eckhart Tolle. It was a utopia for me. I met hundreds of people who were into talking about their addictions, their processes, and the progressive therapies they were practicing to heal.

It was at Omega that I met my mentor, Glenn Black, a human movement, yoga, and BodyTuning* specialist. Glenn's knowledge of human embodiment, yoga, movement, massage, and meditation make him unlike any other teacher I have ever met. Even twenty-three years later, I still have not met a teacher whose journey, practice, and experience surpass Glenn's. He got

under my skin at a very early age and helped me see through my own blindness. He gave me my first non-shiatsu-style massage and taught me his hands-on massage techniques and, over the years, just about everything he knows about movement, breath, and meditation. His work changed my heart and the course of my life. I owe him a debt of gratitude, especially since, during my first summer with him, at age 19, my need to throw up vanished. Forever.

As I learned to tune into what I was really craving in my heart and soul, my bulimia dissolved, and I was on the road to recovery. I began teaching others the movements that soothed me, strengthened me, and helped me know myself better. Glenn taught me how to see issues in tissues, and I shadowed him while he gave sessions to his clients, often assisting during BodyTuning treatments.

During these sessions, Glenn's potent combination of bodywork, yoga, and innovative movements worked on every single person we

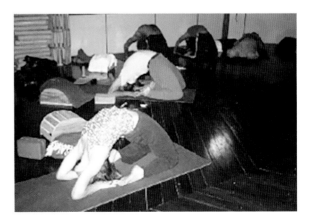

---

* BodyTuning is a style of orthopedic medical massage created by Shmuel Tatz, a brilliant physical therapist in New York City (www.nyphysicaltherapist.com).

saw. Whatever aches or pains a client walked in with, she walked out pain-free. Glenn was able to locate the genesis of imbalance in a person's body, fix it with his hands, and then teach the person exercises that reinforced the newfound ability to move without pain. He did the same for me, changing the way I walked, stood, and breathed. I had ingrained some bad body habits from years of running improperly, dancing daily at school, and pushing myself beyond normal ranges in yoga. I was obsessive about exercise, and luckily he intervened at a time when I was metabolizing massive emotional and structural change. It was the perfect prescription to launch my life and climb my way toward health. Among the thousands of gifts he gave me, the greatest was opening my ability to "see" postural issues in people's bodies—and to think creatively to help them help themselves. He taught me to become a body whisperer.

I continued to train and apprentice with Glenn for four years and amassed countless hours of teaching, observing, and building hands-on skills. I assisted him with his classes and his sessions with private clients. We had a very old-fashioned mentor/apprentice relationship—what I like to describe as "wax on, wax off," à la *The Karate Kid*.

For my own professional development, I made a big move and left for Los Angeles. Glenn wasn't there to work on me when I hurt. There were no eyes as keen as his to help me make corrections and connections. Without his watchful eye on me, I fell off the wagon at age 23. But this time it was not about abusing food; instead, I discovered Ashtanga and flow yoga.

These classes became a double-edged sword for me. My yoga practice became my refuge, but also a place to hide from deeper psychological suffering while trying to start a new life. The stress of being a 20-something in a new city inflamed my fears and awoke my inner demons. I was running from voices inside me that told me I wasn't good enough, pretty enough, or sexy enough and that I needed to try harder and be better. I abused yoga the way I had abused food. It was self-flagellation. I dove into practices that tore my body from end to end. I was always the most flexible student in class, and teachers *loved* using me as

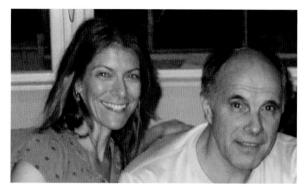

My longtime mentor, Glenn Black, and me in Los Angeles, 2011.

a body demo. I allowed myself to be compacted, twisted, and wrapped around like Gumby's child, and I paid a price for it. I remember waking up at age 24, unable to straighten my knees when I got out of bed. I walked to the bathroom like a woman whose kneecaps had been knocked out with a hammer. Although I was swinging my own hammer, I was in denial about pushing my body beyond its safe limits. I was a yoga junkie. I had to once again reckon with my addiction and work my way out of the emotional pain that I thought I had conquered—and now the physical pain I was creating from compulsive over-stretching. This addiction was destabilizing nearly every joint in my body.

I visited lots of different body therapists and never could find one who helped me the way Glenn had. So I started experimenting with self-treatment, along with every tool I could get my hands on, trying to find a way to replicate the hands-on work I used to receive from him. I used the corners of couches and countertops, sticks, foam and wood rollers, dog toys, gadgets galore, and, yes, dozens of different balls. I was on a mission to become completely self-reliant and put into practice the mentoring I'd absorbed from Glenn.

I also realized that the movement-based training I had learned from him was much more in line with who I was than the yoga practices I was now studying. So I began to teach classes in order to continue to practice movements and processes that I knew were healing for me. And it just so happened that I brought my balls into class. First, I'd see what worked for me, and then I'd introduce those tools and techniques on a wider scale in my classes. My classroom became a well-known self-care laboratory, and it was astounding to witness the results my students were unrolling. This book is filled with many of their stories!

My students always commented that my teaching was not like the yoga they were familiar with. My classes and workshops were a combination of self-massage, embodied anatomy lessons, and conscious corrective exercise, and students from all walks of life came to resolve their aches and pains. My open-minded students uncovered movement issues that had been body blind spots for them. These blind spots were destined to create additional pain or injury, and my classes helped get their bodies back on the path of physiological balance. I taught from my experience, sharing the movements and processes that had healed me emotionally and physically and gave my body a feeling of strength, precision, and connectedness. I continued to push the boundaries of what was possible in a yoga or fitness classroom, and I started a new movement. No one was doing this type of work in groups. I was breaking through walls of formality and class structure that had clearly been obstacles in the past. My self-care fitness therapy format was born, and I settled on the name Yoga Tune Up®.

EMBODY: *To willfully, tangibly, and consciously participate in the physical cognition of oneself and one's body parts.*

ANATOMY: *The study of the structure and parts of the body. From the Greek word* anatemnein, *which means "to cut up." "To cut away" –Gil Hedley*

EMBODIED ANATOMY: *A process of heightening one's self-awareness of the body as an integrated and interrelated tool for mapping the experience of the body's parts, physiology, and sense.*

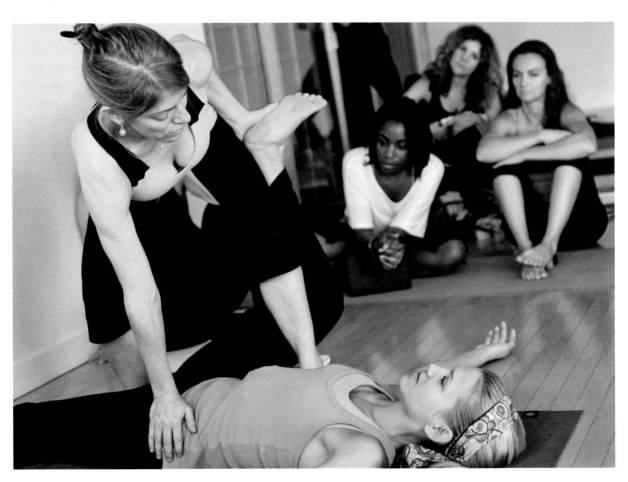

Poses Are Not Pills:
Yoga's breaking point, and why I chose to Tune Up and go "balls out"

Yoga, in a broad sense, seems to be endowed with the allure of being an "ancient healing art" just because it is "ancient." But the reality is that our bodies today are intensely sedentary and have adapted to a completely different lifestyle than the bodies of the pre-industrial world. The art form of yoga had unfortunately done some damage to many of the students who came to my classes to "Tune Up." I saw so many broken bodies enter my classroom from popular yoga formats that hid behind historical myth and mystical anatomy. Undereducated yoga (and fitness) teachers were pushing people through sequences of repetitive motions that were not being performed with biomechanical accuracy. *When you repeat movements with bad form over and over again, your body eventually breaks.* My classroom became a sanctuary for those students and their teachers to get honest about their bodies' limitations.

Although my format was called Yoga Tune Up, my classes soon started to attract personal trainers, massage therapists, Pilates masters, fitness infomercial superstars, and medical professionals as well as athletes, actors, and dancers. I talked straight human biomechanics as opposed to the Sanskrit found in most yoga classes. My classroom was a welcoming environment for anyone who was truly ready to reckon with their physiological imbalances and wanted to unlearn the habits that had gotten them into trouble in the first place.

Eventually I found professionals in other body arts and science spaces: physical therapists, chiropractors, anatomists, pain medicine doctors, and fascia researchers who welcomed my inquiry and influenced my creative development. (Learn more about fascia in chapter 4.) Soon thereafter, my teacher training programs were born, and educators, fitness professionals, and those seeking an embodied understanding of anatomy found a home in my coursework. They felt empowered to speak out about what they saw going wrong in their movement-based communities. All of them felt that there were missing links between some of the conceits that their fields represented and the day-to-day realities of their clients' healing processes.

Sadly, there is a global issue that many in the fitness community overlook or ignore. The easy sell of "weight loss" or "fast results" drives people and dollars toward unhealthy biomechanical practices. Students flock to classes and trainings because of these lures, and studios, gyms, and clubs repeat exercises and drills that fail to address foundational imbalances, weaknesses, or postural faults. Students walk in with bad posture and aches and pains, then work out in a way that reinforces their poorly coordinated blind spots, unknowingly perpetuating their imbalances. Their workouts set them up for further weakness and injury until one day their bodies give out. This is not a dig at any specific format or method, just a statement that embodied anatomy is a fundamental part of training that any teacher or coach working with human bodies should learn. Memorizing moves or choreography is, in my opinion, far less helpful than developing an understanding of functional human movement and using that lens to educate students.

I have taught at many conferences and conventions with rooms full of movement educators. When I ask them where a certain muscle is, they can point to it on a chart, but they are often unable to locate it within their own bodies. This disconnect is unacceptable. What kind of modeling are they offering to their students? It is not okay for movement educators to overlook the inner workings of human anatomy; they must take control of their own self-care and body habitats to be better examples of fitness and health for their students. Anatomy is not a concept that lives in your head; it is the matter that minds your body. *To not know your way around your own body is to lack self-knowledge.* We have lost our way inside our own skin. We are dissociated and *disembodied* from our own structures. Our collective reliance on others to take care of our own basic needs cripples us, perpetuates our dependency on drugs and doctors, and is simply disempowering.

But this body ignorance goes far beyond the fitness community. *Everybody* needs to have a basic understanding of how to hold oneself to maximize health and minimize damage. Along with that, you need a basic toolkit that helps you find and then fix the "issues in your tissues." You need to stop behaving as though posture, breath, movement, and lifestyle don't matter to your overall health. We as a society need to stop reacting to issues and move toward proactively treating ourselves.

It may sound daunting, but you do not have to be an anatomy expert to fix yourself. It really is as simple as flossing your teeth, which I hope you do on a daily basis for personal hygiene. While the book includes lots of pictures of muscles, bones, and other anatomical goodies, you don't need to memorize them or even read those pages if anatomy isn't your thing. Most of the Roll Models in this book are just folks who somehow found their way to the Therapy Balls, were provided with a little bit of instruction, and let their bodies tell them what they needed. They rolled with their own intuition and transformed their painful conditions.

The process of becoming embodied is simple. Start here:

1. **Be aware of your posture.** Alignment matters. Keep your head over your ribs, your ribs over your hips, and your hips over your ankles (more on this in chapter 3).

2. **Recognize that everything in your body is interconnected.** Your fascia provides the living seam system and soft-tissue scaffolding for your body. This means that quite often, the root cause of a pain in your low back is probably not going to get fixed if you just address the musculature of your low back (more info on fascia in chapter 4).

3. **Value your breath; it is a highway to your brain and mental health.** Your breath is observable and trainable and can be changed instantly, so breathe deeper and more frequently (more on this in chapters 7 and 9).

What Is the Roll Model® Method?

The Roll Model is a simple self-treatment method that teaches you to use a variety of grippy, pliable rubber balls to eradicate your aches and pains and reform your body from the inside out. The Roll Model Method helps you identify your body blind spots: those areas of your body that are catalysts for pain and injury. These areas are overused, underused, misused, abused, or totally confused and need to be felt, seen, and heard by you. What you don't see inside your body can and will hurt you unless you skillfully integrate your blind spots into your global movement patterns.

One of the greatest causes of aches, pains, and degeneration (all part of the larger category of musculoskeletal disorders and diseases) is a lack of total body awareness. I have found fail-safe ways to help people from all walks of life and of all fitness levels find and heal their body blind spots. My techniques awaken your body sense and heighten your awareness of your own tension, pain, and coordination. This body sense awareness is called *proprioception.* Your body relies on proprioception to move through space in a coordinated way; it's like an inner GPS system to help you navigate your way through your own tissues and the world around you. Proprioception exists because of specialized nerve endings peppered throughout your body. These nerve endings are found in deep joint capsules, in the surrounding muscles, in the multiple fascial layers within muscles, and in the fatty tissues underneath the skin. (For more on proprioception, see chapter 4.) The tools used in the Roll Model Method interrupt your destructive movement cycles and demand that you become accountable for the way you carry yourself.

My mission is to help you get to know your body better. You'll do so by using a combination of corrective exercise, breathing strategies, and specialized tools like the Roll Model Therapy Balls to help you locate, assess, and fix your body blind spots. Improving your body's sense of itself will help you make better positional choices no matter what tasks you tackle. When your proprioceptors are not firing correctly, you become poorly coordinated *and* injury prone.

Most people know their way around the streets of their hometown better than they know the map of their own body. But this is a teachable skill. All of the fitness programs that I've created, including the Roll Model Method, Yoga Tune Up, and Coregeous, are built around proprioception, as it is the foundation of self-care. Whether you are an elite athlete, you are a yogi, you are just starting a movement program, or you have a chronic neurological disease, understanding how to map your body so that you can find and heal your body blind spots is critical to good posture and, more important, to a long and healthy life.

MUSCULOSKELETAL DISORDERS AND DISEASES

The Centers for Disease Control and Prevention defines musculoskeletal disorders as "injuries or disorders of the muscles, nerves, tendons, joints, cartilage, and disorders of the nerves, tendons, muscles and supporting structures of the upper and lower limbs, neck, and lower back that are caused, precipitated or exacerbated by sudden exertion or prolonged exposure to physical factors such as repetition, force, vibration, or awkward posture."

Musculoskeletal diseases include osteoarthritis, osteoporosis, rheumatoid arthritis, fibromyalgia, connective tissue diseases, neuropathies, inappropriate bone growths, and too many others to list here.

It's in Your Hands

You have enormous potential for healing yourself and fixing the issues that plague your tissues. I believe that it comes down to simple body behaviors that are often overlooked as causes of aches, pains, dysfunction, exhaustion, and emotional unrest. How you stand, sit, walk, and breathe has a ripple effect throughout your entire being. Every move you make should be an attempt to normalize the tissues of your body so that they are strong and balanced enough to hold you in good posture within optimized positions. Optimized positions are the ones that put the least physiological strain on your body, which is especially critical when you load yourself with weight or move rapidly.

Without good proprioception, it's easy for your body to become complacent. Instead of progressing in health, your body begins to regress, injure easily, and manifest a constant stream of aches and pains. Look around and you'll see necks, spines, hips, and feet in all manner of incongruent positions as "baseline" postures. Watch the folks ahead of you in line at the grocery store, constantly shifting their weight from one hip to the other, finding "balanced" positions that unknowingly overload certain tissues while weakening others. (For more on posture, see chapter 3.) Your skull, ribcage, and pelvis and the spinal bones connecting them are shaped harmoniously by nature. But when you interfere with their sense of poise, the soft tissues that stitch these bony structures together (ligaments, tendons, and fascia) are overshortened or overlengthened with excessive tension, becoming compromised and dysfunctional. This results in soft-tissue imbalances, trigger points, and pain.

// *Our lack of movement input is slowly suffocating us on a cellular level. Motions that used to be incidental to living (read: occurring all day long) and cellular loads that used to be built into everyday life have been doled out–to computers, machines, and other people moving on our behalf. There is no way to physically recover the specific bends and torques, no way to recreate one hundred weekly hours of cell-squashing in seven, and no technology, at this time, smart enough to override nature. Illness is typically looked at as physiology gone wrong. I assert here that in most cases, our physiology is responding exactly as it should to the types of movement we have been inputting. Instead of thinking of ourselves as broken, we should recognize our lack of health as a sign of a broken (mechanical) environment.* //

–Katy Bowman, *Move Your DNA*

Your posture follows you like a shadow. Believe me, you don't want it skulking around like a ghoul. A slumping posture negatively affects your breath, digestion, heart rhythm, and nervous system. Your trunk and ribcage are often the weakest links, so it's no wonder that back pain is the largest health complaint besides the common cold. Your ribcage houses the most primal physiological muscular tissues in your body: the dome-shaped diaphragm and the heart that sits atop it. Wherever your ribcage goes, your diaphragm and heart follow. Fuel your body with a sense of its posture, and you'll honor the way nature designed you.

As a fitness and yoga professional with a background in massage and dance, I was lucky to have teachers who mandated extensive warm-ups and self-care. After all, as a teacher, I am the poster child for my own methods and practice. As the creator of the successful Yoga Tune Up format, I am blessed to be in high demand, and my travel schedule is brutal. I lead more than fifty trainings, workshops, conferences, and retreats a year, all over the globe. All this travel includes multiple press appearances and video shoots–and maintaining a fantastic marriage and family to boot! I also mentor more than 300 Yoga Tune Up teachers and am in constant development processes with my company, Tune Up Fitness Worldwide. I marvel at the fact that I get only one or two colds a year, rarely have muscle aches and pains, and manage to get eight hours of sleep most nights. I am in the driver's seat of my own stress levels at all times. I can let my tasks overwhelm me, or I can apply my own brakes by taking excellent care of myself. Happily, the practices that I teach are exactly what keep me in tune. My movement medicine cabinet keeps me sharp and "on the ball."

Now it's time for *you* to get the ball rolling, onto your feet, and then into the first of many inspiring stories of genuine Roll Models.

Break in Your Balls: Play Footsie

By now, I bet you're itching to sample the sensation of the balls. Hopefully you've got a couple of Roll Model Therapy Balls on hand. I recommend using the Original Yoga Tune Up Balls for this "ball break-in session." (They are available for purchase at www.tuneupfitness.com.)

If you've never rolled before, or if you're working with brand-new balls, the nicest way to break them in is by smushing them under your feet–giving yourself a nice foot massage at the same time! The 26 bones of your feet will appreciate being massaged and mobilized by the grippy, pliable rubber of the Roll Model Balls. Your feet take a beating from footwear, pavement, and posture (for more on posture, see chapter 3), and relieving them precipitates a relaxation ripple effect throughout your body.

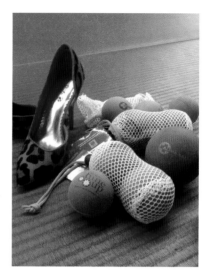

The sequence below is very simple, and you are welcome to expand on this basic outline as your feet desire. There are detailed foot sequences with more exact cues later in the book (beginning on page 194), but I want you to "play ball" now so that you are empowered to experiment as you read further into these pages.

PLAY FOOTSIE:

Remove both balls from their Snug-Grip Tote and place them on the floor near a wall or a chair. Place your hand on the wall or chair to stabilize yourself.

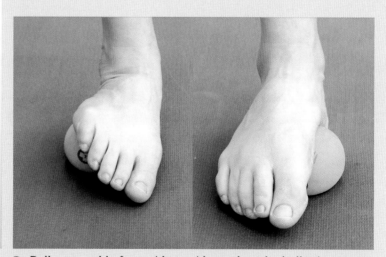

1. Stand with one Original Yoga Tune Up Ball under the most arched part of your instep.

2. Roll your ankle from side to side so that the ball crisscrosses and massages the arch of your foot. Repeat 10 to 20 times.

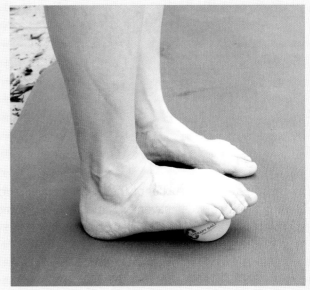

3. Move the ball to your heel, smush your heel into the ball, and briskly rub your heel with as much force as you can from side to side 10 to 20 times.

4. Place the ball at the base of your toes, keeping your heel on the floor, and allow the bones of your foot and toes to drape over the ball. Roll the ball from side to side 10 to 20 times.

5. Roll the ball up and down the length of your foot 10 to 20 times.

Now take a brief stroll and feel the difference between your feet. Then switch feet, grab your unused ball, and play footsie again!

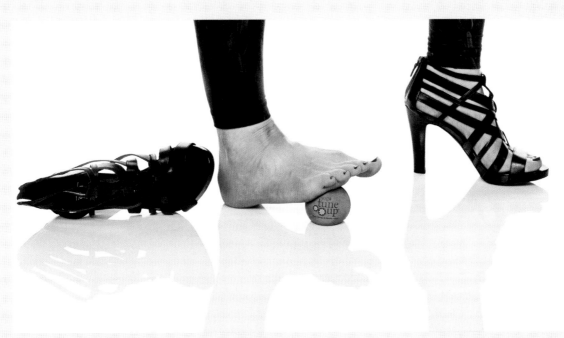

If high heels are killing your feet, try healing your heels with some ball therapy!

Healthcare Reform Begins in Your Own Body

Diane "V" Capaldi, 51
Entrepreneur, Business Owner,
Social Medicine Reformer
Venice, California

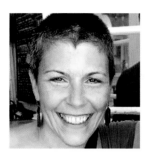

In November 1986, at age 23, Diane "V" Capaldi woke up one morning with a strange tingling sensation in the toes of her left foot. As an aerobics instructor and a respiratory therapist, she knew her body well, and knew that something was up. A few days later, her car broke down during a snowstorm, and she was forced to walk half a mile home in deep, heavy snow. As she walked, she could feel the numbness in her toes traveling up her left leg. Within a day, she had lost all sensation in the left side of her body.

Initially, doctors diagnosed an inoperable brain tumor. But V didn't think the tumor diagnosis was right. After traveling to New York for an MRI and a spinal tap, she received the correct diagnosis: she had multiple sclerosis. With MS, a person's immune system attacks his or her own myelin, the sheath covering the nerves in the brain and spinal cord, which creates scarring and damage not only to the myelin covering but also to the nerves themselves. This brings on a host of physical symptoms that vary massively in severity and onset from person to person.

"To be honest, I threw a big party!" exclaims V. "Because it wasn't a brain tumor, so it wasn't a death sentence. I knew what living with MS might be like, and that it wasn't going to be easy, but it was a better alternative than death."

Multiple sclerosis is categorized into four symptomatic phases, each increasing in severity and duration. V was diagnosed with the first phase, called relapsing-remitting MS, in which symptoms flare up for a period of time and then either partially or entirely disappear.

V learned to pay attention to the small warning signs that an attack might be coming—fatigue, tingling, her mind racing. The MS would take whatever it wanted without rhyme or reason, and she never knew what was going to be next. She would be driving and suddenly see triple out of her left eye and double out of her right. Or she would try to get out of bed in the morning and collapse to the ground. One day she woke up completely blind in both eyes, which lasted for a terrifying three days. Her arms and legs would jump and twitch, she couldn't walk, and she would experience the "MS girdle"—"like someone hugging you to death."

From 1987 to 2001, V endured seven violent flare-up periods. She also developed a constant burning sensation in her arms and began to suffer from rigidity (sometimes called spasticity), another common but debilitating MS symptom. Her muscles would seize up in a painful contracted state, holding her body hostage in immovable armor. While eating, V's throat would go rigid, which made every meal a minefield of possible choking hazards. Repetitive motion triggered her hand rigidity, which meant that she couldn't perform regular day-to-day activities like typing, shaking hands, or driving a car. One particularly terrifying incident happened while driving her 4-year-old daughter home from school, when her hands froze on the steering wheel and she couldn't get them off.

In 2001, V was pronounced legally disabled and required a permanent live-in helper to manage her life. She could no longer drive, walk her dog, cook, or clean her own house. But the real hardship was being unable to write calligraphy cards, play piano with her daughter, or even cuddle, because she couldn't turn her head to talk intimately with a partner. She could dress and feed herself, but that was it.

V had become a successful entrepreneur, but in 2001 she had to stop cold. Her condition quickly stymied any attempt to retain a job. Never one to complain, V kept the disease invisible from those around her. She was isolated from friends and family and began to feel that her disease had become her life partner, swallowing up her every waking moment.

Throughout the ordeal, V never permitted herself to feel depressed or angry, but for V, this was never an option. After fifteen years of watching her body deteriorate, her neurologist finally asked V, "When are you not strong? When do you let yourself get angry about this?" But for V, fighting the disease is her emotional outlet. "The less likely I am to succeed with something, the more motivated I am, so succeeding over my symptoms is my release. I don't ever say uncle."

V became a board member of the National MS Society, lecturing and raising funds all over the United States. She signed up for trials of every new MS drug that came on the market. Eventually V was taking twenty-four different medications daily, some for almost twenty years. She took drugs for the rigidity and the MS girdle symptoms, Provigil for narcolepsy (because of her fatigue, she was constantly falling asleep), interferon for her immune system, heart muscle-strengthening drugs, hormones, allergy medications, antacids, laxatives, blood pressure medication–the list went on and on–and then more drugs to manage all the side effects. She went to physical therapy religiously, had bodywork done, and practiced yoga when she could, determined to slow the progress of her disease.

But beneath it all, V had a nagging fear that could not be quieted. People with multiple sclerosis are the second largest and the youngest population placed into institutions, a possibility that horrified her. V's illness had progressed to phase two, in which symptoms remain relatively constant, suggesting that she would end up bedridden. Her quality of life was rapidly declining, and there was no indication that the downward spiral was going to stop or even slow. "I was

told that nothing good was going to come my way, and I just had to hope that it was a slow progression. I was an exemplary patient, I did everything I was asked and more, but it didn't make any difference.

In 2006, V moved from Philadelphia to Venice, California. For years, she had been running through her hard-earned savings on home healthcare and insurance premiums. V refused to consider living out the rest of her life in an institution, and the specter of homelessness loomed over her for years.

V continued with her healthcare regimen nonetheless, and in 2009, at a weekly physical therapy session, she saw a flyer for Yoga Tune Up teacher Trina Altman's classes. V and her therapist, Dr. Dawn McCrory, were intrigued by the possibilities of the Roll Model Method and began to play around with the Therapy Balls. V had used foam rollers and other self-massage implements, but they just aggravated her condition. The Roll Model Balls felt different–like real healing could occur. Something about their texture and the way they molded into her body tapped into both her tissues and her psyche.

V started with her tight chest muscles (pectoralis) and her upper-shoulder and neck muscles (levator scapulae) and was amazed at how quickly they responded and softened under the Therapy Balls. She was inspired to work on her tight, tough hands, so Dr. McCrory came up with a few different techniques, and V started rolling the balls between her fingers and into her palms. She could hear them breaking up tough adhesions that had developed from years of lack of mobility. It wasn't long after the success with her hands that V began to use the Therapy Balls on every part of her body. Dr. McCrory was thrilled with her patient's quick results, and even though she is admittedly "yoga averse," she promptly signed up for my certification training and has been incorporating Yoga Tune Up techniques into her therapy prescriptions ever since.

V developed a new strategy, focusing her healing on her diet, a steady yoga practice, and use of the Roll Model Balls. The end result is nothing short of miraculous: over the past five years, she has gotten her hands and, by extension, her life back. The Roll Model for V has not just been about recovering from injury or going back to a sport or pastime that she had to give up; it has enabled her to live on her own again and be self-sufficient. She used to wake up and allow whatever symptoms she was feeling to determine her day. Now, she listens to what her body is saying and rolls on the balls for thirty minutes–all three sizes, depending on what her body craves–to ease her pain, remove rigidity, and get her body ready for activity. Because of the nerve symptoms, certain parts of her body, like her calves, are extremely sensitive, so she sometimes starts in one area with the ALPHA Ball to warm it up before switching to the smaller, more precise Original Yoga Tune Up or PLUS Balls. Even when she feels like she can't walk, V pins an Original YTU Ball under her foot and feels sensation returning.

For a woman who only a few years earlier could barely dress herself, simple things like walking the dog, cooking meals for friends, and even cleaning the house fill her with joy, pride, and profound gratitude. "I mean–I can file my nails again!" she says with delight. The left side

of her body has regained sensation, which she also attributes to her adherence to a strict Paleo diet created by Dr. Terry Wahls, a fellow MS sufferer.

V's dexterity has improved so much that she has begun chronicling her story of food and movement as medicine. She cooks mouthwatering meals for herself, has a popular social media following under the name "Paleo Boss Lady," and recently published a cookbook. All this was unthinkable just a few years before she discovered the Roll Model. Years of muscle rigidity have evaporated, and her self-sufficiency is completely restored. "I used to see it as me against MS, but now I know it works best if we peacefully coexist," she says with a smile. "I'm 5'7", but now I stand 7'5"–I'm not a victim in waiting anymore."

Best of all, V is living almost entirely drug-free, taking only one thyroid medication. She recently earned her master's degree in community psychology, impressing her professors and classmates with her ability to type her own notes in class, and she's pursuing a PhD in healthcare reform, passionate that the incredible results that she has achieved should be made readily available to everyone living with chronic conditions.

V intends to use her hardworking hands to promote healthcare reform.

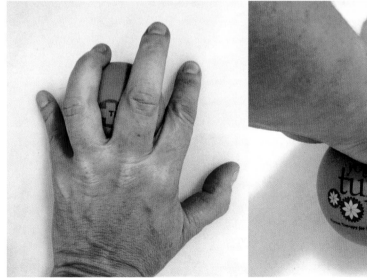
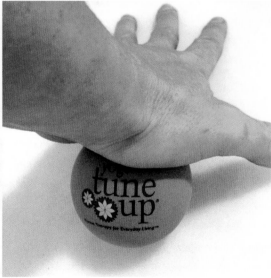

// What breaks my heart is that I'm fortunate. I get another chance, but a lot of people out there don't get this opportunity. One in three Americans will be considered legally disabled by 2018, and we're just told to live with it. But if we get them the information, they don't have to be victims of their condition. With Yoga Tune Up and the Roll Model Balls, it doesn't have to be about waiting–it's about getting up and getting moving! That's your healthcare, take control of it! The Therapy Balls cost nothing compared to the costs of the medical system, and they work for everyone across age, gender, and economic status. The Roll Model is the movement revolution. //

–Diane "V" Capaldi

1 A New Model of Self-Care Healthcare

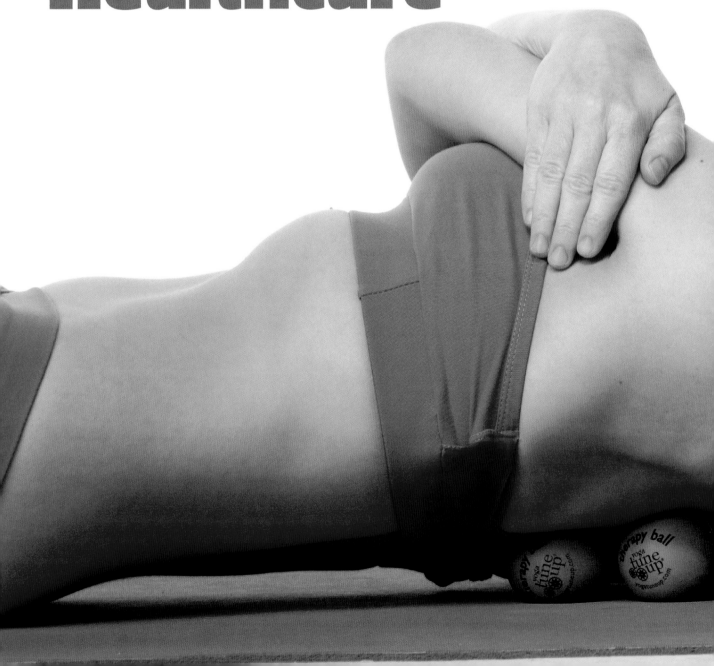

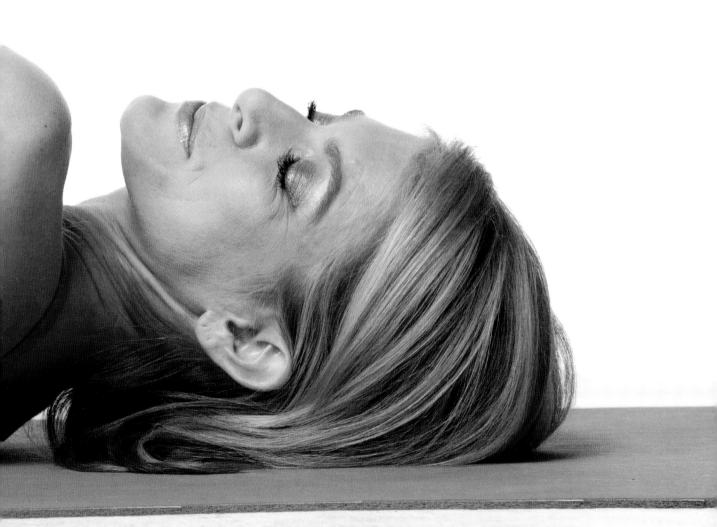

People should be able to perform basic maintenance on themselves. Whether you're sitting at the table, flying, traveling for hours in a car, or lifting your kids, you're going to be in compromised positions and you need to be able to treat yourself. It's YOUR HUMAN RIGHT.

–Kelly Starrett, DPT

I see aching people making movement mistakes constantly. All the slumping, leaning, walking like a duck, and bad breathing habits add up over time. They lead to pain, injury, and, if left unchecked, surgery, medication, and more pain. Let's put it this way:

If you _knew_ that you could prevent a disease from crippling you twenty years from now, wouldn't you do everything in your power to get on the right track and avoid the triggers that result in that disease?

Whether you are a top athlete who wants to improve your performance, a new mama with sore shoulders, a chef suffering from back pain, a vet with hardware inside your body, or a yogini with constantly sore hamstrings, the treatment is the same. Dysfunction is dysfunction, and the human body is the human body. Whether you're doing downward dog, pressing a barbell overhead, or lifting a laundry basket, the issues in your tissues need comprehensive, integrated strategies to restore optimal performance so that you can do what you want to do, better and pain-free.

For the most part, musculoskeletal injuries and diseases—including wear-and-tear on your joints, osteoarthritis, bone spurs, stenosis, osteoporosis, fractures, and more—are *entirely preventable*. If you *know* that wearing high heels hurts your feet by the end of the day, why do you continue to abuse the twenty-six bones, thirty-three joints, ligaments, nerves, and soft tissues that form your foundation? Do you think that you can buy a new pair of feet like you would buy a new pair of heels? It's time to take responsibility for what you are doing to yourself mechanically.

You already know what the consequences of a daily junk food binge would be, so you likely avoid or minimize that behavior. But the majority of people are bingeing on junk movement habits that are slowly whittling away at the integrity and functional ability of their bodies. (Find examples of "junk movement" habits in sitting and standing on page 88.) In this book, I give you tools to take care of your soft tissues in ways that you would normally find only inside the sanctum of a clinic or doctor's office, which also comes with considerable expense.

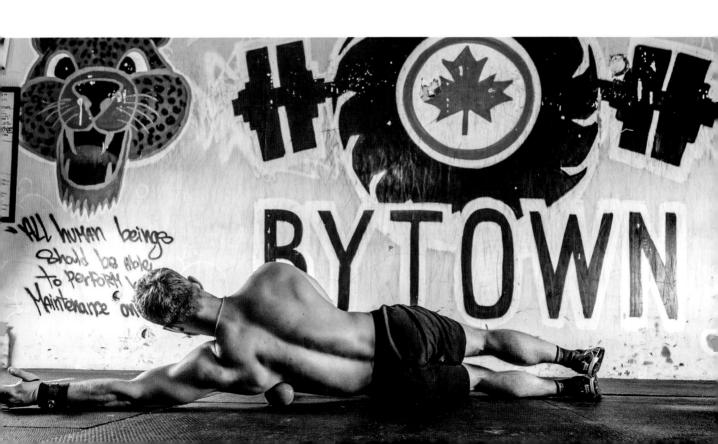

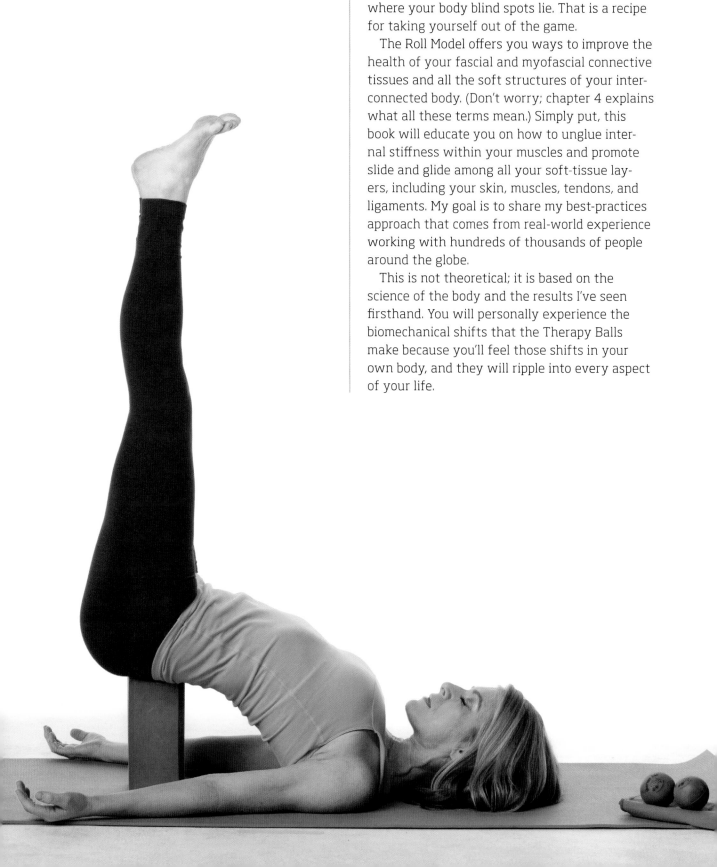

It's just not okay to ignore your pain or push your body to its limits without discovering where your body blind spots lie. That is a recipe for taking yourself out of the game.

The Roll Model offers you ways to improve the health of your fascial and myofascial connective tissues and all the soft structures of your interconnected body. (Don't worry; chapter 4 explains what all these terms mean.) Simply put, this book will educate you on how to unglue internal stiffness within your muscles and promote slide and glide among all your soft-tissue layers, including your skin, muscles, tendons, and ligaments. My goal is to share my best-practices approach that comes from real-world experience working with hundreds of thousands of people around the globe.

This is not theoretical; it is based on the science of the body and the results I've seen firsthand. You will personally experience the biomechanical shifts that the Therapy Balls make because you'll feel those shifts in your own body, and they will ripple into every aspect of your life.

What Is Self-Care?

I've given this premise of self-care a lot of thought. As a child, it seemed there was no ill or condition that my father couldn't fix, whether it was doling out a prescription for strep throat, removing splinters from my hands, or applying Band-Aids to my knees when I fell. But as I matured and came to reckon with my own demons, I recognized that the greatest degree of healing happened when I administered my own doses of care and activated my own prevention of illness or injury. I empowered myself with my own solutions for hurt or harm and brought myself calm.

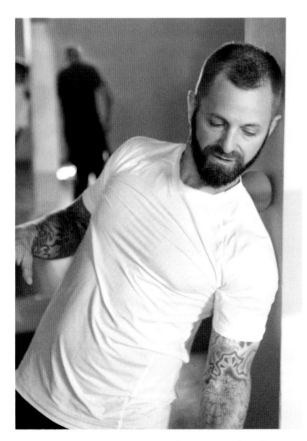

Create your own conditions for renewal and recovery. Reduce stress and treat your emotional and physical well-being in a way that restores you and resets your body's ability to function.

In my worldwide seminars, I always ask the trainees what self-care means to them. Here are some of their answers:

- naps
- meditation
- deep breathing
- massage
- walks in nature
- sleep
- relaxing
- exercise
- prayer
- creativity
- stretching
- good nutrition
- play
- journaling
- wine
- manicure/pedicure
- community/friends
- pets

Here's my definition of self-care:

"Empowering myself to intuitively and authoritatively address my needs as they arise. Reducing my pain, irritation, or emotional suffering in a self-compassionate and long-lasting way."

Whether your background is yoga, Pilates, massage therapy, personal training, sports, coaching, or none of the above, you have likely found your way to this book because you recognize the importance of adding a self-care practice that revitalizes your whole body and keeps you healthy. Eating right, getting enough sleep, and exercising correctly are not enough to keep your body in balance. A self-care practice must also include concentrated doses of relaxation, and that actually takes some skill.

Intentionally entering into states of relaxation is critical to help regulate your parasympathetic nervous system (see chapters 7 and 9). It is well known that meditation induces the relaxation response and ushers in clearer thinking, decreases stress hormones, boosts immunity, and improves emotional resiliency. Massage has similar effects, with the added benefit of improving circulation and perfusion among the internal and external surfaces of your tissues. When your tissues are clear of the cellular debris that accompanies aches and pains, your muscles function and "breathe" better on the inside. You have the power to care for your insides in the simplest and most direct way. This book shows you how.

> **PERFUSION:** *The body's process of transferring fluids, nutrients, and waste into and out of tissues and blood vessels.*

The Roll Model is your own self-care prescription that is always on call. This preventative medicine helps you by relieving stress and aches without popping an ibuprofen or downing a cocktail. You can lower your incidence of preventable disease by empowering yourself to take your care into your own hands!

How the Roll Model Therapy Balls Help with Self-Care

No one can walk a mile in your shoes. You earn your keep in your body with your dedication to maintaining yourself. Your movements can pound you down or lift you up. Thankfully, you come biologically equipped for self-healing. The Roll Model Balls are your new "rubber drug," and when you roll them into your life, they will catapult your ability to heal yourself and prevent further damage.

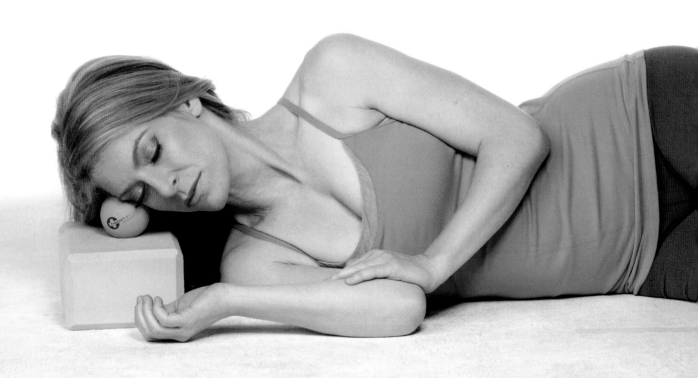

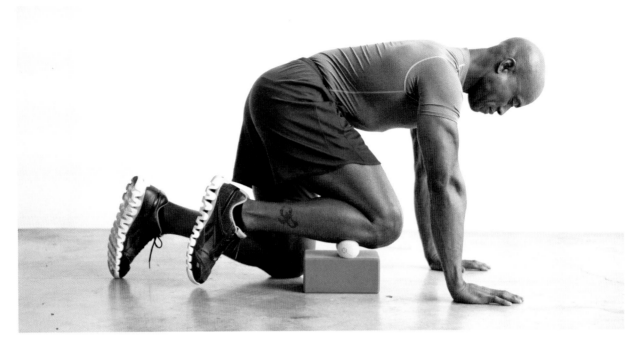

They Relieve Aches and Pains

Muscle aches and pains can often be attributed to overuse, underuse, or misuse of a particular area of the body.

- **OVERUSE:** Overuse—that is, using one muscle group more than another—can develop from a habit like being right-handed or from compensating on one side of the body while avoiding the other. For example, when standing, most people tend to lean to one side, cocking out one hip more than the other. This lean may seem insignificant, but that side of the body bears more weight, those muscles get stronger (and shorter and tighter!), and, over time, continuing to lean on that hip can cause massive imbalances from one side of the body to the other. The Roll Model Balls help alleviate these aches and pains by rolling into the overshortened muscles that have become cramped and tight.

- **UNDERUSE:** Underused body parts are perpetually ignored by your movement habits, whether in your daily life or in your expression of fitness. They are often bypassed or overlooked due to an old injury, a lack of training, a lack of sensing (see page 109 on proprioception), or a failure to realize that these tissues are needed for proper mechanics. For example, the diaphragm is your primary breathing muscle, but very few people are instructed in how to breathe so that their breath mechanics serve them in every aspect of life. Excessive tension from underusing the diaphragm (as outlined in chapter 7) not only leads to breathing problems, but also is an underlying cause of back pain, acid reflux, certain heart conditions, and more.

- **MISUSE:** So many muscles are used inappropriately. Misuse occurs when you use a certain muscle for a task and it becomes hard-wired for those movement patterns. For example, the shoulders often "shoulder" a bigger burden than necessary. Many people trap their phones between their ear and shoulder while speaking. This misuse taxes the upper trapezius and levator scapulae muscles and throws the rest of the head, shoulder, and upper back into a fury of compensation. Don't you ache just thinking about it? A better way to manage that call is to cradle your phone in your hand and bring it directly to your ear while carrying your head in good posture. Better yet, use a headset.

They Enhance Breathing Function

Shortness of breath can frequently be attributed to a lack of strength and flexibility in the respiratory diaphragm, intercostals, and neighboring muscles of respiration (see page 155). The dome-shaped respiratory diaphragm attaches to much of the inner ribcage and the lower spine. Breath muscles, like all other muscles in your body, can become rigid due to lack of use, carrying excess weight, or protecting an injury. These locked-up muscles dramatically reduce the ability of the diaphragm and ribcage to move well during "normal" breathing. And when your body is stressed, as in walking up stairs or trying

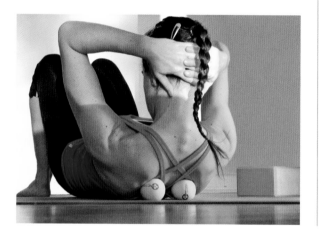

to break a personal record, a chronically weakened diaphragm has to work harder than ever to assist the breath's flow and exhausts quickly, resulting in shortness of breath and whole-body fatigue.

On top of that, when you get short of breath, panic sets in as your endocrine system floods your body with stress hormones in an effort to dilate your air passageways, speed up your heart rate, and inject your system with adrenaline. When it's working well, the respiratory diaphragm is a gateway to deep relaxation. The more your diaphragm moves, the more easily your body can relax and rid itself of that stress response. A tight and weak diaphragm leaves you trapped in a catch-22!

When the Roll Model Balls roll through the muscles of the upper back, they palpate, stretch, and knead into the chronically clamped muscles that limit respiratory flow. The balls roll and relieve the layers of muscle that tether and tie into the ribcage, which helps your spinal bones work in harmony with the underlying respiratory diaphragm. Your back muscles relax deeply and completely, and the joints of your back and ribcage become more hospitable to the respiratory muscles that are screaming to become more supple and functional.

They Increase Your Mobility and Energy Level

Unfortunately, the factors that lead to decreased mobility are often the very things that cause it to continue. When your body hurts, you don't want to move. Being stagnant makes you feel sluggish, and when you feel sluggish and in pain, you don't want to move! It's a vicious cycle that continues to weaken the body as it perpetuates poor circulation, muscle and joint stiffness, and inertia. Conscious movement is the way out of this trap!

The Roll Model Balls coax motion into tissues that are tired, achy, and "depressed on the inside." These moping muscles need to be refreshed, mobilized, and revitalized with the grippy pressure that the balls provide. The balls compress and elongate dormant and tired tissues and introduce

circulation back into the most recalcitrant areas. After a few minutes of rolling, these loosened areas will *feel* like moving and encourage you to use more of your body in everyday actions, eventually catapulting you into a more formal exercise regimen, as described in chapter 11.

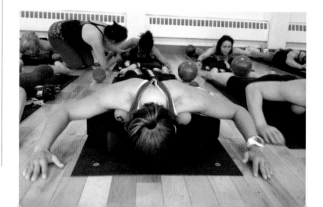

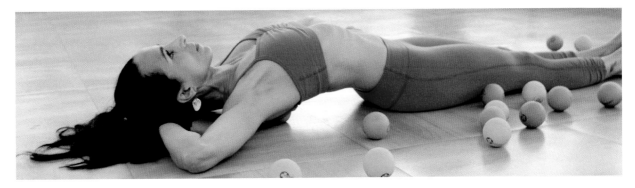

They Reduce Stress

Stress wreaks havoc on every system of the body. A chronically stressed body is stuck in the fight-or-flight response. This is a body whose nervous system is on sympathetic overload (see chapters 7 and 9). Long-term exposure to high levels of the stress hormone cortisol creates inflammation, impedes circulation, and reduces muscle function by stiffening muscles. Stress taxes your heart and breath (as described previously) and can even affect your sight and hearing! Over time, it weakens your systems and sets you up for accidents, disease, and general misery.

The Roll Model Balls induce the relaxation response and take your body into the rest/digest/recover mode of the parasympathetic nervous system. This response is the *exact opposite* of everything that happens when your body is stressed out. The balls help flip the stress switch "off" by increasing circulation and stretch wherever they are rolled. The rolling and kneading action unglues persistent myofascial restriction by unwinding knots, sticky lumps, and adhesions.

A muscle stays contracted because the nervous system is telling it to do so. Deliberate ball work coupled with a mindset of being willing to let go can alter your nervous tone. The pressure of the balls offers a micro-stretch to the tissues they touch. This recalibrates the muscle's resting length by switching off nerves that were maintaining unnecessary tension in that muscle.

And finally, this muscular relaxation helps your body breathe better, which further reduces nervousness and anxiety (see chapters 9 and 10).

They Improve Your Posture and Performance

Many of your pain issues are connected to other challenges you face because your musculoskeletal system is inextricable from the other systems of your body. You are one big integrated organism. When you begin to address one issue, quite often you will see improvement in others. Similarly, when you neglect one area of your body, you will begin to see breakdowns in other areas and in your overall health.

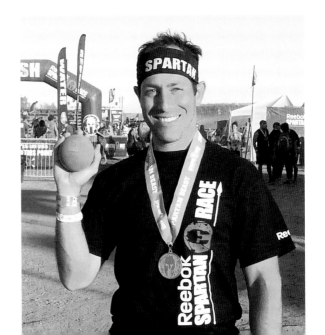

Posture issues are often caused by poor habits such as slouching, leaning, or a lack of awareness of proper alignment. They can also be caused by an accident or surgery that has left scar tissue in the body. Scars almost always lead to compensatory patterns in the way a body moves. Posture issues can also be a form of emotional expression—for example, if you are depressed or sad, your head often droops, making it harder for your back and neck muscles to support its weight. Eventually your fascias, muscles, ligaments, and bones *adapt* to your personality, and you become physically limited by your emotionally induced posture!

The Roll Model Balls will help dramatically improve your posture by loosening up muscles and connective tissues that have become locked and tight because of either a habit or a structural issue. This helps restore balance to the tissues and makes you feel better about living in your body and facilitates better alignment for the activities you pursue. When you stand and move with grace and poise, you are better positioned to take on the challenges that life presents to you! (See chapter 3 for more on the importance of good posture.)

The Backbreaking Story of a Bodybuilder Who Rebuilt Himself

Greg Reid, 51
Personal Trainer and Former Bodybuilder
Los Angeles

There's nothing average about Greg Reid. His successful bodybuilding career spanned fifteen years ("I've been picking up weights since I was 12," he says) and many championships and titles, including the Long Beach Power Lifting Championship in 1984, the Cal Gold Cup Champion in 1985, and Mr. Los Angeles in 1991. But at the height of his career, Greg walked away. As a movement purist, he was in it for the love of the sport, and he didn't want to engage in the political maneuvering that was required of him to continue to succeed. Instead, he focused his years of expertise on training clients in Los Angeles.

Now, at age 51, he has been working to improve his clients' health and fitness for thirty years. "Everybody at the gym, they know me, and they know this is what pumps my heart. This is what puts breath into my lungs," he says with gusto. His energy and charisma make his age hard to believe—he's on the floor with his clients six days a week, eight hours a day, educating their minds, bodies, and souls to move better. Fitness is not just a job for Greg—it's his life calling. Greg calls himself a "physique connoisseur," and given his long career of bodybuilding and weightlifting, it's the ultimate title, eclipsing any medal or statue on his mantel.

He's also—incredibly—been the victim of seven car accidents. So when the seventh crash happened early one January morning in 2010, Greg knew what to do. "I was driving west on Ventura Boulevard to go to a client session. As I was crossing over Coldwater, this car coming the other way made a hard left like there was nothing else going on. It smashed into the driver's-side corner panel of my car and I got spun around. All I could do was close my eyes and not get tense—and what took the brunt was my lower back."

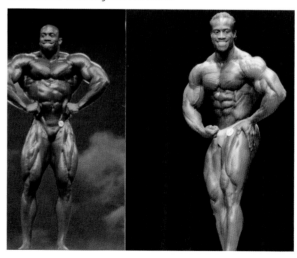

Greg at the peak of his career in 1992 and in 1994 with his top National Bodybuilding placing.

An MRI showed that Greg suffered a huge 5-centimeter bulging disc between his L-4 and L-5 vertebrae–an injury in which the soft-tissue cartilaginous disc protruded from between the bones of his spine and pressed against his spinal nerve roots, creating a condition called nerve root impingement. What it meant for Greg's body was vicious and debilitating pain. Now, Greg is an incredibly strong man who knows how to handle the kind of pain that you experience when lifting enormous amounts of weight. The man can leg press a jaw-dropping 1,700 pounds! But the pain of that effort was nothing compared with the searing pain traveling up and down his spine, and with that pain came the terrible realization that there were a lot of things he was no longer going to be able to do with his body or his life.

This was without a doubt the worst injury that Greg had ever experienced. He's a man who puts great thought into his movement and alignment, and throughout his long bodybuilding and power-lifting career, the worst thing he'd ever done was pull a groin muscle that he had to work around for a week or so. Nothing had prepared him for not only the physical limitation but also the psychological frustration he was to endure as he tried to heal from this devastating accident.

He spent about six months receiving chiropractic care, at first six times a week and then gradually dropping down to three. The chiropractor gave him therapeutic exercises to do for his spine that avoided certain twisting and side-bending movements, but he confirmed Greg's worst fears: that he should avoid these kinds of movements not just in this initial period of healing, but for the rest of his life. Even the lawyer handling Greg's case confided that he too was living with a bulging disc, and that Greg would learn to live with the limitations and the pain.

But Greg wasn't about to just "live with it." His identity was wrapped up in helping others achieve greatness, and while out of commission and flat on his back, his spirits began to crumble. It's hard to conceive your life as you know it ending because of an accident. Training others and himself is his entire skill set (well, he does make a mean BBQ sauce and is famous for his fried chicken...but that's another story). When your

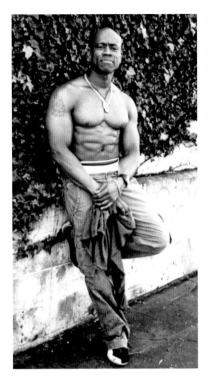

Greg lost years of sleep and happiness as he succumbed to constant pain after multiple car accidents.

livelihood depends on your well-functioning body, an accident like this is not just a setback; it's a complete life overhaul–unless you beat the odds and find a way to heal completely.

Greg continued to work with clients but had to modify how he taught them. Unable to demonstrate movements, he had to sit much of the time, which he hated. "Everybody knows I'm the guy who shows you how to do things correctly, egos checked at the door, because it's not about that. I don't ever want to ask my clients to do something that I can't do, and I want to give them my best. But there were a lot of things I couldn't do. And I would think to myself–I barely make it to 50, and this is it? In that moment [of the accident] there was nothing I could do, and now there's a ton of things I can't do. It was really breaking me down." Though the severity of the initial pain decreased somewhat over the first six months, Greg still had to go home every night, lie down on the couch with ice on his back, and try to stay positive. He continued to investigate different kinds of movements and therapies and through trial and error developed a vocabulary of what was okay versus what laid him out for two days, but he was no longer able to lift weights and had to stay far away from any kind of high-impact movement (like jumping) that had the potential to put compression into his lower back.

Greg's social life took a huge hit, too. He is an established 200+ league bowler with five 300 games and two 800 series, and he has competed at the nationals annually for the past eight years. "I was a champion bowler, and I didn't want to stop, but that summer at nationals, six months after the accident, I had a very tough time. I couldn't even negotiate how to throw the ball because just standing there trying to hold the ball radiated pain up and down my spine. I couldn't focus or concentrate; the pain totally derailed me. I'm not the kind of person who runs and gets a shot or pops a pill when there's any pain, so even taking Advil like I had to was a big deal for me."

Greg doesn't like to admit it–seven years in the Marine Corps trained him to be mentally strong–but the unending frustration of being what he calls "basically comatose" and at the mercy of pain that he couldn't control or predict, all because of an accident that wasn't his fault, left him wrestling with anger and depression. "I was so angry at what had happened, how my life in an instant was changed, but not for the better. Sitting hurt, lying down hurt, sleeping hurt. I would wake up in the middle of the night in pain. My whole body would just clench up. And this went on for years."

As coincidence would have it, my husband happened to work out with another trainer at Greg's gym, and the two had seen each other around. Greg remembers seeing a pair of Roll Model Therapy Balls that Robert had left at the gym one day and wondering, "Who left these here–and what the heck are they?" Then Greg saw Robert rolling on the balls, and his curiosity was piqued. He started talking to Robert, and their connection quickly grew. Robert showed Greg some simple techniques–how to roll the balls on his lower back while standing up against a wall–and gave him a pair of Therapy Balls to practice with, explaining that they would help break up the densely bracing fascia. Greg was suddenly flooded with a memory: he had heard about fascia many years before from a trainer who manipulated it to help her athletes build bigger muscles, but he hadn't given it any more thought until now.

Greg decided to take my Roll Model Therapy Ball training so that he could absorb everything I was teaching. He was fascinated by my descriptions of fascia and was convinced that this would be his way out of pain. Greg truly was a Roll Model, so I asked if he wanted to participate in a new DVD that I was making with Kelly Starrett. So Greg got to spend two days straight rolling the Therapy Balls over his entire body for hours on end. This intensive work jump-started his quest for self-care, and for the next six months, he rolled religiously at least three times a week, concentrating on finding deeper areas in and around his hips and lower back. He even began bringing the balls with him to the bowling alley so that he could roll between frames, amazed by the way that rolling out his lower back would stop it from tightening up.

Then, in September 2013, more than three years after his car accident, Greg had a life-changing moment. He was rolling the balls on either side of his sacrum, when an up-and-down hip movement produced what he calls "a crack and a crunch that made my eyes pop open"–like something that had been stuck for a long time was moving again. He knew instantly that this was a huge breakthrough. "When I got up I was like–I did it. I fixed myself! That all-the-time tightness and frequent radiating pain that happened because of the accident–it was gone."

For a man who has dedicated his life to what he calls "down to the bone" training, this breakthrough was a huge deal. He continued to practice rolling several times a week and was ecstatic that he was no longer at the mercy of one potential wrong move. "I've had the squat rack on my back again, I can do explosive movements again. I'm able to do side-bending movements without being tight for the next two days," he says proudly. He has even enrolled in ballet classes and is jumping again.

Greg's adoption of Therapy Ball work into his self-care routine has been wholehearted and enthusiastic. He's found that rolling the bottom of each foot for fifteen to twenty minutes causes a profound release all the way into his hips, and when he rolls his feet at the end of a long workday, he's ready to bowl at night with renewed energy and precision and, most important, without pain!

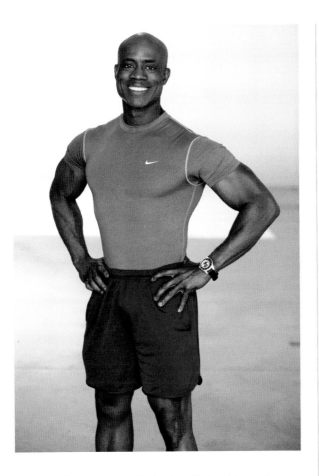

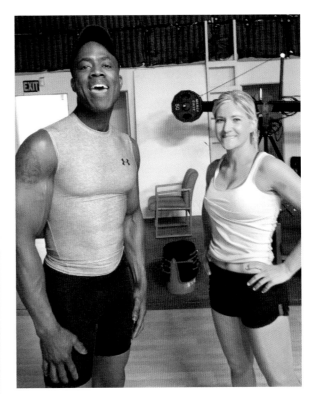

The "glistening within" Greg I know and love on the set of *Treat While You Train,* which also features our "cover girl" Roll Model, Sarah Kusch.

The results were not limited to fixing his body after the accident. His years of bodybuilding had left him with unexplained nagging pains in various places and a great deal of dense, tight tissue throughout his body. His dedication to ball work has eliminated the pain in those little niches, and his range of motion and suppleness are far more complete. He's come to understand that the movements he was doing were good for building muscle, but that to release the stuck areas that were causing pain and stiffness, he needed to talk to his fascia. "To get underneath and know where the real engine of pain and discomfort and lack of range is coming from? I feel like I won the lottery!"

Not only did the self-myofascial release from the Roll Model Balls bring an end to the pain from Greg's car accident, but they were also the missing link in the holistic self-care that he both practices and preaches. They are the tool he was looking for to improve as a trainer. He offers his lucky clients impeccable instruction on the Roll Model Balls that resculpts their physique as only

a connoisseur could. It keeps his weekly "filled to the brim schedule" of forty clients healthy, injury-free, and out of pain. He's able to walk the walk with his clients once more, leading by example of how ball work keeps his body supple and strong, even as he is growing older within what is often a young person's profession. In addition, the hands-off nature of ball work saves his forearms and hands from premature wear-and-tear. He's seen clients' movement visibly improve from their ball-rolling sessions, and this success keeps him in constant demand among the Hollywood elite.

Greg's backbreaking journey was resolved through dedicated self-care. He is thrilled to have found the missing puzzle piece. "I have been given more knowledge on how to take care of myself through the Therapy Balls. I don't know that there is anything invented that can do the work as immediately as they have done with the amount of ease, comprehension, and application. I have the keys to help my body heal itself. I don't need anything else."

Recovery and Self-Care

// An ounce of prevention is worth a pound of cure. //

–Benjamin Franklin

Constantly pushing yourself to the brink in your workouts necessitates that you give your body a reprieve from that stress. For healthy growth and healing of tissues to occur, you need to take time to create an internal environment that optimizes adaptation. In other words, if you play hard, you need to rest hard.

But stress accumulates in your body whether you run an ultramarathon or burn the midnight oil finishing a presentation. Life is stressful. As a little girl, I remember everything being closed on Sundays. You didn't get your shopping done on Saturday? Too bad! Sunday was a Sabbath for all. Now, you can shop 24/7, and many stores are even open on major holidays like Thanksgiving and Christmas.

Society is demanding more of our attention than ever. TV is constant, the Internet is always available, and cell phones seem to have no boundaries. These days, no matter what you do, it is exceptionally hard to clock out.

So what's the answer? If your work/life balance seems to tip heavily toward work, then how are you supposed to recover?

Years ago, my mentor, Glenn Black, gave me some excellent advice about managing my time and health as my career started to become insanely demanding and I noticed that I was taking care of other people more than myself. He said, "Condense your practice and magnify its effects at the same time. It should become potent like a teaspoon of orange juice concentrate versus a full glass of watered-down OJ." In other words, I needed to make every moment count and execute everything I did impeccably.

My Therapy Balls have become my go-to tools that symbolize my ability to take a time-out. Whenever I use them, I enter into a state change. The balls work swiftly and refresh me like that teaspoon of orange juice concentrate. I get immediate results when I nuzzle a Therapy Ball into my body. If my left ankle is hurting, I can

immediately make a change. On an even more global level, *nothing has to hurt for the balls to work*. They act like a sedative to help tamp down my stress response and accelerate calm into my body and mind. It's like having a glass of red wine without the calories or the wooziness.

The balls hasten recovery. Here's how:

Working out tends to leave your nervous system in a heightened state of arousal called *sympathetic overload*. In order for your body to heal and restore itself, it is vital to switch to a parasympathetically dominant state to foster cell repair, growth, and rest. (For more on this, see chapter 9.) If your muscles and their associated connective tissues are not given adequate time to rest, they are more vulnerable to tears, other injuries,

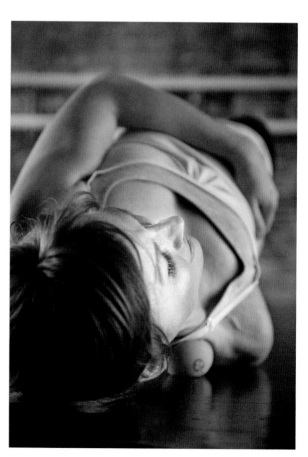

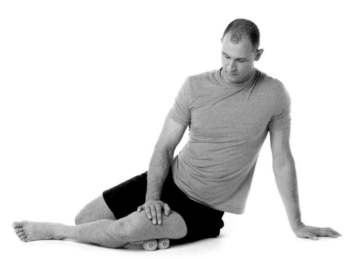

and loss of force production. That means your next workout will not give you the results you are seeking and could lead to pain and injury that take you out of the gym for *real* recovery.

Deep-tissue massage can aid and enhance recovery. In fact, a recent study conducted by Dr. Mark Tarnolposky at McMaster University proved that it takes only ten minutes of deep-tissue massage post-workout to enhance the effectiveness of cell mitochondria (the energy generators) while creating a natural pain-relieving effect and diminishing inflammation.* In other words, post-workout massage speeds up recovery and reduces pain—no Advil needed! With the Roll Model Balls, you've got your own *rubber drugs*.

The Roll Model Balls are like small rubber scalpels that help restore the sliding surfaces among the interfaces of muscles and their fascias (connective tissues). Self-myofascial massage (SMM) with the Roll Model Balls also plunges pressure and turbulence into the depths of individual muscles and helps pry apart adhesions that are commonplace when tissues are loaded with knots and trigger points. Muscles that are loaded with knots, trigger points, and adhesions are unable to fully contract or stretch. These locked-up tissues start to create dysfunctional compensation

patterns that lead to more imbalances throughout the body. Aches, pains, injuries, and diminishing returns in performance are inevitable side effects that accompany those imbalances.

Your muscles depend on nutrition to generate their contractile force. Muscles that have become locked up due to stress, injury, or poor movement patterns create an internal dam effect, where nutrients are not delivered into hungry tissues and waste products are not filtered out. This is one of the reasons why knots are tender to the touch; the inflammation locked into the tissues irritates the nerve cells within the environment of the knots, causing wincing pain. SMM is one of the best ways to help restore a correct fluid balance and perfusion to the myofascias so that nutrients and waste are distributed efficiently.

One other major benefit of SMM, particularly with the grippy, pliable Roll Model Balls, is that it helps heighten body sense, or *proprioception*. The balls take a hold of all tissue layers, from the surface of the skin into the depths of the muscle. The friction created by their grippy surfaces generates massive shear within the tissues, exciting specialized nerve cells that ultimately improve the body's mapping of itself. (Seeee page 49 for more on shear.) In short, the balls reduce pain, improve nutrient flow, and improve coordination.

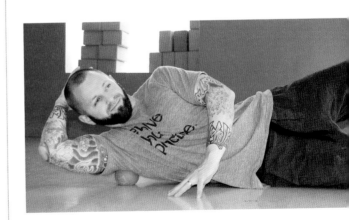

* J.D. Crane et al, "Massage therapy attenuates inflammatory signaling after exercise-induced muscle damage." *Science Translational Medicine* 4, no. 119 (2012): 119ra13. Also see www.npr.org/blogs/health/2012/02/01/146216300/massage-eases-inflammation-in-worn-out-muscles.

My Thousand-Mile Pilgrimage with Self-Care Instead of Suffering

Dear Jill,

In the past five years I have walked several different pilgrim routes across Spain and France. My first one was the Camino Frances de Santiago, a walk of almost 800km (500 miles), and I got serious tendonitis in my ankle and often suffered from shin splints. The second time, when we walked the Le Puy route, another 750km walk, I got debilitating Achilles tendonitis and had to stop walking for a couple of weeks. However, just last spring we walked almost 1000km, and I never got tendonitis or shin splints once. The difference, I believe, was the Therapy Balls.

After being introduced to this therapy in a yoga teacher training and later taking the Therapy Ball course with you in Ottawa, I decided to carry a set of Original Yoga Tune Up Balls in my backpack. At first my husband thought I was crazy to carry the extra 8 ounces of weight in my pack. I assured him that he would eventually be thankful for them because our Camino would be so much better if I didn't have to endure searing pain that would slow us down and involve whining. I also promised to share them with him if and when he got shin splints. The added weight was worth every ounce and more. Every morning and night I rolled out my feet and shins and this time never suffered from shin splints or tendonitis. We had a totally injury-free Camino, and I recommend the Therapy Balls to everyone! As a matter of fact, I just gave a little mini-workshop on the balls to a lady who is right now on the Camino, and she has emailed me that they are a blessing at the end of every 25km day.

I have advised so many other Camino walkers to include these Therapy Balls in their backpack, and every single one has come back from their trip and thanked me for the advice and the lesson in using them. They totally changed my pilgrimage: absolute miracle workers to keep your feet happy on a month-long walking trek.

Karen Hypes, 69

Retired High School Physical & Health Education and Dance Teacher

London, Ontario, Canada

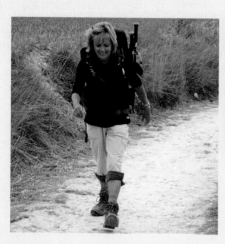

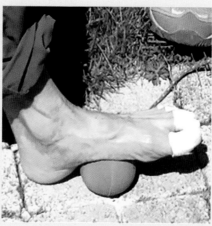

A pilgrimage implies suffering, but carrying all your belongings in a backpack and walking 30 to 40 kilometers a day is already a grind! No need to add foot and ankle injuries to the mix.

OTHER BASICS OF SELF-CARE HEALTHCARE

GO TO SLEEP TO DREAM

During sleep, your body plays out its regenerative processes at every level. If you want stronger muscles, higher cognition, less stress, and a better sex life, get your ZZZs. It's not debatable.

So many studies say that seven to eight hours of sleep a night is adequate. I know that when I fall below six hours, I cannot perform at my best, and I start to lose short-term memory, crave stimulants, and get very irritable. So I make a point of factoring eight hours of nightly sleep into my life.

I don't know many people who get *too much* sleep these days, but the ideal scenario is to have a consistent bedtime and wake time to maintain balanced body rhythms. Some people require longer durations of sleep at different times of life, depending on body growth. For example, teens need more sleep than adults, and pregnant women (growing another body!) need more sleep, too.

DRINK YOUR WATER

Water is the most prevalent component in your body. By mass, you are 78 percent water. On a molecular level, if you subdivide all your molecules into types, you are 99 percent water!* Every single system in your body relies on water to function. Keeping your fluid intake high is a necessity for health. I have seen family members develop chronic diseases from being chronically dehydrated. Dehydration affects everything from blood clotting to sperm count to saliva and sweat production. Don't cheat yourself! Drink up!

Rolling on the Roll Model Balls churns fluids into and out of your connective tissues and enhances your tissues' ability to "drink" the fluids they need for regenerative processes. Make the most of this turbulence by staying hydrated.

CHECK YOUR BREATH TO RECOVER

Proper breathing is the most underanalyzed and least popular component of recovery. You breathe 20,000 times a day. If you take these breaths while your body is poorly organized, whether you are standing, sitting, or working out, you reinforce an inefficient breathing pattern that creates layers of knotty myofascial tension in the innermost lining of your birthday suit. Imagine doing 20,000 push-ups incorrectly, every day, for a lifetime!

Deep breathing that correctly engages the diaphragm and intercostals while permitting the core muscles to stretch reflexively is critical to total body relaxation. In my practice, I consistently see clients and students who are unable to escape a faulty breathing pattern that is contributing to pain, stress, and loss of performance and joy in life. Deep breathing sets the stage for deep relaxation, and when it accompanies self-massage with the Roll Model Balls, you have a potent recovery cocktail that beats any doctor's prescription. And best of all, you empower yourself by managing your own care.

* Gerald Pollack, *Cells, Gels and the Engines of Life*, by (Ebner & Sons, 2001).

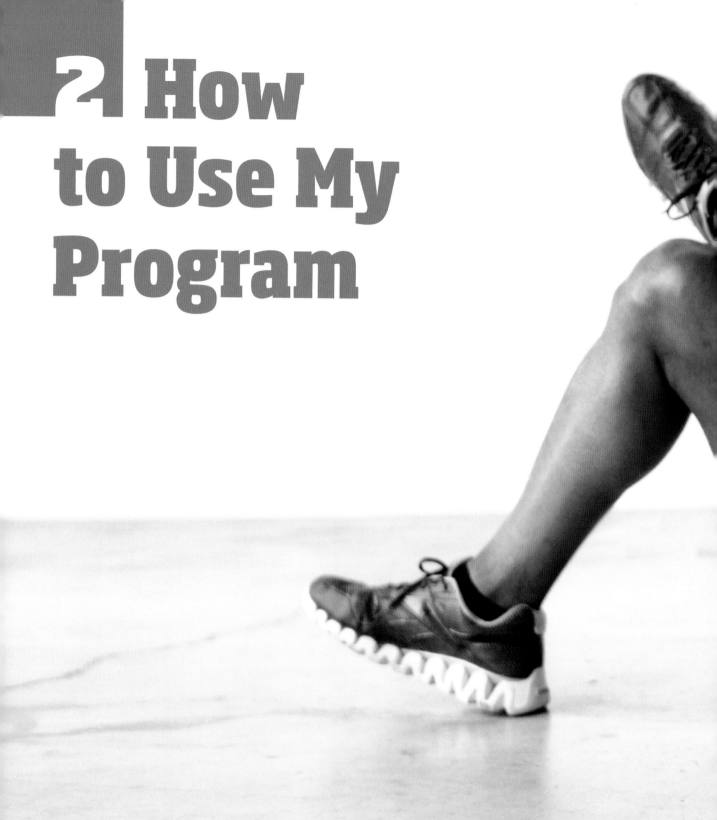

2 How to Use My Program

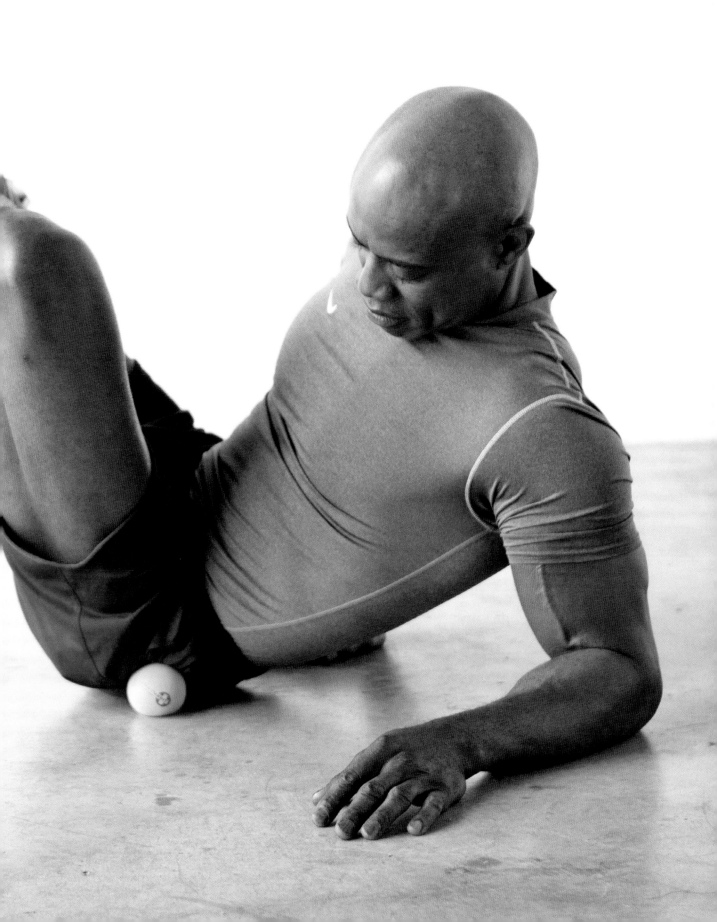

"There's a key for every door, and if you can't find it, you can make one."*

—Pharrell Williams,
singer, songwriter, mogul

The Roll Model Method helps you become a key-maker to your own pain relief. The balls transform you into a pain locksmith. You will learn how to treat yourself if you are hurting, or to troubleshoot sticky movement patterns before they blow up into issues. Taking care of your own pain is an empowering process. It doesn't mean that you have to abandon all the help and input that your therapists, doctors, and medications can provide. It just means that you make yourself the agent of action behind your own care rather than feeling out of control and at the mercy of pills, potions, and others' opinions.

As the cost of healthcare climbs, many people are turning to self-care as the most reliable and cost-effective solution. It's true, prevention is the best medicine. Don't get me wrong, rolling on balls will never replace the skills of a brain surgeon if you've had a catastrophic aneurism, and chemical-based medicines are a life-saver for many of our ills. But using the Roll Model Balls is a powerful complementary treatment for your own health, recovery, and wellness. You'll see from the stories in this book that the Roll Model program has enabled people to manage and heal a variety of symptoms, conditions, and illnesses that conventional treatments bypassed.

* Mary Kaye Schilling, "Get busy: Pharrell's productivity secrets," *Fast Company* 181 (December 2013/January 2014).

Meet your new best friends.

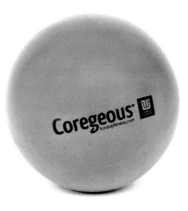

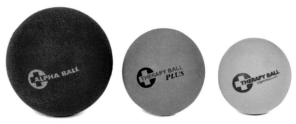

Hundreds of my students and clients were headed toward surgery because of chronic back, hip, knee, or neck pain but managed to alter the course of their lives by using the Roll Model Balls. These simple implements enabled them to reform themselves from the inside out. They remodeled their body habitats so that they were no longer accelerating their own tissues' demise. Movement is medicine, and with the correct dose, you might just save your own life and end up with more money in the bank to boot.

As the public is becoming exposed to more and more modes of self-massage, we truly are at the genesis of a new era of proactive healthcare. This book's title, *The Roll Model*, encompasses this new wave of empowered self-treatment pioneers. It is no longer acceptable to turn your body over to someone else to be treated when you can fix so much of what ails you yourself. Depending on others to fix your problems weakens you mentally, physically, and financially.

Finding Her Way Back to Normal After Breast Cancer: Sidelining Side Effects

Jennifer Jennings, 47
Part-Time Vision Therapist and Mom
Denver, Colorado

Jennifer Jennings and her three sisters grew up on a farm in Nebraska setting hay bales, feeding chickens, and taking care of a huge vegetable garden. From an early age, she developed a hands-on, no-nonsense approach to life, tackling challenges as they came and not allowing herself much room to worry about things. As an adult, she built an active life for herself, and she now lives with her husband and son southwest of Denver. They love the outdoors and go skiing, hiking, and camping whenever they can. Jennifer also played ultimate Frisbee for years and learned to swim as an adult. Her can-do attitude extended to her health: both

her mother and grandmother suffered from breast cancer, so she was always vigilant about her own self-care, religiously getting sonograms and checking for lumps, staying well on top of the situation.

After a May 2010 mammogram came back clean as usual, she was surprised to discover a lump in her breast a few months later. "It was a terrifying moment, finding that lump, and it seemed so obvious, like it was right under the skin," she says. "I knew with my family history I might get it, but I never thought it would happen in my 40s." An added painful irony: she and her husband were leaving that morning to visit her mother, who had

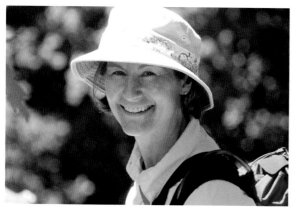
Jennifer pre-diagnosis: she has always loved the outdoors.

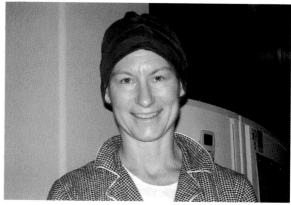
Jennifer tackled chemo and multiple surgeries at the same time.

just been diagnosed with a recurrence of her own breast cancer, fifteen years after her first diagnosis. Jennifer decided to go ahead with the visit, knowing that her mom needed help with doctor appointments and scheduling, and planned to check in with her own doctor when she got back. She hoped that the lump in her breast was just a fibroid. Given her family history, she knew in her gut that it probably wasn't, but at the time she had to concentrate on taking care of her mom, and she pushed it to the back of her mind.

When Jennifer returned home and had an ultrasound, the surgeon confirmed her growing fear that the lump wasn't a fibroid. "I knew at that moment it was going to be a tumor, and it was going to be malignant," she says. A biopsy confirmed that it was a stage 1 tumor, just over 1 centimeter in diameter. Though the cancer had not yet spread to her lymph nodes, there were precancerous cells throughout her breast tissue. Jennifer sprang into action and followed her doctors' recommended treatment plan without hesitation: a mastectomy of her right breast and chemotherapy to reduce the chance of the cancer spreading. Prior to her diagnosis, Jennifer had suffered from endometriosis and was already considering a uterine ablation due to painful periods, so on top of everything else, she decided at age 44 to have a hysterectomy at the same time.

Once the plan was in place, Jennifer's surgery and treatment happened at a whirlwind pace—the tumor was diagnosed in September 2010, and she had the mastectomy, hysterectomy, and oophorectomy in October, followed by four rounds of *chemotherapy from November through January. Then she started taking the estrogen-blocking medication Femara, as her adrenal glands were still producing small amounts of estrogen and were likely signaling her tumor to grow. The Femara would reduce the possibility of a recurrence, though it came with its own ugly side effects that she would have to manage as she took it for the next five years.*

Throughout this ordeal, the hardest moment for Jennifer was the night before her surgery. She went into her 4-year-old son's room to watch him sleep and began to cry. "He was still so young, and he wasn't really able to understand what was going on, but we were honest about it, and when he asked at one point if you can die from it, we just emphasized that we caught it early and that the doctors know what they're doing," she says. At the beginning of each round of chemotherapy, Jennifer would send her son to her sister's house, wanting to protect him from seeing his mom at the worst of her sickness. She and her husband would go for walks, timing them during the lull of her chemo side effects, so they could squeeze in some time together before she was down for the count again. They relied on their faith to get them through this dark period, as Jennifer grieved the loss of her breast and her uterus. Her husband was the director of pharmacy for his company and traveled frequently for work, so she relied on support from her neighbors—they live in a patio home community with a lot of friendly retirees and empty nesters who always rally around a family in need. One neighbor had recently gone through breast cancer herself, so she sent emails organizing food delivery to the Jennings.

But no one could help Jennifer process the onslaught of what her body had gone through and the painful, ongoing side effects of the chemotherapy and the Femara. She found the entire experience so frustrating, having built a life that she felt really good about and then having to watch that life screech to a halt, as she was no longer able to ski and hike with her family. During her treatment, she suffered from nausea, hair loss, and a metallic taste in her mouth that made her lose her appetite, along with constipation from the anti-nausea medication she was taking in an attempt to regain her appetite. Even after the chemo ended, she experienced a great deal of fatigue and brain fog (sometimes called "chemo brain") as well as nerve pain. She developed carpal tunnel and tendonitis in her elbows and forearms from reading in bed during the administration of the chemo drugs. The chemo also seemed to go after old injuries and bring those symptoms back–flaring up back pain from a sledding injury in high school, for example.

The Femara made it hard for Jennifer to sleep and added to the emotional roller coaster she was already on from the hormonal deficit that her body was suddenly dealing with. Her whole body hurt; it was reeling from the war that had been waged against her cancer. "I don't know what fibromyalgia feels like, but I imagine it's like this–my muscles were tight and I couldn't stretch well, [and] my joints ached all the time," she says. Many breast cancer patients stop taking Femara because they can't handle the side effects, but Jennifer persisted, relying on her natural toughness. She'd seen her mother live through a recurrence, and she was not willing to gamble. "There have been times that I wanted to stop taking it, but if I quit taking it and the cancer comes back–am I going to regret it?" she wondered.

During those first few months, she tried to return to simple movement, taking walks and swimming, and she did a few physical therapy sessions with a cancer specialist, but she found it hard to carve out the time to get back and forth to appointments when she was so busy with her young son. She looked for something she could do at home and found a few breast cancer rehab DVDs, but she wasn't crazy about them and didn't feel much benefit.

And then, during an online search, Jennifer came across Yoga Tune Up. She liked the self-massage aspect, as her aching body could have used professional massage therapy every week, but there was no way she could afford it. She ordered the Roll Model Therapy Balls and DVDs and began religiously rolling out her body, alternating upper body one day with lower body the next. In the beginning, she couldn't believe how tender her body felt; it was so riddled with knots, aches, and stiffness that she could barely use any pressure at all. At the same time, she experienced some relief, and that motivated her to keep at it. Her first "aha!" moment came when she was able to roll more deeply on the muscles around her armpit, shoulder, and chest, especially into her pectoralis muscles that had been affected on both sides, the right side by the mastectomy and the left by the port for her chemotherapy. When she got up and tested her shoulder range of motion, she was blown away by the difference! Jennifer has also found that the Roll Model Balls have helped ease some of the pain she felt in her

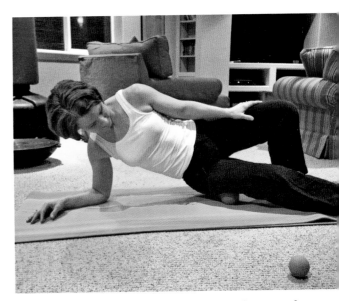

Jennifer pulls out her Therapy Balls to take care of her needs as they arise.

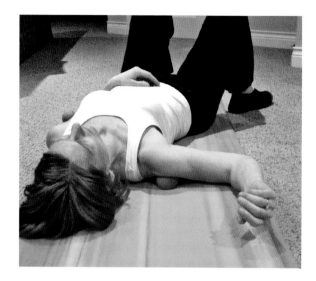

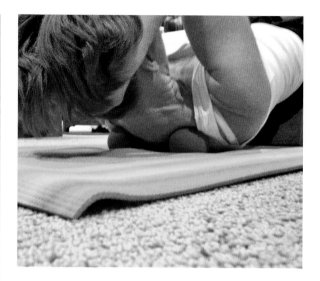

piriformis and gluteus muscles from the hours she spent lying in bed during and after chemotherapy. Her carpal tunnel symptoms and nerve pain are far more manageable, as she can apply a ball directly on whatever spot is flaring up and relieve the pain immediately. As a busy mom, she appreciates how she can split up her routine into five- and ten-minute chunks interspersed throughout her day rather than having to commit to a long class or DVD routine. While relaxing in front of the TV at the end of the day, she pulls out the Therapy Balls and rolls on whatever body part is calling out for attention. Having learned the Roll Model routines, she feels confident in her intuitive ability to take care of her tissues' needs as they arise.

Jennifer also began using the Coregeous Ball for her abdomen to help break up the scar tissue from her hysterectomy and rebuild strength throughout her core. She loves how the Coregeous work starts deep down, in contrast with old-fashioned core training that targets only the surface muscles. Her swimming instructor has noticed a big difference in how Jennifer uses her core to make more efficient strokes in the water.

Jennifer's regular Roll Model practice is both giving her more energy to get through her days and helping her manage her emotional ups and downs so that she can relax and sleep better at night. "It's that feeling of–I have cancer and it's not because of anything I did, and there's nothing I can do about it. Using the Roll Model Method has helped me hugely boost my energy for the day, even if it's just five or ten minutes of rolling. As much control as I can take back with this, I feel like I'm able to do it now with the Therapy Balls," she says.

Now, three years after her surgery, Jennifer feels that she's finally processing both physically and emotionally the war her body waged–successfully–against her breast cancer, and she can get back to enjoying her life with her family, skiing and camping like they used to before her cancer hit.

❚❚I tell people all the time–you can feel better, but you have to put the time in and do it. Recovery from the trauma of cancer and the treatment isn't going to magically happen on its own, and I may never go back to where I was, but I'm getting to a new, much improved normal thanks to the Roll Model Method.❚❚

–Jennifer Jennings

Your Movement Medicine Cabinet: What Are the Roll Model Balls, and How Do They Work?

Any object you use to knead, compress, stroke, or prod your body without breaking the skin is a *stress-transfer medium*–a massage tool that attempts to mimic the touch of another human being. Throughout history, people have used objects to rub out their aches and pains. The oldest device found to date, a Neolithic jade ritual blade from China, is thought to be from 2000 BCE. Special sticks, stones, ropes, vibrating tools, and fabrics have been used for self-soothing for generations. It seems that everything old is new again, and self-massage implements continue to be popular, slightly redesigned according to the medium of the day. In fact, there are models of vibrating chairs (easily found in Sharper Image stores today) that were in use in Greek and Roman times; the first electric version appeared in the late 1800s.*

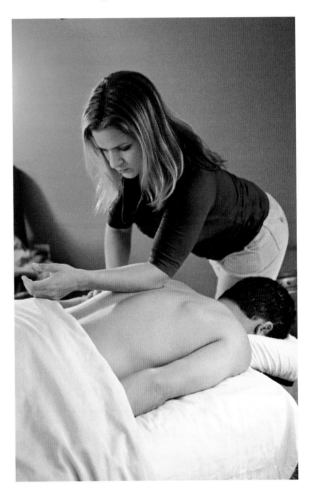

I used to think that no one and no *thing* could replace the hands of my mentor, Glenn Black. I spent a lot of money on therapists, objects, machines, and more, trying to re-create the genius touch that had established my baseline for the platonic ideal of massage. After years of trial and error, I found a ball made from the right grippy rubber coupled with a pliable density with just enough squish to tumble into all the issues in my and my students' tissues. The balls' grippiness maximizes their ability to create shear, and their pliable density allows them to conform without injuring the tissues on knobby bony prominences.

This grippiness adds a valuable component to the stress-transfer medium: it makes the balls a *shear-transfer medium*. This means that they create a lot of local turbulence in the layers of your body as soon as they make contact with your tissues.

> **SHEAR:** *A mechanical action or stress that involves using the balls to grip the skin and slide the pinned tissues in any direction, which causes motion among contiguous, connected body parts in a direction parallel to their plane of contact.*

* For more on these tools, read *The History of Massage: An Illustrated Survey from Around the World*, by Robert Noah Calvert (Healing Arts Press, 2002).

DYNAMIC IMAGING OF FASCIA AND THERAPY BALLS

My colleague Dr. Steven Capobianco is a huge fan of the Roll Model Balls. I introduced him to the balls at the International Fascia Research Congress. Luckily for him (and me), his wife, Robyn, began training with me a few months later and became a Yoga Tune Up teacher who uses the balls with her students. Together they have been performing dynamic ultrasound diagnostic imaging before and after use of the Therapy Balls. Their preliminary findings are significant and exciting:

"In analyzing before and after images using Mind Ray DP-30 musculoskeletal dynamic ultrasound, we noticed a significant difference in the space between the superficial and deep fascial layers after 90 seconds of rolling and shearing with the Roll Model Therapy Balls. One of the most significant demonstrations of this shearing effect was captured in the medial gastrocnemius. In our opinion, we believe that preparing the fascial system prior to movement can facilitate optimal tissue gliding."

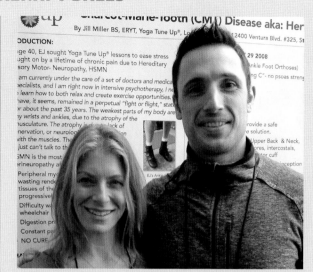

I met Dr. Capobianco at the International Fascia Research Congress in 2012.

According to Dr. Capobianco, "We can, at this point, strongly suggest that there is some fascial traction that occurs with Roll Model Therapy Ball treatment." Further studies are underway.

These images enable you to see beneath the skin.

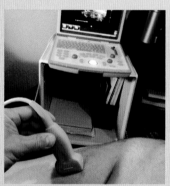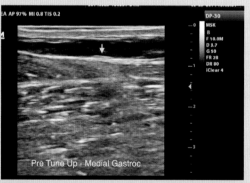

Pre Tune Up - Medial Gastroc

The inner calf is being tested.

Before Dr. Capobianco applied three different rolling techniques for a total of 90 seconds, the tissues of the inner calf show a lack of gliding potential, with a compacted appearance.

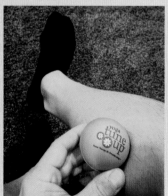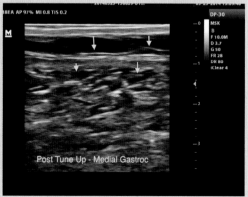

Post Tune Up - Medial Gastroc

The Yoga Tune Up Ball is rolled for 30 seconds of stripping, 30 seconds of CrossFiber, followed by 30 seconds of skin-rolling/shear.

The arrows point to changes in the superficial and deep fascia. The tissues appear off-loaded, decompressed, or what I call "fluffed," similar to fluffing a couch cushion. This may indicate an increase in slide & glide potential and mobility.

The Roll Model Therapy Balls: Your Toolkit

While the Roll Model Therapy Balls are by no means going to resolve every pain you may encounter, they provide options for handling a wide range of myofascial issues. The goal is to keep your tissues healthy so that you stay out of the doctor's office and avoid a bigger breakdown down the road.

The Roll Model Balls have three significant features that make them incredibly effective:

1. They are *grippy.*
2. They are *pliable.*
3. They are *portable.*

The balls' grippiness enables them to take a hold of your skin and the underlying superficial fascia and slide and transition it over the deeper fascias and muscles beneath. Their grippiness maximizes their ability to create shear in your tissues. This shearing effect awakens proprioceptive nerve endings that benefit your central nervous system by calming it down and improving its mapping of the area. Tools like tennis balls, golf balls, and slick rollers are unable to create this grip-plus-shear effect on multiple tissue layers at a time.

The balls' pliability creates a springy cushion as they roll up and over bony prominences. The soft rubber yields to the hardness of bone, reducing the risk of bruising, pinching, and irritation. The balls have just enough "squish" so that your bones can sink into the rubber. Because a ball can nuzzle against, tumble across, and surround bony prominences with ease, its grippiness can then grab the delicate tissues in and around bony junctions that a harder object like a lacrosse ball, golf ball, wood implement, or hard foam roller can't even find.

Lastly, the balls are lightweight and portable, so you can easily throw them into your gym bag, carry-on, glove compartment, or briefcase. They give you on-demand pain relief wherever you are.

BONUS BENEFIT: THE ROLL MODEL BALLS ARE BUDGET-FRIENDLY

The Roll Model Balls feature one last benefit worthy of mention. I love the harmony of groupings of three, but there is a fourth feature to add:

1. Grippy   2. Pliable   3. Portable   4. **AFFORDABLE**

With the Roll Model Balls, on-demand pain relief is available to you anytime, anywhere, without costing you up to $200 per session. And no messy oil or undressing in front of strangers! You won't have to wait weeks to see your doctor or file a claim with your insurance company. The balls are also much easier to "refill" than a prescription for Oxycontin. Some Roll Models even claim that the Therapy Balls are their own private health insurance.

A BASIC BALL-ROLLING MINI PHYSIOLOGY LESSON

If there is restriction or adhesion in a certain part of your myofascia, the muscle cannot function fully, and neither can the joint(s) to which that muscle attaches. Therapy Ball rolling and other self-massage techniques squeeze, knead, compress, and pry loose muscle fibers and their associated fascial tissues that have become adhered to each other. All this turbulence and beneficial commotion within the tissues increases local blood circulation, consequently bathing and ultimately rehydrating the area (known as *perfusion*).

Rolling teases apart the "sticky" or adhered parts of the tissues, thereby separating the individual fibers within the muscle so that each fiber can literally pull its own weight instead of its neighbors'. Your muscles are then better able to fully contract and release as your movement dictates. The Roll Model Balls help herd unruly tissues into better alignment with your bones so that you move with efficiency and ease.

Roll Model Ball work makes corrections and connections in tissues that daily exercise, stretching, and yoga often bypass. A Therapy Ball provides a micro-stretch into areas of myofascia that have become adhered because of damage, lack of use, poor nutrition, scar tissue, emotional holding, or other reasons. Because the ball has so much grip and grab, it does much more than just apply pressure to an annoying knot. To understand how the Roll Model Balls work so well, you must understand a little muscle knot physiology.

TRIGGER POINTS: HOW TO UNTANGLE A KNOTTED MASS

When doing the Roll Model sequences, you will often stumble across knots or clumps of adhered tissue that feel hard, unyielding, and rather painful. These are often referred to as *trigger points*. In his book *The Muscle and Bone Palpation Manual,* Joe Muscolino describes them this way:

> *"A skeletal muscle tissue trigger point is a hyperirritable focal area of muscle hypertonicity (tightness) located within a taut band of skeletal muscle tissue. Furthermore, as with all trigger points, it is locally sensitive to palpatory pressure and can potentially refer pain or other symptoms to distant areas of the body."*

Using the Roll Model Balls directly on trigger points can help alleviate those knots and adhesions, but you must also consider the perimeter tissues of the affected area. Instead of placing the ball directly on a hotspot (sometimes the pressure is intolerable), try moving the ball a bit "uptown" (above) or "downtown" (below), and begin to tease length, stimulation, and circulation into the tissues being drawn into the vortex of pain. Areas "across town" (on either side) of the trigger point may be locked into their own compensation patterns and may need a rubdown as well.

View your body as a whole, an interdependent ecosystem, because every part of you is interconnected. *Your whole body has created an environment for trigger points to form.* You need to manage your whole body, along with your breath, attitude, and intention, in addition to that specific pain point.

Size Matters

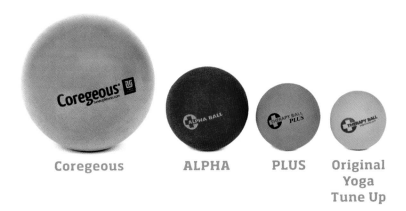

Coregeous   ALPHA   PLUS   Original Yoga Tune Up

The Roll Model Therapy Balls come in a variety of sizes to target different regions of the body for your desired pressure effect. You are always your own most trusted guide to determine which ball satisfies your own personal "kneads" and needs. Your tolerance for deep therapeutic touch will change the more you practice and experiment, and you may find yourself using many of these tools interchangeably for different effects.

All of the solid rubber balls, the Original Yoga Tune Up, PLUS, and ALPHA, come in pairs tightly secured in a Snug-Grip Tote. As you'll see in the sequences, they can be used in pairs in the tote or individually. The tote is made from a mesh fabric that allows the grippiness of the balls to reach through its fishnet cells. The mesh fabric also has its own grip to add to the impact of rolling. The toggle at the top helps keep the two balls rolling in sync when secured inside.

The largest ball is the Coregeous, which is filled with air and made of a soft, stretchy, grippy, skin-like rubber.

The various sizes and densities of the balls provide different stimuli for different parts of your body. The Original Yoga Tune Up Ball is like a thumb compressing its way into your tissues. The PLUS is similar to the pressure of an elbow working its way in, and the ALPHA is like a fist. Finally, the Coregeous Ball is like having a friendly bear paw take hold of large sheets of tissue at once, but with less depth of pressure than the solid balls.

Become familiar and comfortable with all four balls and how they feel on different body parts. You can use them interchangeably for the most part; I'll show you lots of options throughout the sequences. I'll also show you how to use the balls both inside and outside of the tote to give you even more depth-of-pressure options.

The big idea here is that you need different-sized tools to fit different parts of your body. The Roll Model set is designed to provide the most variety with the biggest impact.

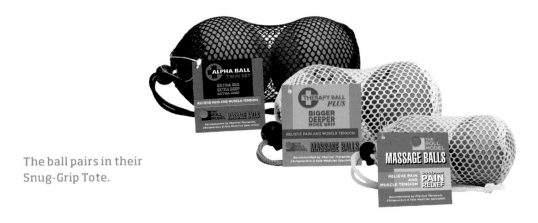

The ball pairs in their Snug-Grip Tote.

Maintain Your Balls and They Will Maintain You

New, solid Roll Model Balls are coated with a thin mist of oil that will rub off right away. To develop the grippy suede texture, scrape them briskly on your jeans or the carpet or give them a quick wipe with a towel. You'll find that they get tackier and grabbier with each use. The first thing I do to break in a ball is to smush it underneath my foot. I get a great foot massage, and then the ball is grippy and ready to go.

New balls are also very firm, but they become more pliable with use. If they feel too firm at first, try doing your rolling sequences on a wall until your body gets used to the deep pressure. The balls will soften over time. Rigorously grind and squash them with your bare feet to soften the rubber, tenderize them, and develop their pliability.

To keep your balls both grippy and pliable, keep them out of direct light, as direct light and open air will dry them out and change their texture. Store them in a gym bag or covered container. Keep the Original Yoga Tune Up and PLUS Balls in their Snug-Grip Tote when not in use; they'll be less prone to roll away.

The solid rubber Roll Model Balls do not last forever. They are made of natural rubber that breaks down over time. Depending on the ball type as well as how and how often you use them, they should last about six months to a year, though frequent foot-rolling with the smallest set will cause them to break down much faster. You know that the balls are kaput when they don't quickly spring back to their spherical shape after being flattened. Save your well-worn balls, though, as they are great to use on delicate bony prominences such as your face, elbows, knees, ankles, and feet. The tenderness of those well-loved balls is the perfect match for your most sensitive areas.

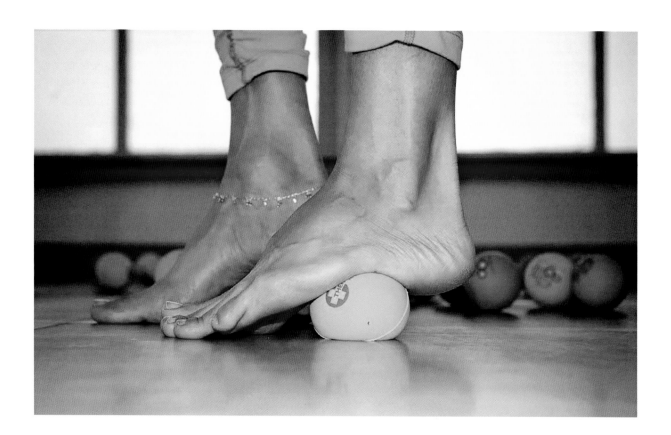

Thirty Years of Numbness Reversed in Two Weeks: Healing from Knee Reconstruction

Lori Wieder, 44

Principal, Wieder Communications Graphic Design

State College, Pennsylvania

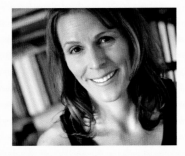

Dear Jill,

When I was 14, I had reconstructive surgery on my right knee. For a couple of years my knee had been dislocating—the patella would slip under the ligaments and over to the lateral side of my leg. Sometimes I could get it to slide back, but on two occasions I had to go to the hospital to have a doctor do it. I remember the feeling pretty vividly—weirdly, when it dislocated it was not very painful as long as I stayed very still. It was just uncomfortable, and afterward my leg would feel very weak and sore. Aside from dislocating while playing field hockey (pivoting on the grass is what did it), it would dislocate at very strange times—twice in the air while performing a dive, once while rolling over in bed. It scared me because it was such a strange sensation and it looked *awful* with the kneecap jutting over to the side of my leg.

At the time my orthopedist thought that the "looseness" of my ligaments and abnormal tracking of the kneecap were possibly due to two things:

1) I was born with turned-in feet, and at that time the solution was to put toddlers in casts up to their knees for a number of weeks (my mom can't remember how many).

2) Around age 10, I was involved in gymnastics and remember doing a backbend and hearing a lot of popping along the side of the knee. There wasn't any pain, but I remember my leg feeling funny and weak for a few days. I continued on with my activities, and the dislocations did not start until a couple of years later.

I had "physical therapy," which basically consisted of two isometric exercises. They also gave me a neoprene brace with a hole to keep the patella from slipping, but it didn't work; it kept dislocating even with the brace on. My parents were pretty stoic and reassuring since the orthopedic doc had told us he could fix it via surgery if it kept going out. And go out it did, so they scheduled reconstructive surgery. I remember the doctor talking about "tightening" the ligaments and "reworking the tracking." They also scraped the underside of the patella because there had been some wear-and-tear due to the dislocations. I know they did not do anything to the ACL (it was fine). The doctor said they did cut muscle, and I remember a *lot* of pain in the lower IT band area and outer quadriceps area for months after the surgery.

The protocol then was to be in a hip-to-ankle hard cast for six to seven weeks, then an immobilizer for three more. My leg atrophied so badly that my thigh is *still* not the same circumference as my other leg. While I was in the cast I experienced a *lot* of shooting nerve pain. The orthopedic nurses kind of blew me off for a couple of weeks, then finally the surgeon determined that the cast was too tight around the kneecap. So they cut a hole in the cast, and I remember the pain lessening.

I'm not sure if it was due to the hole they cut in the cast or if the nerves finally just went numb, because from then on I had no sensation in the skin all around the knee, and the numbness went way below the skin in the area below the knee (the patellar tendon). Because there was no "pain," the doctor said not to worry about it. It was strange, and for many years my knee would often buckle—I think because I couldn't sense that area very well, but I figured that's just the way it would always be.

The numbness created a general feeling of "the leg" not being a part of me, a feeling of separateness. My leg was so unbelievably weak and shriveled from being in a cast and an immobilizer for so long, I literally had to learn to run again. I remember being back on the sidelines during basketball practice and learning to try to trust my leg again. The numbness in particular did not preclude me from anything. The surgeon told me no downhill skiing, but there were no other restrictions. However, for many more years than I needed to, I wore a brace to play any type of sport and also while running out of fear of reinjury. Well into my late twenties I had recurring dreams of my knee dislocating again, but I never talked to anyone about it.

It wasn't until I started exploring mind-body activities that I began to reclaim my leg. Because I had the surgery so young, I developed bone spurs under the patella and arthritis that was causing a lot of swelling and aches and pains. I knew in my late 20s that I needed to give up running for good, so I began to pursue tae kwon do pretty seriously. At the same time I started to explore yoga. I had a revelation when a teacher said, "We need to stop labeling parts of ourselves as bad or good"—I realized how long I had been speaking and thinking about my "bad" leg and how that was contributing to feelings of brokenness and separateness. Over the next decade, as I continued martial arts, yoga, and other mind-body practices, not only did my leg strengthen and the arthritic pain in my knee go away, but I developed a much greater feeling of body-wholeness.

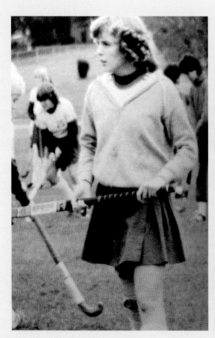
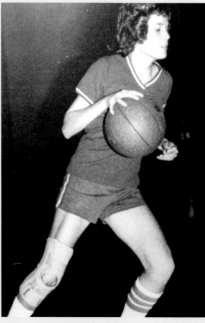

By age 15, Lori had resumed playing sports, but she wore a knee brace at all times to prevent her kneecap from dislocating and prevent further injury.

Today, Lori has full feeling in her knee and leads her athletic lifestyle without hesitation.

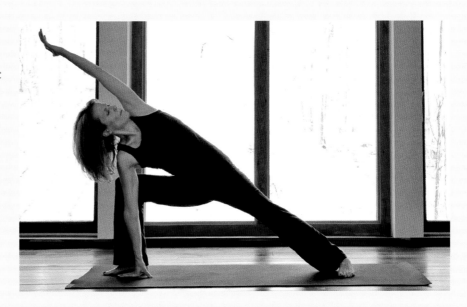

And then something really extraordinary and unexpected happened. I went to a Yoga Tune Up training and was introduced to skin-rolling with the Therapy Balls. I started rolling the skin around and below my knee, and within *days* feeling started to seep back into those tissues, in a good way, not painful. Almost immediately I felt some tingling sensations. I was *amazed* that there could be feeling in those tissues again after all those years! And I just felt happy that the area wasn't lost or a "dead zone" as I had thought of it before. It only took a couple weeks of skin-rolling for *all the feeling to come back*. The ball work seemed to wake everything up—after 30 years of numbness, it now feels almost normal.

Physically the one difference I notice is less "buckling" of my knee. Since I have feeling back, it hasn't buckled once. I have not shared the return to feeling with any docs or therapists. Fortunately all I've needed lately, aside from my Yoga Tune Up Ball work, yoga, and fitness classes (cycling and TRX), is occasional adjustment from a chiropractor.

While this work recovering from numbness has been wonderful, equally profound has been the work with the balls around my hips and the other Yoga Tune Up body rebalancing techniques. My body spent *decades* compensating for the trauma to my right knee, and as a result my hips are often extremely tight in spite of an almost daily yoga practice. This is what led me to Yoga Tune Up—I started searching for something I could do beyond traditional flow yoga and found the *Lower Body Quick Fix* DVD, which gave me such immediate and deep relief and openness that I wanted more, so I enrolled in the Yoga Tune Up training, where I was introduced to the Roll Model Therapy Balls. The balls allow me to unwind my tight connective tissue much more deeply than yoga alone. And the Yoga Tune Up moves are enabling me to rebalance where I've been compensating, stay strong, and keep sufficient space in the knee joint.

Today the combination of ball rolling, Yoga Tune Up moves, and flow yoga allow me to stay strong, maintain healthy feeling in the tissues, manage aches and pains, and keep doing the things I love! I've been privileged to share this ball work, and Yoga Tune Up, with others and to hear how it's helping them alleviate pain and keep doing the things they love to do—thank you, Jill, for all you are doing!

Other Tools of the Tissue Trade

Of course, I am biased toward my Roll Model Ball collection. I tout their benefits over many of the tools listed in this section, but I also firmly believe that your own body discernment is the best teacher in the long run. If you can, experiment with any and all of these tools until you find the right mix of stress-transfer mediums or shear-transfer mediums for you!

Here is a short list of popular self-massage tools and a few others that are worth exploring. Nowadays, you can purchase these tools at your local Walmart, drugstore, or sporting goods store.

Foam Rollers

Foam rollers have become ubiquitous as self-myofascial massage has risen in popularity. They come in different sizes, shapes, and densities. Foam rollers can be great tools to create global shear (see page 144). They apply pressure to broad regions of tissue and can help create sensations of temporary relief and stretch.

Because of their large size, however, foam rollers lack nuance. They cannot provide precise contact with specific trigger points, nor can they easily navigate around bony prominences into the hard-to-reach tissues at joint junctions. Their broad shape also renders them unable to burrow into the depths of your tissues. And foam rollers are not very portable—you can't easily throw one into your gym bag or take it on a plane.

Most foam rollers are incredibly dense, hard, and slick and thus lack the ability to absorb your body's bony protrusions, which can lead to skin pinching and bruising. Hard rollers are made of dense foam or foam surrounding PVC pipe, wood, more foam, or even metal. While some have extra features such as nubs or tire-like tread, the firm core does not allow for the yield and tender touch that is needed to prevent muscle guarding and bracing.*

While softer foam rollers are less common, they are made from a pliant foam, so they

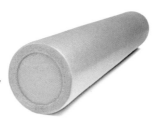

> **MUSCLE BRACING:** *Exactly the opposite of the effect you want to create while rolling. Muscle bracing occurs when the muscle spindles (stretch receptors in muscles) sense that too much stretch is happening. Instead of allowing the stretch to occur, the muscle contracts to protect itself, locking into a hardened, tensed state. This can happen when a tool is perceived by that myofascia as too hard, the stroke against the body is too fast, or the body is in a state of global tension. Hard instruments such as lacrosse balls, tennis balls, and hard foam rollers can trigger this unwanted effect.*

are not injurious to your tissues. While they lack the nuance to untack smaller areas of the body or rub into areas around a joint, they can be a great supplement for global shear techniques. I love to lay my entire spine lengthwise on top of a soft foam roller while I practice breathing.

In short: Many foam rollers are too large and too hard to navigate around bony prominences, joints, or delicate tissue junctions into which the grippy, pliable Roll Model Balls can easily navigate.

* Leonid Blyum and Mark Driscoll, "Mechanical stress transfer - the fundamental physical basis of all manual therapy techniques," *Journal of Bodywork and Movement Therapies* 16, no. 4 (2012): 520.

Sports Balls

Balls designed for sports are perhaps the easiest tools to find and can be very budget-friendly. I have "played ball" with softballs, baseballs, tennis balls, racquetballs, golf balls, lacrosse balls, bocce balls, soccer balls, and volleyballs. But these balls all share something in common other than their spherical shape: they are designed for sports, not for the human body. While they come in handy when nothing else is available, they are not crafted to perform soft-tissue conditioning.

Tennis balls are practically household items, and many people use them when they start self-massage. Thousands of chiropractors and physical therapists can be found on the Internet suggesting that you place two tennis balls in a sock to perform self-massage. But there are a few challenges with this approach:

1. Tennis balls are harder than the Roll Model Balls. They lack the cushiony pliability that permits the Roll Model Balls to sink into bony prominences while still contacting all the soft tissues relating to that junction.

2. Tennis balls are covered in fabric, which makes them slick rather than grippy. A hard ball covered in felt can provide pressure, but it is unable to grab at all tissue layers and create the amount of shear that a Roll Model Ball can.

3. Tennis balls are not designed to absorb your body weight. They burst easily and split at the seams.

A lacrosse ball is an inexpensive tool that has many of the same properties as a tennis ball, with two major differences:

1. Lacrosse balls have absolutely no yield. They are dense and hard and unable to conform to the bony structures they roll against. Their density and hardness also prevent them from maneuvering into the smaller joint junctions in the hands and feet and along rib joints. Their lack of pliability can lead to skin bruising and irritation at these bony prominences.

2. Lacrosse balls have one advantage over tennis balls: they have a grippy surface, so in a pinch, they can be used for topical skin-rolling to create shear. Just be careful not to allow the balls to pinch and collide your skin up against bony nubs and create bruises or nerve damage.

Golf balls are slick, harder balls that can do significant damage to soft and hard tissues. This small ball might easily tuck into the sole of your foot and find its way into the deep bony grooves, but it cannot absorb pressure, so it drives intense force up into the delicate fascias, nerves, ligaments, and blood vessels and can easily cause harm.

In short: Sports balls play better on the field than on your tissues. Use them only when nothing else is available. Keep your sports balls and body-based balls apart to prevent a turf war.

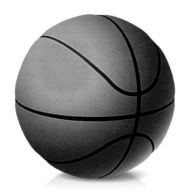

Inflated Balls

Inflated balls come in different sizes, are made from different densities of rubber, and have different levels of pliability. They are not all designed to bear the weight of a human body and can pop. A basketball may be around the same size as a child's Gertie Ball (or my Coregeous Ball), but it does not interact with your soft tissues in the same way. I have a friend who actually broke a rib rolling on a basketball. That's enough for me to issue a legitimate warning about hard inflated balls.

Softer inflated balls that have a grippy texture can be excellent tools to induce global shear and for positional stretching. You place the ball somewhere on your body and then lie on top of it. Your body weight plus gravity creates a deep stretch in the area of the ball and beyond into the fascias connected with that area. Inflated balls do not necessarily plunge deeply into specific trigger points, but they are excellent at providing stretch for large areas of the body.

In short: Avoid hard inflated balls; instead, opt for soft-skinned inflated balls that offer softer, gentler pressure. Depending on their diameter, they provide different degrees of positional stretch. They also facilitate shear but are limited in their depth of point-specific penetration.

Wooden Massage Roller

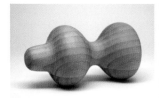

This old-school tool was my first self-massage implement. I was a teenager when I received one as a gift. It looks like a small dumbbell made of solid wood and is designed to roll on either side of the spine. Wooden rollers that have nubs, ridges, and novel shapes also fit into this category. The stiffer your tissues are, the harder the wood feels. As with any harder implement, if you are unable to relax your tissues deeply as the strong pressure of the roller pokes into you, your body and your nervous system will brace unconsciously against this extra-hard tool.*

In short: Ask yourself, "Does this tool help my body feel better? Am I becoming more pliable, or is it making me harder and more wooden?"

* Blyum and Driscoll, "Mechanical stress transfer - the fundamental physical basis of all manual therapy techniques," *Journal of Bodywork and Movement Therapies* 16, no. 4 (2012): 520.

Additional Specialized Tools That I Love

Based on your needs, goals, and body type and the areas you'd like to treat, a plethora of unique self-myofascial massage tools are available to help. The folks who create them are just like you and me; they're looking for ways to resolve their pain and craft products that suit their issues. The tools range in cost and configuration, but their creators typically invest a lot of thought and time in them to help people from all walks of life manage pain. Aside from my own tools, here are my favorites:

1. **MobilityWOD tools:** Kelly Starrett's specialized rubber tools, the Supernova, Battlestar, and Gemini, are engineered for superior shear.

2. **MELT Foam Roller:** Sue Hitzmann's super-soft foam roller is the only foam roller I trust on my body. It is very pliable and will not irritate bony prominences.

3. **Sharper Image Percussive Vibrating Handheld Self-Massager:** What can I say? Sometimes a pricey gadget that requires a little electricity makes a gal happy! Glenn Black gave me one of these massagers as a gift thirteen years ago, and while I don't use it often (because I prefer the precision of rolling over having to hold something), it's awesome for stimulating blood flow and mobilizing lymph with the press of a button.

This is a very short list, and I apologize if I have left out your favorite tool. Feel free to share it with me on social media!

Ultimately, you'll need to be your own soft-tissue judge. Whichever tools you use, look for ones that help induce deep relaxation and detangle the knots and stiffness that keep you from feeling great. I have experimented with nubby balls, sticks, plastic stones, rocks (oh, did that hurt–thanks, David Lepp, for experimenting with rocks on my IT band!), vibrating gadgets, doorknobs, window cranks (see below), couch arms, chair backs, walls, gearshifts, airplane armrests, barbells...the list goes on and on. Look, if you were a dog or cat, you would not be at all self-conscious about rubbing your body on any object that looked like it would placate the inner itch that needs a deep soft-tissue scratch.

Use your tools to remodel yourself so that your body runs more smoothly and efficiently and is less apt to collect aches and pains in the first place.

THE TOOL THAT WAS TOO HARD: A CRANKY TALE OF A SOFT-TISSUE HANGOVER

Years ago I picked up a friend at the massage clinic where he worked. He was running late, so I sat by the window in the waiting room and leaned back in order to let the base of my skull rest on the conveniently positioned window crank for a little suboccipital rubdown. I burrowed the back of my neck into that metal crank for twenty minutes. Like a cat trying to scratch an unreachable itch, I nudged that metal crank into every nook and cranny at the base of my skull. I used that crank like a miniature crowbar, attempting to traction my skull away from my neck. At the time it felt awesome, and it certainly helped pass the time.

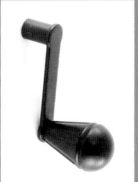

This window crank made my neck cranky.

But for days afterward I paid dearly for it. The next day, I was hit with the equivalent of a soft-tissue hangover! The base of my skull was irritated and exceptionally tender–I could hardly touch it. Stretching my neck was also out of the question. By day 2, the sensation was even worse; it felt like a cross between the flu and whiplash. I was not visibly bruised, but that hard metal crank had certainly aggravated deeper tissues.

There is a reason why using hard objects for self-massage hurts. You may not necessarily feel the "bad pain" while chipping away at your tension, but there will be a price to pay later. It's difficult for your muscle spindles to turn off when they are pressured with tools that have no yield. That's why I don't endorse the use of hard balls like lacrosse, golf, or tennis balls. And that's why the Roll Model Balls are grippy and pliable and designed to soften with use.

The misery I created in twenty short minutes took at least a week to evaporate, and I have never forgotten the results of that experiment!

Remember, your soft tissue likes a soft tool.

Who Can Roll on Balls?

Everyone can find their soft and hard spots with the Roll Model Balls. If you are uncertain whether rolling is right for you, check with your physician. In the more than twenty years that I have explored this work, I have never encountered anyone who was unable to roll some part of the body for at least a brief period. From 104-year-old great-grandmas, to parents who discover their babies crawling on top of their balls, to Olympians and professional athletes, and everyone in between, there is something for everyone.

As you leaf through the stories in this book, you'll find individuals who have used the balls to help their bodies recover from acute injuries, diseases, and conditions. Naturally, it is not my place to declare that this method will work for all individuals facing these circumstances, but these Roll Models are inspiring examples of how the various sizes of Therapy Balls can help.

When Should You Use the Roll Model Balls?

Hardly a day goes by when I don't "knead my balls." It's hard to resist the physical and mental refreshment that they provide. (It's also hard to resist the bawdy humor that they naturally elicit in classrooms, in gyms, and with strangers on long flights.) Whether you feel like a knotty mess or you feel wrinkled in body, mind, or spirit, the balls iron out your soft-tissue seams so that you can "ball-lieve" in yourself again. The following are five great ways to use them in the course of your day.

Where Is the Best Place to Roll?

The beauty of these small, portable balls is that you can take them anywhere. They are small enough to fit in your purse or backpack. They fit in your car's glove box, your gym bag, or your diaper bag. You can make any space your venue for self-care. If you wish to create optimal conditions for rolling, I suggest the following:

- Find a clean floor, clear wall, or firm chair. Wood floors and gym floors are great surfaces for rolling on the balls. You can also place a yoga mat on top of the floor or on carpet.
- Dim the lights to decrease the glare in your eyes.
- Play soothing music if that calms your senses.

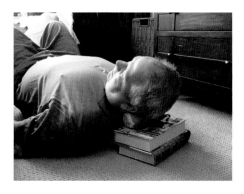

When You Are Aching

The balls are faster-acting than ibuprofen or Tylenol. According to a study by Michael Kjaer, MD, DMSc, and Albert Banes, PhD, cited by Dr. Banes in his keynote address at the 2012 International Fascia Research Congress, the strongest stimulation to any cell is mechanical stress, and mechanical load acts more quickly than a drug. According to Dr. Banes, it takes approximately 90 seconds of consistent pressure for the organelles within cells to excite and respond to pressure changes. It takes a lot longer for a pill to dissolve and make its way into your bloodstream.

The motion created by the balls immediately affects your body's stretch and pain receptors and recalibrates how you process your hurt. I elaborate on this on page 67, where you'll discover that aches are fickle; sometimes you can erase pain by rolling directly into your knotty trigger points, while at other times you'll solve your issue by placing the ball on adjacent areas or working the ball around the perimeter of the ailing tissue.

The fastest way to get a response in your body is through touch. Not through a pill, but through motion. *Motion is lotion.*

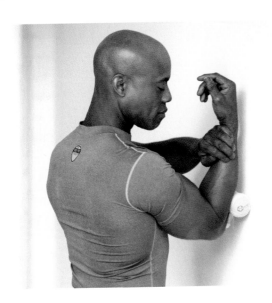

Before Exercise

The rolling sequences outlined in chapter 8 are excellent pre-exercise warm-ups. They heat up and lubricate joints and connective tissues while increasing blood flow to the area being targeted. They also usher in proprioception to areas of the body that may be prone to injury due to poor circulation, chronic tightness, old injuries, or scar tissue. The penetration of the balls also activates the fascial, joint, and muscle proprioceptors that help with awareness for physical performance. Think of your balls as a "precovery" tool.

After Exercise

The rolling sequences are helpful as post-exercise "warm-downs," as they help stretch out muscles and connective tissues that may have been heavily targeted in a workout session. The balls work to unwind knots and adhesions that develop as a result of overuse, underuse, misuse, or abuse. All of the sequences induce deep relaxation, a much-needed element in *any* physical discipline to help the body enter the parasympathetic phase of down-regulation for rest and repair (see chapter 9 for more on relaxation). Many rollers do the sequences just before going to sleep, as it fosters tranquility.

As you progress in your workouts and move into areas of your body that had been dormant or deconditioned, soreness for a day or two is quite common. Before jumping into your next workout, ramp up by doing some self-massage to bring fluidity and warmth back to your tissues so that they are not "running on empty." Soreness is sometimes associated with knots from overworking, or it could be that the fascias and muscle cells are still in a delicate state of regeneration. If you're excessively sore, respect that—never try to break a personal record! Give your body a chance to recover fully.

When You Want to Relax

Your ball-rolling time is not always about erasing pain and enhancing your mobility. The Roll Model Balls also flip your stress switch off. Use them when you want to give yourself a time-out and escape from emotional trauma or pressure that keeps you in overdrive. Let the balls coax relief and stillness into your mind and body. You'll find that within moments of using them, your day will feel new again. It's like pressing your internal reset button and starting fresh. (See chapter 9 for more on rolling for relaxation.)

When You Are Traveling

The balls are perfectly sized for travel. They are a must-have in cars, trains, planes, and more. You can use them discreetly in restaurants, libraries, theaters, classrooms, and other public places. The smaller balls make for easy stealth self-care on the go, wherever you go. You'll feel so much better than everyone around you!

HAVE BALLS, WILL TRAVEL: ON-THE-GO PAIN RELIEF

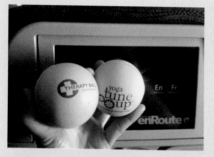

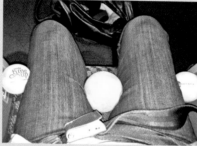

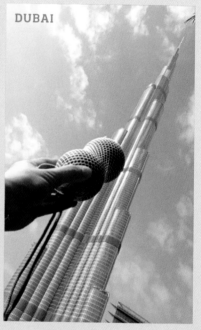
DUBAI

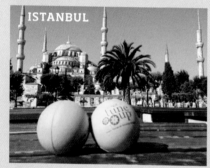
ISTANBUL

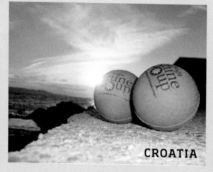
CROATIA

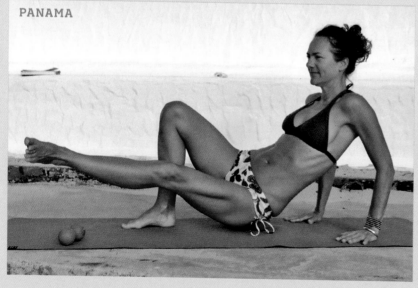
PANAMA

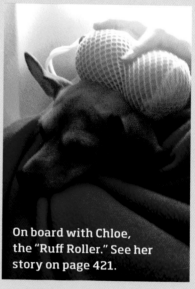
On board with Chloe, the "Ruff Roller." See her story on page 421.

How Often Can You Roll?

I recommend rolling every day. A little goes a long way—you will feel change in as little as two minutes. If you can, carve out ten to thirty minutes in your schedule each day for dedicated self-care.

If you don't have twenty minutes to do a concentrated practice, then try to incorporate the balls into your daily routine:

1. Place them under your feet while you do the dishes.

2. Sit on them in your car, or place them on your back.

3. Put on your headset and lean against them on a wall while you take a phone call at work.

4. Turn on your favorite TV show and lie on top of the balls while you watch.

5. Wherever and whenever you are stationary, slip a ball into the mix to introduce movement and stimulation into your position.

The balls don't need to disrupt your life or demand great tracts of time. Figure out how to add "roll nutrition" into your day, just like you do by drinking water to remain hydrated. You will reap great benefits from "dosing" throughout the day.

Pain: Differentiating the Good from the Bad

There is one final topic to cover before the balls roll your cares away: *pain.* Once you get on the balls, you will likely find areas of glorious relief—spots that have been waiting for your attention for decades. You'll tumble into regions of your body that will seem to sigh with pleasure and unwind with ease. On the other side of the soft-tissue spectrum, the balls will find sections of tissue that feel like stones, walls, or barbed wire that scream out "DO NOT ROLL HERE!" This brings us to the very important question: *How do you differentiate "good pain" from "bad pain"?*

The Roll Model Balls are notorious for eliciting widely varying degrees of comfort or discomfort. One person's "aaaah" is another person's "yeeoow!" Levels of sensation are different for every individual. Many factors are involved with the perception of pain and discomfort, and I aim to clarify this for you in the coming pages, but ultimately *you* are the decider, and *you* must

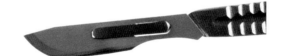

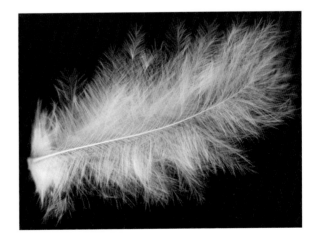

discern whether the discomfort you are experiencing is tolerable or intolerable. The general rule is that if the tissue feels better after rolling, the discomfort was healthy and therapeutic ("good pain"). If it feels worse after rolling, then that tissue may not be healthy enough to withstand the rigors of self-massage and should be avoided. In that case, seek out a qualified specialist for help.

Pain is a sensation designed to inform your body that it is injured or is about to get injured. Because there are so many gradations of pain when rolling on the balls, it can be helpful to think of it as *sensation* that varies in intensity.

Reserve the word *pain* for when you need to stop doing a particular activity. Use *sensation* and *healthy discomfort* to describe how rolling feels, and you will feel safer and be more apt to continue. In order to receive the therapeutic benefits and feel better, you must *get comfortable with your discomfort.*

It likely took you many years to accumulate the discomfort in your tissues. To erase that pain, some discomfort may be a part of your healing process. The goal of using the Roll Model Balls is not to *create* hurt, but it's probably not going to feel like you're being stroked with feathers, either.

Sometimes the Work Is Gonna Hurt

There is a great divide among therapists, with some believing that treatment should never hurt. I believe that treatment should never induce *pain,* but the reality is that when certain tissues or joints have become riddled with adhesions from lack of use, overuse, or scar tissue, it is necessary to progressively break up those adhesions in order to restore proper fluid balance and movement mechanics. The typical way of medicine is either to prescribe pills that mask pain, inject the site with steroids, which reduces inflammation but does not address the *cause* or *root* of the ailment, or operate, which often sets the stage for more wear-and-tear on neighboring areas and then manifests as issues created by scar tissue.

I am biased on the side of manual therapies that proactively address removing stiffness, dysfunction, and loss of motor control in tissues. This means using hands, fingers, elbows, toes, equipment, or tools to manipulate the affected tissues. And often it is a bit uncomfortable.

With long-standing pain, talented therapists will sensitively palpate and probe into stiffened tissues, joint capsules, and areas of dysfunction to manually break up the adhesions there. He or she will identify the different layers of dysfunction and treat each one individually. This process induces a bit of local swelling that ultimately helps remove the old stagnation and inflammation. It often feels like a tolerably brutal process.

For example, I recently dislocated my pinky toe, and it was excruciating. I was unable to walk correctly because of the pain, swelling, and stiffness. I used the Roll Model Balls on my feet, shins, calves, and hips to help minimize holding patterns in all the areas connected to the toe. Nonetheless, the joint that suffered the blow was too painful to touch. After two weeks, I was finally able to move it somewhat, and then I went to my Active Release Therapy (ART) specialist, Dr. Christopher Tosh, who was able to intelligently manipulate the joint capsule and help break up the adhesions that were forming. I'm not going to lie; it was an extremely painful process, but the swelling decreased immediately, and I was able to make rapid improvements because of this one "discomfortable" intervention.

Many people experience unpleasant sensations the first time they roll on the balls, especially if they have no experience with therapeutic massage or are not used to any form of exercise. Their tissues are so underconditioned that they are very sensitive to any type of touch. But this does not mean that they are experiencing "bad pain." These tissues respond best if they are introduced to the modifications (see page 70) to acclimate them to the balls. Be honest with yourself: if you're not used to deep therapeutic touch that moves muscles relative to one another and manipulates the innards of individual muscles, then you'll likely feel your tissues resist at first, and you may struggle with the rolling routines. Use modifications if the pressure seems too deep.

Bear in mind that the ball routines themselves shouldn't cause pain, but you may feel pain because the balls are revealing where pain already exists in your body.

As you practice self-care with the Roll Model Balls, it is up to you to experiment with these tools and the many techniques outlined in this book in order to learn how to differentiate between types of sensation and to discern for yourself *the good* versus *the bad.*

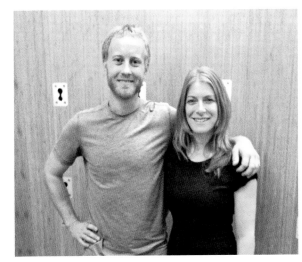

My favorite ART chiropractor and fascia friend, Dr. Christopher Tosh.

Bad Pain

Bad pain, or *intolerable discomfort*, comes in many forms. Your body will issue warning signs that where you are rolling is *not* okay, and that you should back off, modify, discontinue rolling, or seek medical attention. Your body is designed for fluid, pain-free movement. In healthy tissues, movement does not involve wincing or pain. Your job as a Roll Model is to enhance and maximize the physiological potential of your tissues and reset them to normal, optimal function. (For more on this, see "Fascia: Your Seam System" on page 97 and "Proprioception: Your EmbodyMap" on page 109.) Here are the signs that you are encountering bad pain:

1. **It hurts both during and after rolling.** The discomfort may even become worse after rolling. This is a sign that you should discontinue and seek medical help.

2. **Your whole body tenses:** Your eyes lock, frozen open and unable to blink. Your hands stiffen as if you were holding a pistol. Your whole body tightens, and you are unable to let go or modify your position. These are all sympathetic responses that tell you the ball has gone too deep or into the wrong place. Try modifying the placement or pressure of the ball first. If that doesn't change your body's feedback, you may need to see a medical professional.

3. **You can't breathe:** Your breath suddenly becomes stuck and frozen. If you are unable to breathe in or out, you need to modify or stop rolling. Your breath is like a safety detector, and it is intimately connected to your nervous system. Your inability to breathe is a great indicator that you are no longer in a safe zone and are experiencing bad pain.

4. **You experience nerve pain**—either the feeling of electricity or numbness. The reality is that the balls are constantly rolling on nerves. They can't help but stimulate small nerve endings wherever they roll. And this is a good thing. But you want to avoid rolling deep pressure directly into your large nerves (see the warnings on pages 72-73). When the balls nuzzle into those large nerves, they can create bizarre feelings of heat or ice, or areas of tissue may experience numbness. These are all indicators that you need to move the ball away from the spot you are rolling. Moving the ball slightly higher, lower, or to the left or right often remedies this problem. (On the flip side, read Eric Johnson's story of how he came out of nerve pain and numbness by using the Therapy Balls, beginning on page 116.)

5. **Bruising occurs:** There may be times when you roll too deeply and create some bruising. If you do, let it heal before rolling on the area again. Do not roll directly on a bruise from an accident or injury, either; keep your rolling on the periphery of the bruised area.

6. **Your muscles are extremely sore the next day:** Muscle soreness is like invisible bruising. If you've overdone the rolling, you may feel tender to the touch for days. Have you ever worked out too hard or gone running for the first time in months and felt sore for days afterward? You can overdo ball-rolling in the same way. Back off the depth and duration of your rolling in areas of extreme sensitivity, and take a couple of days off from rolling those areas.

7. **You feel emotions that manifest in behavior like screaming or crying out in pain.** Let me begin by saying that emotions are not "bad pain" in and among themselves. I am including this subject here because emotions can be an indicator that we may need to seek professional help to confront and heal our psychological wounds. Emotion is a category of sensation that indicates some degree of release. Emotions vary in intensity; some are helpful and cathartic, while others may suggest that counseling is warranted. Emotions are likely to arise when you roll; you may weep, laugh, or become angry for no apparent reason. These gentler emotions signal that you are processing the feelings connected to the stiffness or stuckness in your tissues. They may also help you gain perspective on past or current issues you're facing. If you are able to breathe fully and stay present,

I would put these emotions on the "tolerable discomfort" end of the spectrum. "Intolerable discomfort" emotions are those that make you feel fearful and out of control. If the balls make you feel re-traumatized in any way, I would encourage you to seek support or counseling. (For more on "soul rolling," see chapter 10.)

If you experience bad pain, try these

modifications:

1. Back off the pressure until you can relax.

2. Move the ball "uptown," "downtown," or "across town" until you no longer feel the bad pain. In other words, move the ball higher, lower, or to the right or left of that spot.

3. Take your balls to the wall: change your relationship to gravity and do your rolling against a wall or the back of a chair, also modifying your pressure as you lean in.

4. If you wish to lie down instead of using a wall, place the ball on a sofa or bed so that a portion of the ball sinks into the softer surface.

5. Use a larger ball on that area, scaling all the way up to the Coregeous if the firmer rubber balls apply too much pressure.

6. Use two balls (possibly in the Snug-Grip Tote) instead of one. One ball condenses and intensifies the sensation; two balls disperse the sensation and minimize the depth of pressure.

7. Stay on the surface with skin-rolling or shear.

8. Contract/relax until you achieve change or stop making change.

ROLLING IN THE PRESENCE OF INJURY

Many variables are at play when it comes to defining "pain," "injury," "safety," and so on. If you are in an acute phase of injury, seek professional help. But pain is scalable and subjective: one person's bruised knee may be another person's unbearable catastrophe requiring crutches. You are the only one who is able to fully perceive your body and its sensations. Your relationship to pain is ultimately knowable only to you. Learn to listen to your body.

In spite of the warnings listed above, you may still be able to roll on areas that are farther away from an active injury undergoing professional treatment. The rest of your body will adapt and compensate for the injury, and often those tissues brace, stiffen, and become quite uncomfortable because they have to bear the responsibility for what isn't working well. Feel free to use the Roll Model techniques to soothe those other tissues and create a better environment for healing.

Stay connected to your breathing, which can be an excellent gauge of whether you can tolerate the pressure of the balls. If you can't take a full breath, you're in too deep, so back off. See chapter 7 for more on breathing.

Good Pain

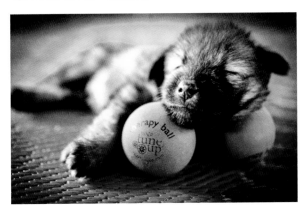

Now let's roll over to the other side of the pain spectrum. I probably shouldn't even use the term "good pain," but rather "tolerable discomfort." This tolerable discomfort reveals a buffet of benefits that you'll see listed here. Happily, your sensation of tolerable discomfort will likely change over time. As rolling becomes a regular part of your self-care and your tissues become more balanced, you will begin to feel *pleasant pressure* rather than discomfort. In fact, you may be so used to living in pain and discomfort that one day you'll start rolling and think that the balls are no longer working because you no longer hurt. The good news is that *it doesn't have to hurt to work.*

Healthy tissues do not poke back at you when you poke at them. The balls mobilize and stimulate both healthy and unhealthy tissues. It's the unhealthy tissues that scream when the balls maneuver deeply within them. They need help resolving their internal stiffness and facilitating a more balanced environment. There is no intolerable feedback from healthy tissues because the fibers and fluids within them are buoyant, nourished, and primed for function. Familiarize yourself with the signs of good pain/tolerable discomfort/pleasant pressure.

When your tissues are conditioned, filled with a healthy balance of fluids and nutrients, the balls will find no obstacles to motion other than your own imagination.

Here's how you know that the discomfort you may be feeling while rolling is good pain that is promoting healing in your tissues:

1. The areas rolled feel as if they are breathing an internal sigh of relief and have a physical lightness; they are no longer held captive to pain.

2. You feel a gentle, fluid heat in the areas rolled, as if you'd been resting on a hot water bottle.

3. You notice improved range of motion in the areas rolled.

4. You feel less pain at the end range of motion in the areas rolled.

5. You feel less pain all over your body, not just in the areas rolled.

6. You feel relaxed; your mood has changed from anxious or stressed to soothed and calm.

7. You have an overall sense of well-being: an emotional lightness and a positivity that were unavailable to you prior to rolling.

8. You experience emotional catharsis: an unlocking and loosening of somatic stress, trauma, grief, or long-held fear masquerading as body aches and pains.

9. You detect an overall change in your breathing: you feel as if your whole body can breathe better and more deeply.

10. Your whole-body tension subsides.

11. You notice that your formerly *stressed tissue* is now a *resolved issue.*

12. You feel more aware of the targeted tissues (see the information about EmbodyMap beginning on page 109).

WARNINGS! OFF-LIMITS AREAS

The Roll Model balls are not a substitute for proper supervised healthcare. If you have any questions about an injury or condition, seek medical advice before using these tools. I can make no legal claims that the Roll Model Method is a "remedy" or "cure." Please use common sense. That said, here are some guidelines:

1. Do not roll on an active injury, which may actually increase damage to the tissue. The balls are effective rehab tools *when used appropriately*.

2. Never use the Roll Model Balls directly on bruised tissue, broken skin, or broken bones.

3. Avoid applying deep pressure to the following areas of the body. You can always use the balls more superficially to skin-roll, or use the Coregeous Ball, but applying deep pressure in these areas is unsafe:

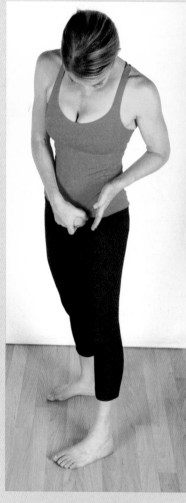

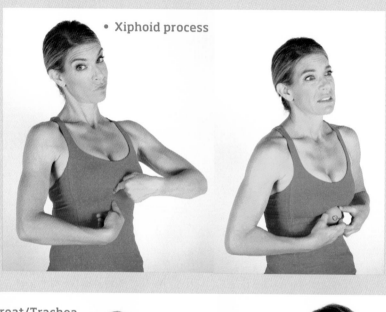

• Xiphoid process

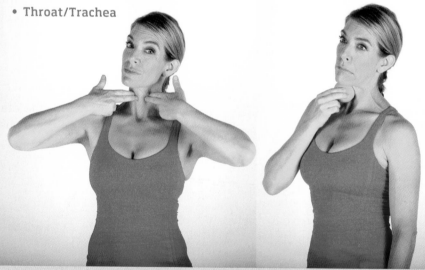

• Throat/Trachea

• Inguinal ligament. Sustained compression can be okay here for some people, but vigorous CrossFibering is strongly discouraged unless you are a clinician.

• Areas near the bones of anyone with osteoporosis. Try lightening the pressure by taking your balls to the wall or using the inflated Coregeous Ball.

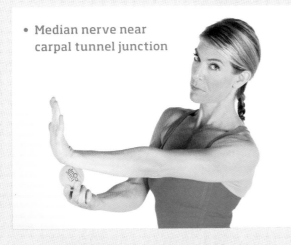

- Median nerve near carpal tunnel junction

- **Median nerve near carpal tunnel junction.** Avoid using a ball to apply deep pressure to your wrist and forearm while your wrist is extended.

- **Coccyx.** Your coccyx is the very bottom of your tailbone. It is easy to break, so don't apply firm pressure with a ball directly on it.

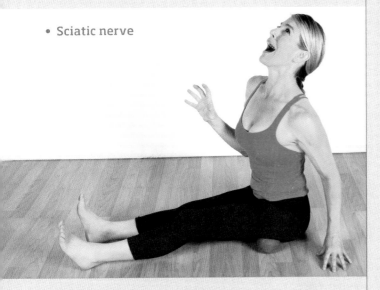

- Sciatic nerve

- **Sciatic nerve embedded within the hamstrings.** It's okay to tackle your hamstrings with a bent knee while you are seated on a bench or stool, and the nerve and surrounding myofascias have considerable slack. But don't sit on the ground with your legs straight out, plop a ball underneath your thigh, and try to "break up" tissue; it plucks directly into the elongated sciatic nerve. I roll my hamstrings while seated during long airplane flights.

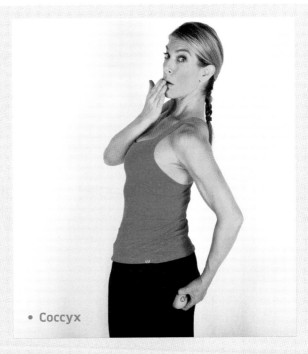

- Coccyx

If you are pregnant, consult your physician before pursuing Roll Model Therapy Ball techniques. As with any exercise or movement program, if you have been practicing ball work prior to pregnancy, you should be able to roll into it with no problem. Here are a few general pregnancy contraindications:

- Unless you've been training in inversions before and during pregnancy, refrain from adopting positions that invert your heart above your head.

- During the late second trimester and throughout the third trimester, modify facedown (prone) positions to avoid placing uncomfortable pressure on your abdomen. Lean against a wall instead.

- During the late second trimester and throughout the third trimester, modify back-lying (supine) positions to avoid placing sustained intra-abdominal pressure on your vena cava and aorta. Roll onto your side or perform while leaning against a wall.*

THE LAST WORD: There is no such thing as a perfect remedy for all people. It all depends on you, your body, and your relationship to pain. Please use caution and pay close attention to your body's signals and your emotions. *When in doubt, don't roll it out!*

For more on pregnancy-related rolling, please see my webinar: www.creativelive.com/courses/healthy-pregnancy-healthy-baby-jill-miller

I Was Lupus, Now I Am Empowered: From Self-Medication to Self-Care

Jennifer Lovely, 39
Pilates/Yoga Instructor
Orange County, California

"I'm one of those people who has an incredibly high pain tolerance," admits Jennifer Lovely, a 39-year-old Pilates and yoga instructor from Orange County, California. *"But really, that's just learning not to feel things."* Abandoned by her mother at age 5, raised by an alcoholic dad and stepmom, constantly moving and changing schools, and molested by her stepbrother throughout her childhood, Jennifer grew up on eggshells, never sure if she was safe, living in constant stress and fear brought on by those who were supposed to be nurturing and protecting her. *"It was one of those families where everything looked pretty on the outside, you know? She was a school teacher, and he had a small business. But my dad would run around the house calling us pigs and hogs, beating his chest and yelling that we needed to respect him,"* she says. One month before her high school graduation, her dad kicked her out of the house, and a year later Jennifer married a man eleven years her senior. Together they had two children, but their eight-year marriage was full of its own issues and arguments. *"Little did I know, I had married my father,"* she says with irony.

In her early twenties, with a young son and another on the way, Jennifer began experiencing radical pain in her elbows and a general malaise that left her constantly exhausted. After the birth of her second son, blood tests came back positive for lupus. Follow-up X-rays showed massive inflammation in her joints, part of what was causing her pain. Lupus is a chronic autoimmune disease in which the immune system cannot recognize the difference between foreign invaders and the body's own healthy tissue, and as a result goes on an all-out offensive, attacking and destroying healthy skin, joints, and organs, causing inflammation and damage throughout the body. The Lupus Foundation of America calls it a *"cruel, unpredictable, and devastating"* disease.

In retrospect, Jennifer thinks that she had been suffering from lupus for almost a decade prior to her diagnosis: after a terrible bout of chicken pox at age 14, she was always running a fever and had sores in her nose and mouth that would flare up during the more stressful times of her high-stress childhood.

Jennifer was put on prednisone, a corticosteroid drug often used to treat inflammation, and Plaquenil, an anti-malaria medication, to attempt to suppress her wildly overactive immune system. She recalls her doctor casually mentioning that she'd have to see an ophthalmologist because she could go blind if the lupus attacked her eyes, *"but I was young and dumb and I didn't really understand the seriousness of it all."* Meanwhile, the drugs were doing nothing to alleviate her symptoms, and she was still suffering from bouts of muscle and joint pain, sores inside her mouth and nose, and hair loss. The pain would come on randomly, in her earlobes, knees, or elbows, like someone was stabbing her with a knife. *"My body felt like it wanted to explode from inside out. It was always so uncomfortable in my skin."*

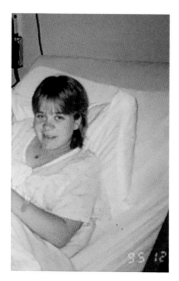

Jennifer was diagnosed with lupus while giving birth to her second child at age 23.

Since the original drug regimen was ineffective, the rheumatologist added methotrexate to Jennifer's roster of medications, a cancer treatment drug that she injected into her buttocks once a week. The incredibly toxic methotrexate did nothing to alleviate her symptoms, but caused almost all of her hair to fall out, grogginess, swollen limbs, and stomach pain. Jennifer's life was falling apart– her unhappy marriage even more strained by her illness, she decided a few months after her diagnosis to take her two kids and leave her husband.

Having been a stay-at-home mom for several years, Jennifer was now stuck trying to find a job and a place to live (her husband kept the house and paid no child support) while managing her disease and raising her kids. Looking back, she shakes her head in disbelief that she managed to muddle through those early years on her own. Eventually she found a job at the YMCA helping special-education kids, drawing on her high school experience working and traveling with the Special Olympics track team. While she stopped injecting the methotrexate after a year, she continued with the other two drugs and would also self-medicate with alcohol, trying to relieve her pain and stress but ultimately exacerbating her symptoms. She could never find the right combination of medications to make the pain go away, but at the same time she was psychologically dependent on the drugs, addicted to the idea of her pain. "I became a victim to these drugs–the story I had was that I have lupus, so I need drugs, that they were what was helping me through, even though they weren't really doing anything. After a while, I began to identify with the disease so much that I was lupus. I wasn't Jennifer anymore."

Her condition elicited a great deal of sympathy and support from her friends, but at the same time, her real character–the inner strength that she had drawn on to survive her childhood and break from her bad marriage–conflicted with her story of victimization from her disease, and every now and then she was reminded of it. "One time a friend gave me a handicapped label for my car, but it seemed so crazy to me–in high school I played varsity soccer, and our team traveled around the world. And now I'm 'handicapped'? Impossible!" she says.

Without insurance, taking care of her health during her twenties was a huge challenge. As it is for many people who are uninsured, the ER was the only solution when Jennifer suffered outbreaks of debilitating joint pain. Hospital doctors would dose her with prednisone and morphine for the pain and send her on her way. She had friends who were nurses and physicians' assistants who would help her with free samples when they could, but their answer was always another drug. The whites of Jennifer's eyes turned yellow from the high levels of toxic medications coursing through her system. "I always felt crappy, like there was a fog in my head. I couldn't see things clearly," she says. At night, she would take Tylenol PM to sleep, convinced that she was going to be in pain, and she always slept with a heating pad in an attempt to soothe her aching body.

Despite her struggles, Jennifer got her life together and found a good job in the automotive industry, but her health continued to plague her, her joints sometimes swelling to the point where she could barely walk. When she was around 30, a new triathlete girlfriend introduced her to an acupuncturist whom she thought might be able to help Jennifer. In their first session, he put more than 200 needles in her over two hours. She continued to see him twice a week and was amazed at her body's response and how the work began to settle down her immune system. While the world of alternative healing was an expensive choice for a single mom, Jennifer knew that this was something she needed to do for herself, as it was the first strategy that had a positive effect on her symptoms.

Around the same time, she decided to become a Pilates teacher, drawn to the practice as it stretched her muscles and reduced her pain. She also began to pay attention to her eating habits, cutting out gluten, drinking more water, and starting hydrocolon therapy. This was a time of huge self-discovery for Jennifer, and she learned that she could take care of her body without drugs and actually decrease her symptoms. She told her doctor that she didn't want to take her medications anymore since they clearly hadn't been helping and she was finding new relief with self-care techniques like acupuncture and Pilates. Though skeptical, her doctor respected her wishes, and over a three-month period Jennifer tapered off her medications completely. Going off the medications was a huge step forward in rebuilding her relationship with herself and her body rather than drowning out the messages with prescriptions or wine.

Yoga was a natural continuation of Jennifer's path, and in 2012 she met Yoga Tune Up teacher Elissa Strutton at a teacher training. Jennifer knew right away that she needed to investigate the Yoga Tune Up method, so she asked Elissa to work with her privately using the Therapy Balls. It was about the same time she put down the pills that Jennifer picked up the Therapy Balls. When Elissa placed them on her tight trapezius and rhomboid muscles, Jennifer experienced complete emotional release, a torrent of long-held-down feelings, and a rush of empowerment that she might be able to truly soothe her aching body. "I remember the feeling when I first lay down on those beautiful balls. It felt like pure relief *inside.* They were able to melt into my areas of pain that I still struggled with, and I was able to get immediate relief."

She knew that there was something special about the Roll Model Balls, and she began to play with them on her own, noticing that when she had joint pain, especially in her forearms or quadriceps, she could place the balls on the point of pain and the pain would disappear after a few minutes. "I don't know how to explain it; it's like I give the pain back to the ball and it absorbs it!" Even with the success of her other self-care therapies, nothing had eradicated the pain the way the Therapy Balls did. Jennifer cries a little at the memory of her realization that she was going to be able to take care of herself from then on, without relying on drugs or alcohol to quell the pain.

She loves all the different sizes of Therapy Balls for getting into different nooks and crannies in her body, and she loves draping herself across the Coregeous Ball. "I cried the first time with the Coregeous Ball under my belly, because I had never felt that pressure on my abdomen before, and I felt so vulnerable." Now, Jennifer even sleeps with the Coregeous Ball in her bed, placing it under her back, neck, stomach, or hips when she wakes in the night to ease whatever discomfort she's feeling (instead of reaching for the Tylenol PM like she used to). She laughs, "My new husband's not crazy about sharing the bed with a ball, but it's been life-changing for me!"

Jennifer's energy and vitality have returned so much that she can now run and play with her two sons, and she is playing soccer again with an adult group. She and her husband travel to Europe every year, and she is once more full of enthusiasm for life and grateful for it at the same time. "If you had told me when I was 22 that I would have my own business, that I would have a circle of support including a wonderful new husband, and I would be traveling the world, I would have called you crazy," she says. For many years, life had not held much enjoyment for her, but now Jennifer feels that she has really started living again and that her life is full of potential. While challenges still crop up and she is not entirely symptom-free, the empowerment she gets from the Roll Model Method keeps her interested in and excited by her triggers rather than cowering from them.

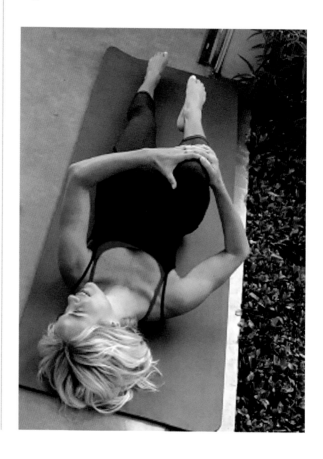

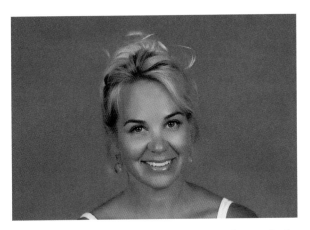

Now, when she finds a sensitive spot, instead of trying to pretend it doesn't exist or dampening it with drugs or alcohol, she plays around with the different Therapy Balls to see what works. Instead of distancing herself emotionally the way she had learned to do as a child, she is learning to feel sensations again, using the placement and depth of penetration of the Roll Model Balls to increase her body's proprioception and self-awareness. "I have taken back the control. When that pain comes on, I rub and twist and roll on those little or big guys, and it goes away! Vanishes!"

She still goes to the rheumatologist to get her blood checked every six months, and each time, "My doctor tells me, 'Jenn, you have that butterfly rash, and your joints are swollen,' and I say, 'I know.' So he prescribes me the Plaquenil and prednisone and says I should be on them for the rest of my life." Jennifer carries her Therapy Balls everywhere with her, and "last visit, when he started talking about medications, I handed him the balls and said, 'I choose these, and I'm glad to share them with you, because this is what helps me.'" Her doctor shook his head in disappointment, called her a non-compliant, bad patient, and said that he'd see her again in six months. But Jennifer just smiled, confident in the results she has experienced, trusting in her own strength and recovery.

In 2012, inspired by her own transformation, Jennifer was certified as a Therapy Ball instructor. She ministers to her students that movement and exercise don't have to be about achieving a particular physique, but about living; getting past the emotional or physical pain that blocks us from living to our fullest. She proudly shares, "Today I have several clients with lupus, and I love sharing my story and also sharing these Roll Model Balls. I love seeing the difference it makes in their life as well."

Jennifer's not limiting herself to teaching just the students who walk into her Pilates studio: on a recent plane ride, she overheard a young woman complaining to her mother about back pain. Jennifer reached across the aisle with a pair of Therapy Balls in her hand and said, "Here, try these."

Jennifer cut her hand badly a few months ago, requiring occupational therapy visits. Thanks to her continued self-care with the Therapy Balls, her recovery was leaps faster than the OTs had ever seen in other patients. They were so impressed with the condition of her entire body due to the soft-tissue conditioning she performs with the balls that they invited her to come to the office to teach the Roll Model Method to the therapists. Among the many moves she'll be sharing with them are the cost-effective and time-saving ways in which she uses the Roll Model Balls to help break up the fascial adhesions in her hand.

For those trapped in a downward spiral of chronic pain, medication, and diminishing returns, Jennifer models a life of renewal, regeneration, and "BALL-ance."

> **//** I have taken back the control. When that pain comes on, I rub and twist and roll on those little or big guys, and it goes away! Vanishes! **//**
>
> –Jennifer Lovely

3 Posture, Pain, Performance:
STAND UP FOR YOURSELF

BY GETTING ON THE BALL

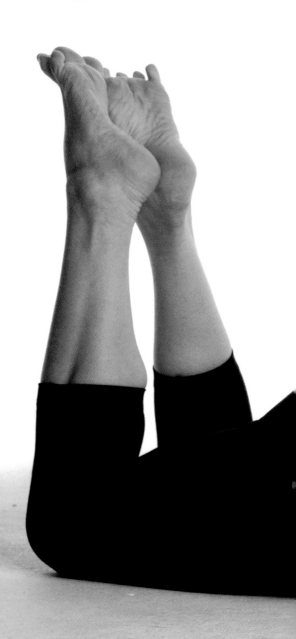

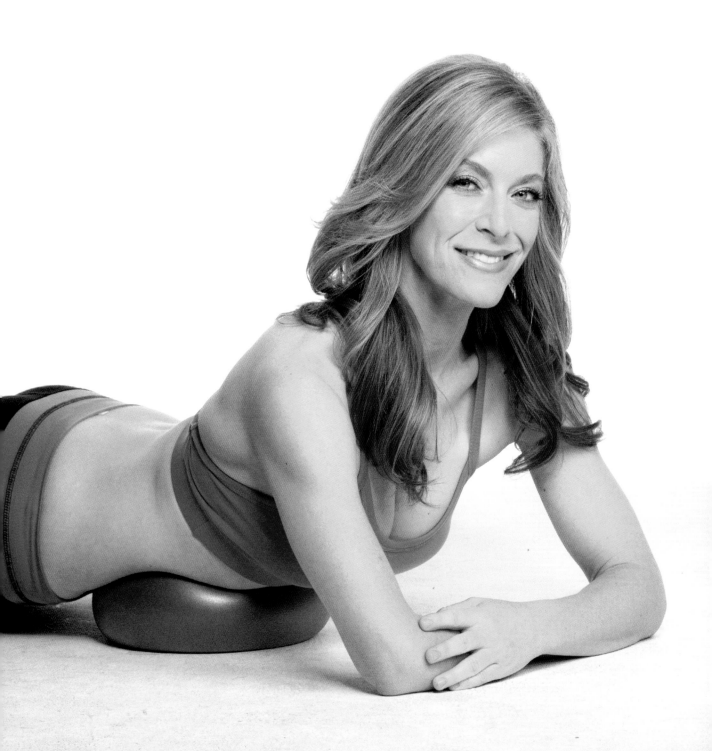

Musculoskeletal disease is the fastest-growing disease category on the planet.*

This book is designed to offset this terrifying trend by deepening your familiarity with your body, its textures, its tensions, and its treatment. While the Roll Model teaches you to self-treat with the Therapy Balls to detangle and loosen up internal adhesions and congestion, ultimately you will use those openings to reclaim *proper posture.*

Posture means "position" in Latin. Make sure that your day-to-day *position* is not an *imposition* on your health.

Before I dig into how the balls work and how they can help you, you need to identify how you hold yourself in life. Your posture follows you like a shadow, and it has a ripple effect into everything you do—how you walk, stand, breathe, and train. Movement is medicine, and at the correct dose, it will improve your quality of life.

Long-term bad posture makes for a very unpleasant existence—just think pain, deformity, surgery, and pills (which then lead to a host of other expensive issues). You have to shine light on your posture in order to make better alignment choices. You may think about exercising your body, toning your butt, or shrinking your belly, but if you do not exercise with good postural alignment, you will actually degrade the structures you're trying to improve. Your tissues function best when they aren't irritated by a lack of attention to how you carry yourself.

From a musculoskeletal perspective, your body conforms to whatever shape you demand of it. Different muscles strengthen, weaken, tighten, and stretch based on your patterns. Unfortunately, many choices lead to degenerated vertebrae, bulging disks, herniated abdomens, torn knee cartilage, or stress fractures in hips, to name a few examples—just ask the many deskbound workers who pay the bills by slumping over a computer monitor for eight to twelve hours a day. These very preventable musculoskeletal ailments are hurting not just us, but also our wallets, our healthcare system, and our economy.

The fact that you picked up this book shows that you're ready to commit to being the driver of your pain-free life rather than letting your condition be shepherded among doctors, diagnoses, and drugs. This book is designed to help you begin a total inside-out makeover. While I will teach you how to use the Roll Model Balls, it is up to you to hold yourself differently day in and day out as you attempt to integrate the new openings that the balls provide. *This process does not work unless you alter your body habits that hold pain in place.* By picking up this book, you have already demonstrated that you care enough to carry yourself with more dignity.

Surviving in a Body Built for You

Your body is a self-sustaining work of brilliance. No matter what your beliefs are about how your physical body came to be, one thing's for sure: it is equipped with the highest form of intelligence imaginable (or unimaginable!). No machine has been able to replicate the regenerative properties or the mental, emotional, or spiritual capacity of the human organism. Think about it: most of your body's functions are automatic (or what neuroscientists call *autonomic*–that is, self-regulating) and designed to keep you alive, sensing and responding to your environment. Most of the day-to-day maintenance of cell repair and renewal is done without you having to lift a finger. Of course, when you start lifting your fingers to type on a computer keyboard, or abandon the natural standing position of the human body to sit at your workstation, travel in cars, and watch the news in a recliner, you start adding different types of stress. But even then, under the radar of your conscious awareness, cells die and are reborn at breathtaking speed.

Your body survives in spite of you paying little attention to it because it has only one job: *survival.* Even if you fill it with potato chips and diet soda for weeks on end, it will find a way to adapt to your choices. Eventually, however, it will exhibit symptoms to try to tell you to do something different. For example, "for no apparent reason" you may start craving watermelon, a fruit loaded with water and fiber, to correct the nutritional imbalance you've created. Left unresolved, these symptoms will magnify in severity as your body attempts to get your attention. If you are severely sleep deprived, your body will eventually fall asleep or create an accident for you so that you have no choice but to sleep in order to recover. Your body is an amazing organism. It will guide you if you listen.

Learning to listen to your body might seem like a woo-woo New Age concept, but it is grounded in the science of the way your body senses itself (read about proprioception in chapter 4). Bad habits tend to erase your ability to hear, feel, and see yourself accurately from the inside out; they dull your perception. But blind, deaf, or numb spots within you no longer need to live without light, sound, or sensibility. They are teachable and trainable.

This book is a survival manual of sorts. It's a guide to developing your ability to hear your body's signals and teaching it new ways of living pain-free. The Roll Model tools help you gain a keen awareness of where you are holding onto *known* and *unknown pains.* These grippy rubber balls locate your body blind spots by helping you detect overuse, underuse, misuse, abuse, and confusion in your own tissues.

Your pain is often linked to your body's fixation on its "normal" posture. With all the intracellular goodness going on in your tissues, the one thing that your body goofs on is maintaining efficient posture. Look around you and see for yourself. Thousands of postural adaptations influence people's bodies. If the body is so good at surviving, shouldn't it give us a better cookie-cutter approach to managing our structure? Why do we have so many aches and pains? Why are knee replacement surgeries, hip replacement surgeries, and shoulder surgeries *skyrocketing*? Why are our bodies so broken?

According to the World Health Organization, musculoskeletal disease, or the accelerated degradation of hard and soft tissues, is the fastest-growing disease category and the second leading cause of disability globally.* Osteoarthritis, rheumatism, osteoporosis, fractures, and neck and back pain all seem to be "symptoms" of people living longer and aging *dis-gracefully*. Musculoskeletal disease is not like the flu or a bacteria; it is a noncommunicative disease. You don't "catch" it. But if you're in pain or you have lived with someone suffering from chronic pain, you know the toll it takes on the body, mind, spirit, and wallet. So why are we falling apart faster and with more pain than at any other time in history?

* *The Lancet,* Global Burden of Disease Study 2010, published December 13, 2012. Accessed via www.thelancet.com/themed/global-burden-of-disease

RUNNING THE NUMBERS ON PAIN AND MUSCULOSKELETAL DISEASE: STATISTICS AND FACTS AT A GLANCE

According to the 2010 study on the Global Burden of Disease researched by multiple organizations, including the World Health Organization, and published in the December 15, 2012, issue of *The Lancet,* musculoskeletal disease is the fastest-growing disease category on the planet. Musculoskeletal conditions include:

- Joint diseases such as osteoarthritis and rheumatoid arthritis
- Back and neck pain
- Osteoporosis and fragility fractures
- Soft-tissue rheumatism
- Injuries due to sports and in the workplace
- Trauma related to traffic accidents

These conditions cause pain, physical disability, and loss of personal and economic independence. They affect millions of people of all ages, in all cultures and countries. Here are the current estimates of people affected worldwide:

- Back pain: 632 million
- Neck pain: 332 million
- Osteoarthritis of the knee: 251 million
- Other musculoskeletal conditions: 561 million

These numbers translate to a war on our bodies that we have created for ourselves. We are under siege. It's time to roll out our best self-defense. Let's *get on the ball!*

The Bitter Truth About Modern Posture

One of the biggest problems with modern living is that our survival "modus operandi" has become terribly "shortsighted." We no longer scan the horizon for food or foe; our computer monitors are inches away from our eyes. We stare at the glow of electricity for hours on end, usually while sitting, stunting the range of motion in our necks and spines as those muscles lock in place and fasten upon the screen. The Internet expands our access to the world while shrinking our physical engagement with it. The technology era has diminished our need to fully engage our bodies. We are passive recipients of a nonstop data-based bounty. In our quest for comfort, convenience, and immediacy, we have handicapped ourselves.

Modern "progress" has perpetuated a life of *immobile reactivity* rather than *engaged proactivity*. Migratory and agriculture-based human tribes were proactive about getting food, building shelter, and running from prey. Now everything is available at the flip of a switch, the click of a button, and the "stress" of turning a key in the ignition (which in many newer models is obsolete; you can now push a button to start your car!). We are stagnating inside our skins, and this passivity is causing a breakdown in our ability to live without pain.

In addition, we sit more than ever. The stress of sitting accelerates the aging and degradation processes in the body. Your body is designed for motion, and when you sit for prolonged periods, you shut down its self-regulating metabolic engines. Recent studies declare that sitting is "the new smoking"* and point to the rise in deadly diseases that non-motion is effecting, including cardiovascular disease, certain cancers, diabetes, depression, and of course musculoskeletal issues.

It's not just that we're sitting more; it's also *how* we sit and the lack of variety within the sitting position that contribute to wear-and-tear on the body. How you hold yourself can either help you or hurt you.

You may be able to find your way around your house in the dark, but do you know how you're sitting right now? Take a moment to check:

1. **Is your head drooping forward, in front of your ribcage?**
2. **Are your shoulders slumped forward?**
3. **Is your low back rounded into a C-shape and collapsed?**
4. **Are your legs crossed?**
5. **Are your breaths shallow, or are you breathing deeply throughout your core?**

What you don't see *can* hurt you, but your posture is one of the easiest things to correct, and you can do it right now. And now. And now again.

* Selene Yeager, "Sitting is the new smoking–even for runners," *Runner's World,* July 20, 2013.

WHY DO SO MANY PEOPLE FAIL TO PRACTICE PROPER POSTURE?

The body likes to take the easy way out. Gravity is hard to resist, and maintaining an organized upright posture takes awareness and strength, especially if your job involves sitting at a desk or performing repetitive tasks. Ironically, people are always looking for a quick fix for fitness or health, and the truth is, stacking your skull over ribs, ribs over pelvis, pelvis over knees, and knees over feet and pointing both feet forward is the absolute quickest fix that helps you last sustainably in your body for the long haul. It takes less time than swallowing a couple of Advil...and it's totally free! Add a dose of proper breathing (see chapter 7), and you are starting to re-tailor your birthday suit from the inside out.

What Exactly Is Good (Correct) Posture?

When you have correct posture, your body efficiently resists gravity in the least stressful way on your physiological and structural systems. Posture is typically thought of as a static and statue-like position. How boring! In truth, posture is dynamic in nature, and managing it is a constant interplay between your moving body and the things you do with your body. Maintaining proper alignment while moving is a challenging balancing act.* For good posture in motion, you must keep your body correctly poised within each movement to minimize the friction on your joints. In other words, activity is *not* pulling you out of good aligned posture—whether it's walking, bending over to pick up the newspaper, lifting weights, running, cycling, or doing yoga.

* My dance studies at Northwestern University exposed me to the wonderful brilliance of Moshe Feldenkrais, movement genius and the founder of the Feldenkrais Method. His analysis of human movement and alignment is a great resource.

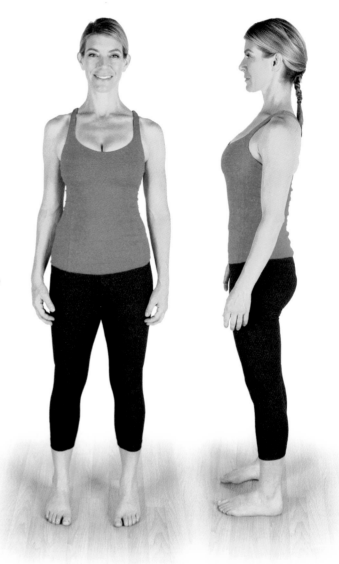

For Standing

Good posture when standing looks like this:

1. Your feet are approximately 8 to 12 inches (hip socket width) apart, and your toes are pointing forward as if you were wearing ski boots attached to downhill skis. (Make no mistake: you would never *ski* with the tips pointed outward; it would damage every soft and hard tissue above your feet. Sliding splits, anyone?)

2. Your hips are over your ankles, and your weight is evenly distributed. You are not putting more weight on one hip or the other, but are evenly balanced on both feet.

3. Add a bit of activation from your gluteal muscles if necessary to stabilize your pelvis in alignment with your ribcage (see #4). This helps give you support while standing still and prevents pelvic tipping or leaning. The amount of gluteal activation you need will depend on your body's habits, tensions, and weaknesses. Your pelvis, often referred to as a bowl, is surrounded by your hip and large buttock muscles. Its contoured shape (which is actually more like a funnel than a bowl) allows things

to flow through it—I hope! The sacrum, the strong bone at the back of the pelvis, serves as the baseboard for the entire spine.

4. Create enough tension in your core muscles so that your ribcage is positioned directly above your pelvic funnel. The amount of stabilizing tension you need will depend on the strength of your muscles and their habit of holding your posture. The upper rim of the pelvic funnel is a perfect match for the bottom of the ribcage that is ideally positioned above it. The bottom of the ribcage is like a bony periscope. Imagine that periscope shining a bright light downward to illuminate the bony funnel. If the ribcage thrusts forward, sways to the side, or pitches back, alignment suffers. You can see and feel the spinal distortions created by a pelvis and ribcage that are not "locked targets" for one another. (This pelvis-to-ribcage alignment is critical to keep all foundational respiratory tissues in reflexive alignment. The respiratory diaphragm's up-and-down movement helps keep the pelvic floor healthy and naturally toned. When the ribcage spins off-axis, the soft-tissue canister

filling this bony canister will have loads of odd twisting patterns, trigger points, and tensions within it. And when the ribcage and pelvis do not match up, the spinal bones between them become improperly loaded and stressed.)*

5. Position your skull and the brain inside it directly above your heart. This is not always easy to perceive. Draw your chin down slightly, as if at the bottom of a small nod, and press your skull into an imaginary headrest (like an early '80s Volvo headrest, not the bucket-seat headrest of a sports car that forces your head forward) to help traction your cervical vertebrae a bit. This places the hole in your ear, known as the external auditory meatus, directly over your shoulders and hips.

6. Set your shoulders directly under your ears. Shoulders tend to roll forward or hunch upward because most of life's work pulls them up and forward. Counteract that tendency by activating the muscles in the back of your shoulders and upper back to help them descend and move slightly back.

* See *Becoming a Supple Leopard,* by Kelly Starrett with Glen Cordoza (Victory Belt Publishing, 2012) for another excellent assessment of midline stabilization and posture mechanics.

THE WAVE-FORM

Your spine has an S-shape that provides a naturally elegant wave-form, with two outward curves and two inward curves. Your low back and neck are the inward curves, and your sacrum and ribcage are the outward curves. For efficient standing posture, you stack your skull over your heart, which is placed above your pelvis, which hovers north of your feet. You must maintain the spinal waves between these larger bony masses with some amount of tension (or, better put, respect) throughout the day. Ultimately, as you maintain this correct form, your body will "form" to this posture and "stand up for itself" with ease! When you are first reforming your posture, it is imperative to resist slumping or leaning, which is what pulls your body out of balance foundationally.

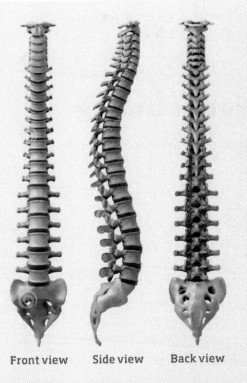

Front view   Side view   Back view

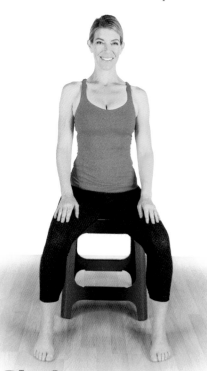
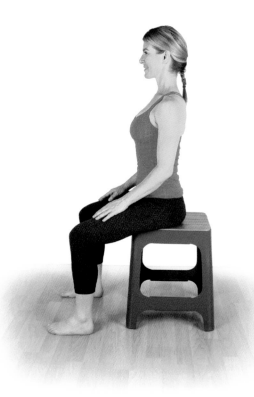

For Sitting

Sitting on a cushy couch? In a car or plane? It's going to be difficult for your pelvis to locate itself if the surface is tipping your pelvis forward or backward or sucking it into a quicksand-like vortex. Sit on a wooden stool or bench to get a sense of the proper pelvic position for sitting. Good posture when sitting looks like this:

1. The two bony prominences called ischial tuberosities, or "sit bones," at the bottom of your pelvis are in contact with the surface you're sitting on.

2. Your knees are a few inches wider than your hip sockets to help passively stabilize your pelvis. Your toes are pointed forward, and your feet are flat on the floor.

3. You are creating enough tension in your core muscles that your ribcage is positioned directly above your pelvic funnel. The amount of stabilizing tension required will likely be much greater than in standing. (It's more difficult for the stabilizing muscles of your core to do their job while you sit. This is one of the many reasons why sitting is so fatiguing to the body. It actually takes more energy to keep these muscles awake!)

4. Your eyes and head are looking straight ahead.

5. Your shoulders are directly under your ears. Activate the muscles in the back of your shoulders and upper back to help your shoulders descend and move slightly back.

SLEEPY BUTTOCKS

As soon as you sit, your buttock muscles are completely stretched, so they lose their effectiveness at supporting the position of your pelvis. They go to sleep because they don't have to work to hold you up against gravity. This weakens your base of support, so your core muscles—especially your spinal muscles—have to work triple time to keep you upright. This is why, after just a few minutes of sitting, you might start to shift in your seat in an effort to find another way to stabilize those hardworking, fatigued trunk muscles.

The Hidden Costs of Bad Posture

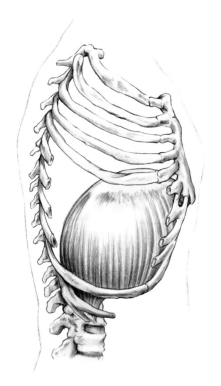

Diaphragm (side view)

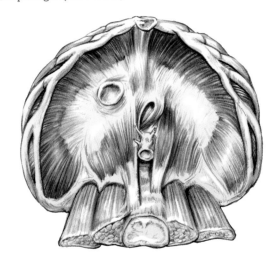

Diaphragm (inferior view)

Bad breath doesn't just ward off vampires; it also sucks the life and integrity out of your posture. Stand up for yourself and breathe better by tuning into your respiratory diaphragm.

In addition to aches and pains, there are real, lesser-known dangers of poor posture.

Poor posture creates distortions throughout your ribcage. This may not sound like a big deal, but these bony changes disrupt vital systems of your body, such as breathing and digestion. Long-term slumping or leaning literally reforms the bones of the ribcage and spine–you end up creating your own scoliosis! The imbalanced ribcage and spinal vertebrae then shift the line of pull on the most central muscle of the human body: the respiratory diaphragm.

The diaphragm is your primary breathing muscle. When it becomes loaded with trigger points, stiffness, or weakness, a host of physiological dysfunctions can develop. The diaphragm is directly linked to your stress response and the emotional centers in your brain. Improper breathing accelerates sympathetic overload, anxiety, and out-of-control feelings in your nervous system (see chapters 7, 9, and 10).

Your diaphragm is also in direct contact with the connective tissues of your heart and its main blood vessels, the aorta and vena cava. Any distortions of the diaphragm can put pressure on the heart and aorta, impacting their function and blood flow over time. The diaphragm is also a soft-tissue partition penetrated by the esophagus, so slumpy posture can weaken the esophageal junction and create gapping of the sphincter within the esophagus. This, in turn, can lead to backflow of food, also known as acid reflux and heartburn.

People who experience any or all of these issues (stress, heart problems, acid reflux, and so on) tend not to attribute them to bad posture. Aches and especially pains are easier to track to posture, but poor posture creates a host of total-body dysfunction. Long-term, the effects of bad posture include pain, limited mobility, and suffering–and in some cases a shortened life span.

Limit the time you spend standing in these shapes:

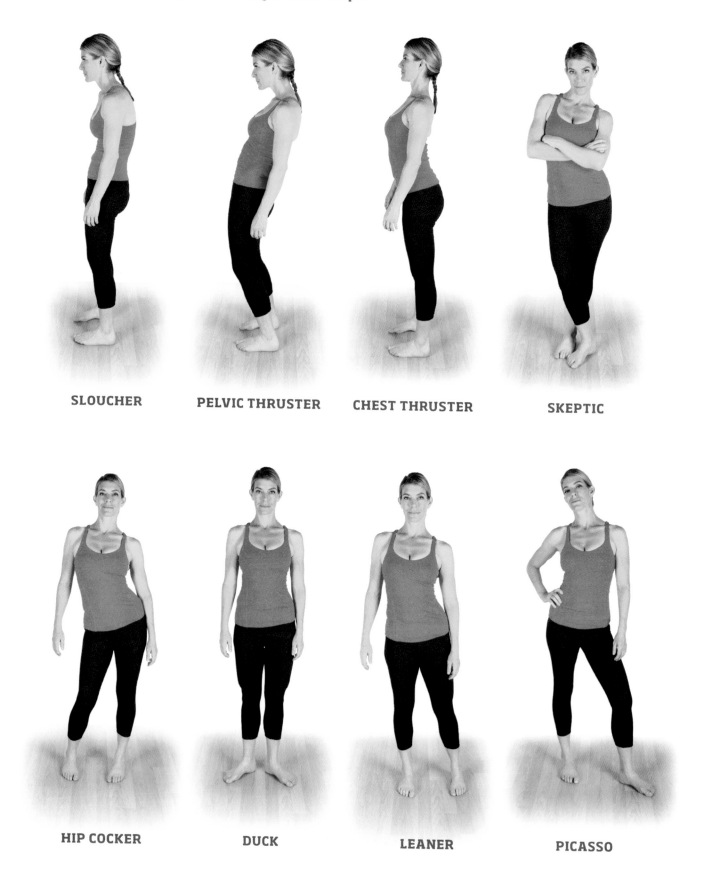

SLOUCHER   PELVIC THRUSTER   CHEST THRUSTER   SKEPTIC

HIP COCKER   DUCK   LEANER   PICASSO

Limit the time you spend sitting in these shapes:

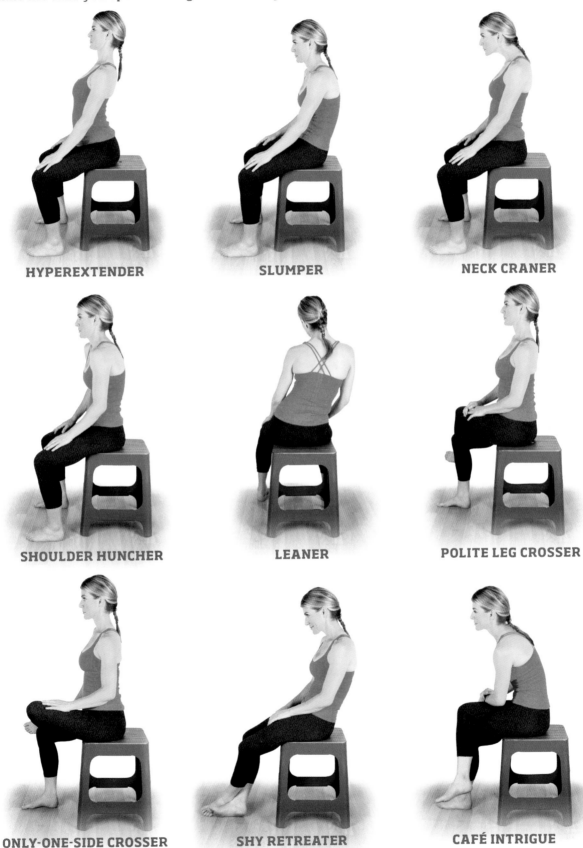

HYPEREXTENDER

SLUMPER

NECK CRANER

SHOULDER HUNCHER

LEANER

POLITE LEG CROSSER

ONLY-ONE-SIDE CROSSER

SHY RETREATER

CAFÉ INTRIGUE

Boning Up Your Posture

Your body adapts to stress, and so do your bones. In the late 1800s, a surgeon named Julian Wolff recognized that *bones adapt to load over time* and actually remodel themselves based on the stresses placed on them. Bones have interesting ridges, bumps, and troughs as part of their design because of their ability to adapt. Bones can get stronger or weaker; their cells can add density or remove mass and become more porous.

There is a genetic plan that helps create the "mainframe" of your frame. But there are also ways in which you can *deform* your form. If you consistently stress your bones in ways they were not designed to be stressed, overgrowths called *bone spurs* develop. These are often accompanied by degeneration of the softer connective tissues surrounding those bones, like cartilage, ligaments, tendons, periosteum, and fascias.

YOU ARE HOW YOU MOVE: MECHANOTRANSDUCTION

Katy Bowman is my friend and favorite biomechanist. A biomechanist studies the way a body is influenced and impacted by the forces placed upon it. I decided to include this excerpt from her new book, Move Your DNA, *rather than paraphrase her wisdom.*

MECHANOTRANSDUCTION: *The process by which cells sense and then translate mechanical signals (compression, tension, fluid shear) created by their physical environment into biochemical signals, allowing cells to adjust their structure and function accordingly.*

EXTRACELLULAR MATRIX: *A complex network of polysaccharides and proteins that provides structure and regulates cell behavior.*

Movement creates a cascade of biochemical processes that alter the state of your physiology. The conversion of movement "input" to biochemical processes is called mechanotransduction.

With apologies to those with robust training in biology, allow me to give you a brief introduction to the organization of the human body. The way academics have organized the body on paper for easier study is this:

1. Your body is made of organ systems which, in turn, are made of organs.

2. These organs are made of tissues which, in turn, are made of cells.

3. But really, your body is just made up of cells, each of these cells being connected to each other via a network of extracellular matrix.

When you move what you probably think of as your body—arms, legs, torso, head—you are rearranging not only the larger structures of your limbs and vertebrae but also your small, cellular structures.

Your Cells Are Loaded

We experience load 100 percent of the time. Gravity is one force our body responds to constantly. Just as your body would collapse if it didn't have bones, cellular organs within your cells would fall in response to the gravitational force if the cytoskeleton weren't there to hold them in place. But even though the gravitational force is constant here on Earth, the loads created by gravity depend on our physical position relative to the gravitational force. For example, gravity is always working on your bones, but the load created by gravity differs depending on how those bones line up with the perpendicular force of gravity. A month of the horizontal positioning common to bed rest can decrease your muscle and

When you consistently place the wrong kinds of stresses on your bones, such as by maintaining inefficient postural habits, you end up degrading your structural support system. That support system soon starts to rearrange itself to the point where the soft tissues decide that this is the "new normal."

When inefficient postural habits remodel your soft and hard tissues, your body is an accident waiting to happen.

Compensation: Not Necessarily a Check from Your Employer

Compensation is the act of transferring one body part's job to another body part that is not designed to handle that job. It's your body's unique way of adapting to structural changes.

Remember that song "Dem Bones"?

The toe bone's connected to the foot bone
The foot bone's connected to the ankle bone
The ankle bone's connected to the leg bone
Now shake dem skeleton bones!

bone mass. Same gravitational force. Same genes. Different position. Different body.

And gravity isn't the only force that loads our cells. External pressures (like the interaction between bone, muscle, and a chair), frictions (like a new pair of shoes against your foot skin), and tractioning (remember, in '80s movies, those old school pulley-on-cast devices used in hospitals after someone broke their leg skiing?) forces all create cellular deformations within our body, as does movement itself. The lengthening and shortening of larger tissues like muscle creates pushes and pulls on the small-scale stuff.

I believe that most of us understand that our body responds to mechanical input. Our optometrist monitors us for high pressure in the eyes to avoid damage to the optic nerve. We're familiar with pressure wounds like bedsores developing in those who sit or lie continuously without shifting much. We discuss, with ease, the new pair of shoes that made blisters at first, and how that one time we had a cast, our muscle wasted away, leaving a noticeable difference. We are quite comfortable with these examples (I hope) but most don't ponder how these phenomena occur. Why, exactly, does the optic nerve die in a high-pressure environment, leaving one with glaucoma?

Mechanotransduction is, finally, being researched as the underlying mechanism of many diseases. Diseases of mechanotransduction are those

ailments arising from an area of cells (then tissue, then organ) troubled by the mechanical environment you've created, both directly and indirectly.

Movement, position, and the resting state of our musculoskeletal system are huge influencers of our mechanical environment. While we think of movement as something we do to train our body into better shape, most don't consider how that "better shape" comes about. Well, now you know. It is via the process of mechanotransduction that our physical self adapts (in shape) to our experience of the physical world. More precisely, the physical expression that is your body is the sum total of loads experienced by your cells.

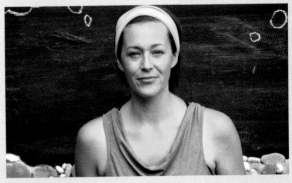

Katy Bowman, MS, is one of my most cherished colleagues. She is educating the world about human movement and its biomechanical meaning in our lives.

Let's say you trip and break your pinky toe. (Did anyone ever tell you that the pinky toe is useless? Well, try breaking yours, and you'll find out just how critical it is!) Your doctor tapes it up (there's generally no splint for the pinky toe) and tells you to wear flip-flops for the next six weeks. (Your doctor told you to wear flip-flops, not me–I, personally, am not a fan of them.) It hurts too much to put pressure on your pinky toe, so you start treading into the inside of your foot, which begins to stress your big toe and ankle in a weird way. This ankle stress travels up the long muscles of your lower leg into your knee, which starts to track in a slightly different manner. Uptown of the knee, the hip joint is also controlling its movements differently to help you avoid the pinky toe, and because of that the muscles in your lower back tighten up to help keep you from driving body weight into that poor foot. In the meantime, you (unconsciously) spend a lot more time leaning onto your other hip, leg, and foot because they are stronger and uninjured. With all this compensation, you start having weird tweaks in your back and pain in your neck. Those back spasms and neck pains are likely the result of all the new tension you've created throughout your hip and spinal muscles by unconsciously compensating to prevent further damage to the pinky toe. Oh dem skeleton bones! And uh oh, the fascial seams that tie it all together! (More on fascia, your body's seam system, in chapter 4.)

Unfortunately, this type of compensation does not add anything to your checking account. In fact, your body's mode of compensating for tissues rearranging into a new normal is often the cause of continued aches and pains, and those knotty bits and creaky joints start demanding your attention–and the costly attention of doctors, massage therapists, chiropractors, painkillers, and so on. Your pain drains your wallet, your time, and *you* of all those things you'd like to be doing if only you didn't have that darn pain. Annual estimated costs associated with pain in the United States are $560 to $635 billion.* Your compensating body has sparked an industry–but you have the power to break that cycle.

* Darrell J. Gaskin and Patrick Richard state in Appendix C of the book *Relieving Pain in America: A Blueprint for Transforming Prevention, Care, Education, and Research:* "We found that the annual cost of pain was greater than the annual costs in 2010 dollars of heart disease ($309 billion), cancer ($243 billion), and diabetes ($188 billion) and nearly 30 percent higher than the combined cost of cancer and diabetes."

How Poor Posture Alters Blood Chemistry

If my scare tactics have not yet convinced you to stand up for yourself and prevent wear-and-tear on your body, perhaps Harvard psychologist Amy Cuddy's studies on "power posing" might. She found that postural choices add up to emotional content in your body via hormones that are released depending on how you hold yourself. She had groups of people hold slumpy, folded-arm postures and found that these "low-power poses" increased baseline stress-inducing cortisol by about 17 percent and decreased confidence-boosting testosterone by about 10 percent. Standing powerfully upright increased levels of testosterone and shrank levels of cortisol (see www.wired.com/wiredscience/2012/05/st_cuddy/).

"We used to think that emotion ended on the face," Cuddy says. "Now there is established research showing that while it's true that facial expressions reflect how you feel, you can also 'fake it until you make it.' In other words, you can smile long enough that it makes you feel happy. This work extends that finding on facial feedback, which is decades old, by focusing on postures and measuring neuroendocrine levels." (See hbswk.hbs.edu/item/6461.html.)

So, if your body is shaped in a frown, you'll not only accumulate aches and pains, but also feel less confident and more stressed than those who "take a stand." Let the Roll Model help you turn that body frown upside down!

Why Does Your Body Let This Happen?

Your body is just going along for the ride, really. Your mind is often the one that decides it wants to slump in a chair, lean on one hip, wear high heels, or refuse to stretch or exercise. Your mindset about your image permeates the way you hold yourself. Your desire to fit in with your friends or fit into restrictive clothing and shoes impacts your structure and your ability to carry your body through space. You are either *aware* or *unaware* of how you stand up for yourself.

Or perhaps your posture was thrust upon you by an accident that caused your body to grow significant amounts of scar tissue that inhibit efficiency, or by a genetic condition has afflicted your structure. Emotional wounds can also lock you into a certain postural behavior, ranging from a recoil from your fears to a positional affectation of bravado. Other contributions come from your environment, such as the design of chairs in offices, restaurants, theaters, and vehicles. Nutrition also plays a role in your structural integrity. If you are not feeding yourself nourishing foods, eventually you will be unable to support yourself to the best of your ability. And, most notably, your structure changes as you age; connective tissues progressively dehydrate, and you lose muscle mass and bone density.

While all this is *common*, none of it is *normal*. You have the power to change your body's behaviors and erase your pain by becoming a Roll Model.

Setting Your Posture Straight

You may or may not be able to pinpoint *why* your posture has become an imposition on your day-to-day structural comfort and enjoyment of life, but no matter the cause, there are things you can do to take control. Once you become conscious of the patterns and habits that contribute to your pain, you will be able to start making choices to reverse it. It's time to reshape your body into a better living environment that serves you, pain-free, for a lifetime.

You're better off doing some simple maintenance yourself than ending up in a doctor's office with a prescription for painkillers or, worse, surgery.

Learn your body, make better choices, and bring your structure back to balance without the middleman. You can do this for yourself, *right now*. Train yourself to master the basics. It's time for an intervention to redirect your growth in a positive and helpful way. The good news is that your body is in a constant state of regeneration. It is possible to look and feel better in your body!

In essence, it boils down to two simple things:

1. **Habits you can consciously control**
2. **Conditions you must consciously work toward altering**

HOW ARE YOU "HOLDING UP"?

EXPRESS POSTURE CHECK:

1. **Your eyes look forward, with your head above your heart.**
2. **Your lower ribcage is positioned over your pelvic funnel.**
3. **If you are sitting, both feet are planted firmly on the floor.**
4. **If you are standing, your weight is evenly distributed and your feet are pointed forward.**

BONUS BREATH CHECK:

Give yourself a "dose" of ten complete breaths daily to reaffirm your posture. Whether sitting or standing, maintain all postural alignment points. Breathe completely into your torso by ballooning your ribcage and abdomen in all directions without lifting your shoulders. Your abdomen and ribs should swell and deflate, but your spine remains upright and unmoving. Your torso will feel supported by your soft-tissue safety vest. It stiffens like inflatable tubing when you breathe in and softens when you breathe out.

4 The Science Section: Fascia and Proprioception

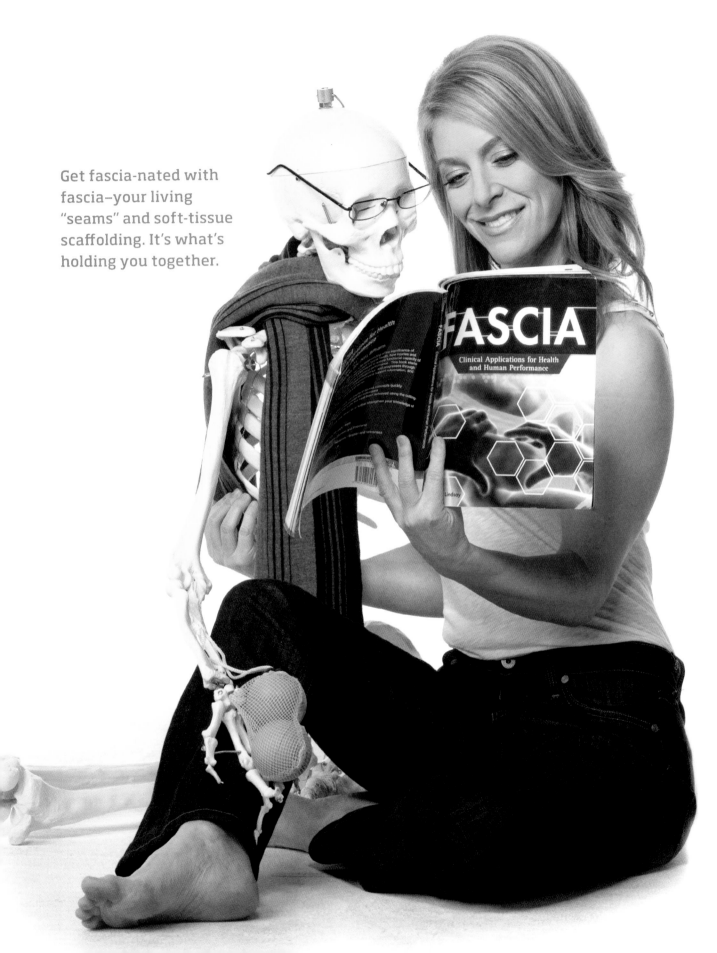

Get fascia-nated with fascia—your living "seams" and soft-tissue scaffolding. It's what's holding you together.

The title of this chapter might be one of the reasons you bought this book, or it might make your eyes glaze over. As I've mentioned before, you can skip this entire chapter and still reap the health benefits of rolling. It is not essential for every morsel of "the science stuff" to make sense to you for your body to *know* that it works.

If you dive into this chapter, though, you just might discover that having unfettered access to your own anatomy and understanding your own body is extremely fun. Using the Roll Model Balls is a way to turn your body into a laboratory. You'll be sampling the anatomy and physiology that I explain in these sections like a skilled research scientist. But in this case, you won't need a lab coat. You'll just "knead" yourself and your balls.

I have distilled the science of rolling into its basic elements so that you understand how the self-care healthcare approach of the Roll Model Method can work for you. There is a lot more to explore beyond these pages, and I hope this chapter inspires your own further research!

Fascia: Your Seam System

We cannot have a thorough discussion about the Roll Model without talking about the soft-tissue scaffolding that links everything inside of you together. *Fascia* is the ubiquitous living seam system in your body that threads your tissues to one another. Wherever the Therapy Balls roll, they impact your body's fasciae or fascias (both of which are correct spellings of the plural of *fascia*). In order to understand fascia, let's take a step back with a brief primer on the subject of *connective tissue.*

The body's connective tissues develop from the *mesoderm*–the middle of the three primary embryonic layers. (Your fascia has been with you since you were fifty cells old!) Connective tissues include the fascias, but this broad category also encompasses all of the other tissues that connect body parts. A wide range of tissues are connective, and they can be broken down into three groups:

- **Hard tissues** like bone, cartilage, and periosteum (the firm tissue surrounding bones)
- **Soft tissues** like fascias, tendons, and ligaments
- **Fluid tissues**, including blood and lymph

Because all connective tissues originate from the same foundational tissue, they are comprised of the same components: cells, fibers, and ground substance.

- The **cells** found in connective tissues differ depending on which type of connective tissue they belong to. For example, blood contains mostly platelets, plus red and white blood cells; bones have mostly osteoblasts, osteoclasts, and osteocytes; and fascia has mostly fibroblasts (plus a few others; see below).
- The **fibers** are the same from tissue to tissue: varying amounts of collagen, elastin, and reticulin.
- The cells and fibers are surrounded by a viscous fluid called **ground substance.**

> **GROUND SUBSTANCE:** *The gel-like component of connective tissue in which the cells and fibers reside.*

The ratio of cells to fibers, coupled with the density of the surrounding ground substance, determines the type of connective tissue and thus its function. For example, blood contains many cells but has no fibers within its ground substance. Bone contains many cells and loads of collagen fibers but has a low ratio of fluid in its ground substance.*

Connective tissue serves many functions in the body. These can be grouped into two main categories: **connection** and **protection.**

The connective functions of connective tissue are to:

- Bind and separate structures
- Support organs
- Provide a scaffolding framework for the whole body's structure
- Fill space

The protective functions of connective tissue are to:

- Store fat
- Make blood
- Fight infections
- Repair tissue damage
- Insulate
- Lubricate

Fascia is just one of many types of connective tissue in your body, but it is the tissue that plays the biggest role in the Roll Model approach. *Fascial* connective tissue has its own specialized functions because of its unique composition.

Before I get granular about fascia, take a moment to digest the following definitions. I've hashed out

* Deane Juhan, "Ground Substance," http://holistichealthservices.com/research/ground_substance.html

three different explanations for you, amalgamated from many sources. The petite one is memorizable, the shorter one will satisfy a blog reader, and the longest one might send you to the Internet.

- **Petite:** Fascia is the body's living aqueous knitting fabric. This seam system is the body's soft-tissue scaffolding that interconnects you to yourself.

- **Short:** Fascia is the fibrous and gelatinous bodywide web. It is a seam system that provides structure, protection, repair, and body sense. It is the interconnected soft-tissue scaffolding that gives your body form and shape. It links muscular proteins and other connective-tissue structures, such as bones, ligaments, and tendons.

- **Long:** Fascia is the soft-tissue component of the connective-tissue system. It surrounds and penetrates muscles, bones, organs, nerves, blood vessels, and other structures of the body. Fascia is an interconnected, three-dimensional web of tissue that extends from head to toe, front to back, and interior to exterior. It is responsible for maintaining structural integrity, providing support, protection, and shock absorption and acting as a home for sensory neurons. Fascia plays an essential role in hemodynamic, lymphatic, and biochemical processes and provides the matrix that allows for intercellular communication. After injury, fascia creates an environment for tissue repair. Fascia can refer to dense plane-like fascial sheets (such as the fascia lata, or iliotibial band) as well as joint and organ capsules, muscular septa, ligaments, retinacula, aponeuroses, tendons, myofascia, neurofascia, and other fibrous collagenous tissues.

Fascia in Latin means "band" or "bundle." Fascial tissue is comprised of

- **Collagen and elastin fibers:** This is the stringy, translucent, cobweb-like stuff that you see when you pull apart pieces of meat.

- **Resident cells:**
  - **Fibroblasts** produce the fibers that form the fascial web.
  - **Myofibroblasts** are contractile cells that create stiffness in injured fascia.
  - **Fasciacytes** help maintain the chemical balance in fascia's ground substance.
  - **Adipocytes** are fat cells that provide not only cushioning protection, but also endocrine function (and more).*

- **Migrant cells:** Macrophages and mast cells participate in immunity and inflammation processes.

- **Fluids:** Hyaluronan, glycosaminoglycans, and water provide the aqueous and slick environment that permits motion (slide & glide) among tissues.

Fascia can be seen as a structural highway for all of the above. It's also laced with multiple types of sensory neurons, as well as pain-sensing neurons. Fascia is so nerve-rich that it can arguably be called a tissue of communication (see the information about proprioception in chapter 4).

Fascia Dynamics: Elasticity and Creep

The collagen fibers in fascia are comprised of collagen molecules that have a triple helix formation. This formation gives fascia its trademark "crimp," which is especially visible in deep fascia. The crimp looks like tiny waves within the fascia (remember crimped hair in the '80s?). This wave formation permits fascias to lengthen to a great extent and then return to their original shape. Think about it: when you stretch within a "safe range," your body always returns to form (unless you've stretched well past your range and torn your tissues).

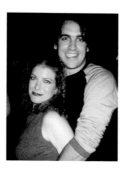

Flashback/Flashdance: As a dancer in college, I occasionally had to crimp my hair.

* Robert Schleip, Heike Jager, and Werner Klingler, "Fascia is alive: How cells modulate the tonicity and architecture of fascial tissues," in *Fascia: The Tensional Network of the Human Body* (Elsevier, 2012): 157.

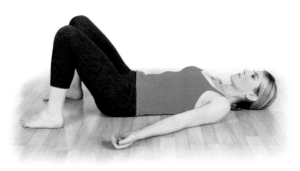

For an example of fascia in action, hold out your left hand, palm up, and let your fingers display their relaxed, natural curl.

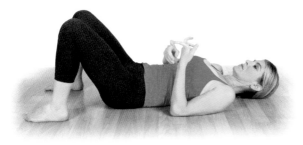

Then, using your right hand, stretch your left index finger as straight as it will go. Hold for 30 seconds, then let it spring back into its curl.

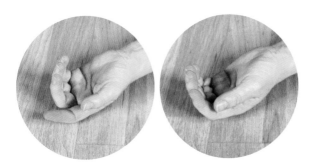

It may take several minutes for your finger to return to its normal resting tone, but eventually it will.

You have not misshaped your index finger's fascia forever. This temporary reshaping is due to the *viscoelasticity* of fascia (*viscous:* like dripping honey + *elastic:* like a snappy rubber band).

The viscoelasticity of your fascia allows your body to morph into different shapes. But when you choose to hold one position constantly, your body starts to re-form to that shape. This is known as *creep.* As Joe Muscolino points out in his book *Kinesiology:* "The concept of **creep** may be negative such as when a client changes the tissue shape and structure over time because of poor posture, or it may be positive when body-work and exercise are done to change and correct a client's poor tissue shape and structure."*

When you roll with the balls, you induce local stretch into stiff and overtightened tissues and improving the flow of their fluids. These taut tissues need your help in restoring their optimal positions. The balls are like little rubber scalpels that can reform you without incisions or stitches. The pressure and grip of the rubber helps you remodel yourself.

* Joseph E. Muscolino, *Kinesiology* (Elsevier, 2010): 64.

Fluidity: You're Goopy on the Inside

Like the Earth, your body consists mostly of water. Seventy percent of your body's water content is suspended within its cells, and another 30 percent is outside the cells, or extracellular.** Your fascia is a bodywide storehouse for much of this water, both inside its cells and soaking throughout its fibrous threads. This extracellular fascial fluid bathes and flows between the cells and fibers of your fascial "wetsuit." You are very, very goopy on the inside. (Luckily, you have skin to seal in all the moisture!) This is one of the reasons why remaining hydrated is so critical to

your health, as fascia relies on water for proper cellular function and replication. Its living elements, the fibroblast cells, need a balanced nutrient bath (the ground substance suspended in the extracellular fluids) to produce the nonliving collagen and elastin fibers that knit together the body parts in need of patching and suturing.

All these fluids also permit your body's structures to move around and among one another. Healthy tissues are pliable; they bend but don't

** Frans Van den Berg, "Extracellular Matrix," in *Fascia: The Tensional Network of the Human Body* (Elsevier, 2012): 168.

break, and they fluff back up after being compressed, like a springy wet sponge. Holding unhealthy body positions day in and day out (like sitting, leaning, or slumping) overtaxes and compresses your fascias and contributes to local fascial distortions. Fascias that are excessively and continuously "oversqueezed" from bad body habits are unable to absorb the water they need to return to their original shape, and as a result they become deformed and dehydrated. Dehydrated fascial tissues tend to be very sticky and stiff. When your tissues are chronically dehydrated from lack of fluids or lack of motion, your fascias literally stick to one another, creating "dams" or *adhesions*. Think of the texture of an old cleaning rag that was crumpled up while still moist and thrown under the sink for a month: it won't return to its original wrinkle-free shape until it's plunged into water.

Unlike an old rag or a dried sponge, your fascias don't automatically plump up when you down 8 ounces of water. If your fascias are stuck together and adhered, no amount of water will help those fibers become better absorbers. The stiffened fascia needs to be coaxed through motion and friction to receive the fluids surrounding them. This is where the Roll Model Balls come in

handy. Using the balls' grippy pressure along with a variety of rolling techniques helps the water molecules bond to the collagen fibers and nourish the fascial web.* Note that areas of damaged fascia may be quite tender due to the inflammatory environment of excessive fluids locked in by adhered collagen fibers. These fluids are often loaded with cellular waste and irritants that annoy the dehydrated and dysfunctional fascia and the nerves embedded within it.

One of the more extreme examples of tissue dehydration is having a cast removed after several weeks or months. Naturally the muscle is very weak, but the fascias associated with the damaged bone or muscle will have adapted to non-movement and will have remodeled themselves into the body's own self-cast of that area. Helping all the fascias return to their springy resiliency takes many more weeks of massage, physical therapy, and painful rehab. There will be abundant trigger points within the muscle, along with toxic buildup from the lack of fluid perfusion in those tissues. Motion is lotion for the human body, and movement is the medicine it needs to reclaim its function. Motion keeps warm fluids circulating, acting as a pump to help fluids enter and exit. Nutrients in, garbage out.

* Sandy Fritz, *Sports & Exercise Massage: Comprehensive Care for Athletics, Fitness and Rehabilitation*, 2nd Edition (Mosby, 2013): 34.

The Categories of Fascia

Fascia is divided into two basic categories, *superficial fascia* and *deep fascia*, with a transition zone on either side called *loose fascia*.

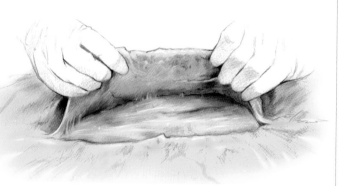

The superficial fascia layer of the abdomen is being pulled away from the layers underneath it, namely loose fascia, which overlies deep fascia.

Superficial fascia lies just beneath the skin and is comprised of loosely arranged areolar (web-like) collagen fibers in a matrix with adipose (fat cells). This layer feels spongy, springy, or fluffy. Ninety-eight percent of your body is coated in fat-filled superficial fascia. In fact, the only areas missing the protective fatty cushion in the superficial layer are around the ears, nose, lips, eyelids, labia, and scrotum. (Gil Hedley notes that "one does not find fatty deposition in these areas, though there may be some representation of the layer otherwise.")

Deep fascia (aka *fascia profunda*) has a tough duct tape–like appearance, with crimp-like waves in different densities. It is highly organized in its arrangement and is found surrounding muscles or as a thickened, broad aponeurotic tendon layer.

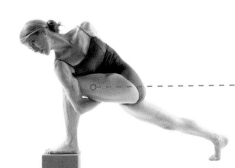

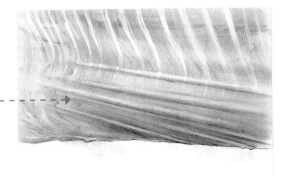

The iliotibial band, considered a deep fascia.

LOCATE TISSUE: TOUCH YOUR SUPERFICIAL FASCIA

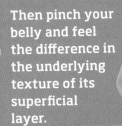

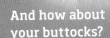

Take a pinch of the skin on your cheek and its underlying fatty layer and roll it between your fingers.

Then pinch your belly and feel the difference in the underlying texture of its superficial layer.

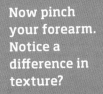

Now pinch your forearm. Notice a difference in texture?

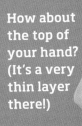

How about the top of your hand? (It's a very thin layer there!)

And how about your buttocks?

Your superficial fascia has different amounts of collagen and elastin, and varying sizes of fat cells, depending on its location in your body. You have more "padding" on your buttocks, for example.

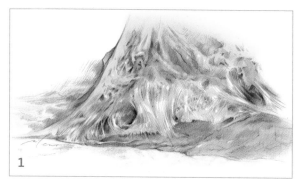

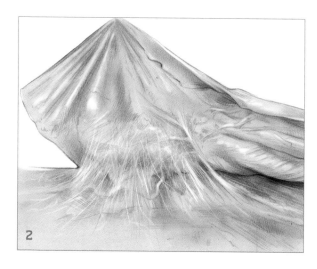

Both images show the loose fascia connections between layers. Image 1 (above) shows superficial fascia tractioned away from deep fascia and the membranous cobweb in between. Image 2 (right) shows deep fascia pulled away from the muscle underneath it; the loose fascia is stretched apart as the deep fascia is removed. Both of these loose fascia zones provide areas of slide & glide.

LOCATE TISSUE: TOUCH YOUR DEEP FASCIA

While seated or standing, bring your hand ▶ to the side of your thigh and attempt to clamp your fingers in a wide grip to penetrate beyond the spongy superficial layer and dig into the wider, flatter, denser, deep, long fascial strip of the iliotibial (IT) band.

Using deep touch, attempt to strum across it and feel its toughness compared with the superficial fascia on top. Now stand up and, maintaining your grip on that IT band, straighten and bend your knee and feel the deep fascia stiffen as you bend your knee and slacken as you straighten it.

Now take your hand to your earlobe and roll it between your fingertips. There is no fatty superficial fascia here; there is skin and a slight layer of loose fascia, which is directly adhered to the deep fascia that gives the earlobe its shape.

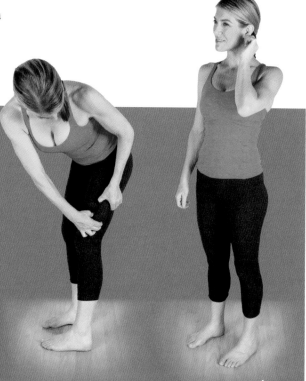

Now travel higher up your ear, where the firmer deep fascia transitions into malleable cartilage. If you rub it, you'll slide the deep fascia over the cartilage, and if you do so with firm pressure, you'll notice that your ear gets hot rather quickly! Heat is released as the collagen molecules temporarily uncrimp and change from a gel-like state to a more fluid state...all because of your applied pressure and friction!

Loose fascia refers to fascia that cannot be categorized as either superficial or deep. It is found as an intervening connecting layer between layers of deep fascia, between deep fascia and myofascia, and between superficial and deep fascias. Structurally, it can be web-like or more like a membrane (known as membranous fascia). *Loose fascia permits the motion of slide & glide all over your body.*

SLIDE & GLIDE: *The ability of motion and movement to occur among fascias and the structures they interconnect.*

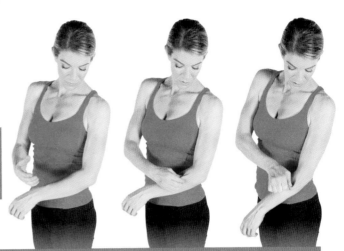

LOCATE TISSUE: TOUCH YOUR LOOSE FASCIA

Loose fascia is not as easy to discern as superficial or deep fascia. One way to get a sense of its location and mobility is to play with the internal slide & glide zone between the superficial and deep layers. It's a slippery seam that keeps the layers tied to one another. To access this transition zone, grab a big pinch of skin on your forearm and the fatty layer that adheres to it and then shift the whole mass within your pinch as far as it will move over the stiffer underlying deep fascia. Then move it in another direction, and another, then pull it away from your body and twist it as much as it will yield. You've just created massive shear (see page 144), which mobilized your membranous fascial layer.

▼ Now try mobilizing this transition layer of loose fascia by skin-rolling your abdomen.

Use both hands and pinch a significant inch on the right or left side of your navel. Go as deep as you can without annoying yourself.

Maintaining that pinch, create a steady rolling action and walk your fingers up and down your abdomen, maintaining the roll at all times.

You'll notice that there is a tighter relationship between the seams in some layers and a looser relationship in others. Attempt to feel the available slide & glide between your superficial and deep fascia layers all over your body.

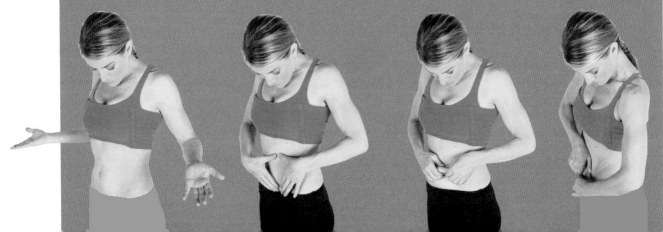

Myofascia

Myofascia refers to the familiar-named muscle structures along with their associated interpenetrating fascias. For example, your biceps is a myofascial structure, as is your gastrocnemius (calf muscle). There is no muscle that does not have fascia winding its way throughout every layer of its cells and fascicles and surrounding its whole structure. Therefore, while we are in the habit of talking about muscles, the terms *myofascia* and *muscle* can be used interchangeably.

Although there can be fascia without muscle in the human body, there is never muscle without fascia. Even your tongue adheres to itself because of its fascias. It boils down to this: every muscle in your body is attached with fascias over 100 percent of its surface, as well as throughout its internal structural components. This means that all contractile tissues in your body are interconnected to one another through your fascias. Make nice with your supportive fascia, and it will support you!

Fascia twines around every cell, cell bundle, and group of cell bundles to create the organ that is myofascia. At every level of wrapping,

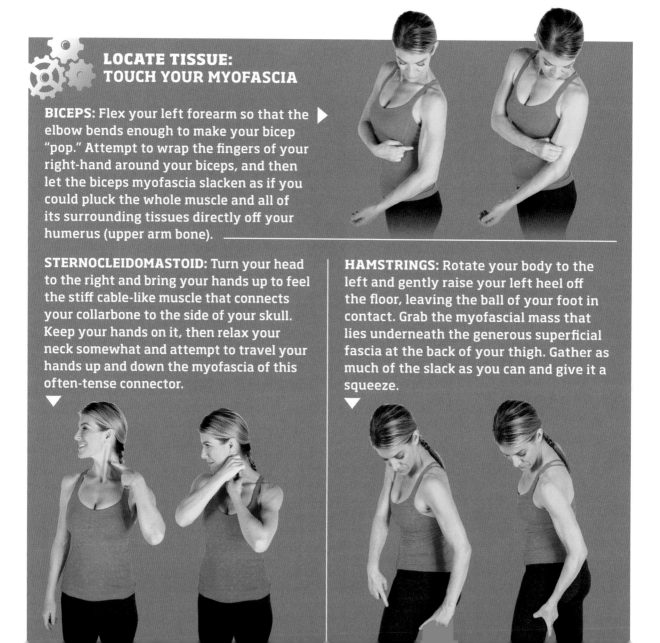

LOCATE TISSUE: TOUCH YOUR MYOFASCIA

BICEPS: Flex your left forearm so that the elbow bends enough to make your bicep "pop." Attempt to wrap the fingers of your right-hand around your biceps, and then let the biceps myofascia slacken as if you could pluck the whole muscle and all of its surrounding tissues directly off your humerus (upper arm bone).

STERNOCLEIDOMASTOID: Turn your head to the right and bring your hands up to feel the stiff cable-like muscle that connects your collarbone to the side of your skull. Keep your hands on it, then relax your neck somewhat and attempt to travel your hands up and down the myofascia of this often-tense connector.

HAMSTRINGS: Rotate your body to the left and gently raise your left heel off the floor, leaving the ball of your foot in contact. Grab the myofascial mass that lies underneath the generous superficial fascia at the back of your thigh. Gather as much of the slack as you can and give it a squeeze.

the fascia has a specific name. It's not critical for you to remember these names, but it is helpful to recognize that your fascias subdivide constantly to provide the optimal interconnected scaffolding for your body's many layered parts.

An orange has a segmented structure that makes fascia subdivisions easy to understand. Here is the whole orange intact (image 1).

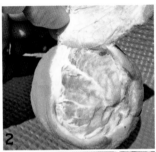

When you peel away the orange's skin (image 2), the underlying thick white pith tends to come with it (image 3). This is similar to how firmly connected your skin is to your superficial fascia. Image 4 has enough pith or "superficial fascia" removed to see the underlying segments. The segments remain held together as a globe by their outermost wrapping of "deep fascia," analogous to human epimysium.

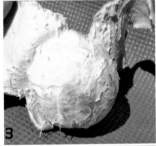

- **Epimysium:** This is the fascial encasement encircling multiple bundles and displaying the familiar shape of the "known muscle." At this level, tendons connect the epimysial fascia into neighboring structures. Structurally, epimysium is considered a deep fascia. In the case of our orange, it would be the bottom layer of pith that stubbornly surrounds the orange. Once you break through that, you see the individual segments waiting to be separated and popped into your mouth.

The membrane surrounding each orange segment contains dozens of juice cells (images 5 and 6). This membrane is analogous to the fascial layer called the perimysium. As it's pulled away (images 7 and 8), you can see that there are fine strands of membrane connecting into the individual cells within. This interconnectedness is similar to loose fascia acting as a "loose stitch" connecting the seams of one layer to another layer.

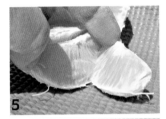

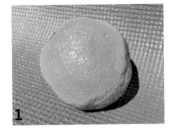

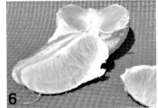

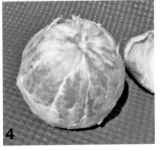

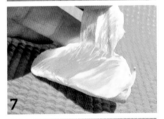

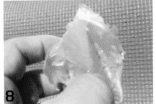

- **Perimysium:** The fascia encircling a bundle of muscle cells. At this level, this bundle is called a *fascicle*. This is also where the muscle spindle sensory neuron (proprioceptor) is located. Picture the membrane comprising a single orange segment. The membrane has a bit more integrity, and if you slice through it, you reveal the hundreds of individual mini-juice units waiting to be squeezed.

The smallest bit of a segmented orange is just a thin membrane surrounding a juice-filled micro-pocket (images 9 and 10). This is analogous to the endomysium surrounding an individual muscle cell.

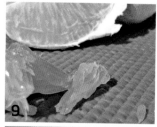

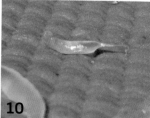

- **Endomysium:** This is the fascia that enrobes individual muscle cells. Think of the thin layer of firm tissue that surrounds the smallest unit of an orange. If you pinched it, juice would spurt out, and you'd be left with a very thin membrane.

All these fascias, endomysium, perimysium, and epimysium are sewn to one another, twining together to give the myofascia its integrity and shape. The tendons that connect the myofascia to the next structure are actually all the fascias woven together without the muscle protein packed within them. The "casings" link into the next structure, whether it's another myofascia, a tendon, a ligament, or the periosteum surrounding a bone. These are the interlinked threads and seams of your interconnected body. It's why the pain you've had in your shoulder for weeks suddenly vanishes as you are rolling on your lower back. Your fascias form a seam structure that is threaded throughout your body, so working on one area impacts the whole. **It's all *interconnected*.**

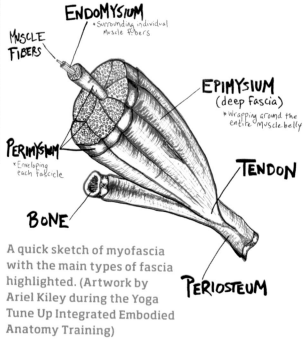

A quick sketch of myofascia with the main types of fascia highlighted. (Artwork by Ariel Kiley during the Yoga Tune Up Integrated Embodied Anatomy Training)

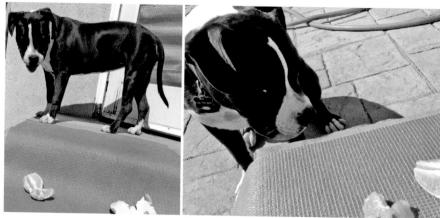

My puppy, Haley, cannot resist the dissection of an orange.

Fascia Remodeling with the Roll Model Balls

Your cells are a renewable resource; cells are being born and dying constantly. It's up to you to foster the healthiest possible environment so that positive changes and adaptations continue to occur in every system of your body.

You are the cruise director for your inner ecosystem. As explained in chapter 3, your body is an adaptation machine, and it responds to stress. It either is stressed to adapt and grow stronger or stressed to adapt toward dysfunction. Taking care of yourself today will pay off tomorrow, but the cumulative effect shows up every seven years, which is the time frame for every cell in your body to renew and replace itself.

It's up to you and your commitment to self-care whether you improve your "interior decorating" or accelerate your own breakdown.

Your fascial tissue and the collagen within it turns over approximately every two years.* That potentially means that two years from now, you will have remodeled yourself from the inside out using the Roll Model Method. You have the power to alter the way your tissues have absorbed years of tension, poor habits, or scar tissue. Now, as you begin to reshape yourself with these tools, you can create the conditions for optimal adaptations to occur.

* www.fasciaresearch.de/Schleip_TrainingPrinciplesFascial.pdf

FASCIA REMODELING AND PHYSICAL TRAINING

Like your bones, fascia responds to the stresses you put on your body to build density or laxity. Due to fascia's lower cell count, it does not repair and regenerate as quickly as muscle or blood cells do. Fascia needs time to repair itself. After exercise, this time frame is approximately 48 to 72 hours (see www.fascialfitnesstoday.com/Images/MassageMatters_Spring2012.pdf). That's why it's not a good idea to try to break a personal record for overhead squatting two days in a row. Your body needs at least 48 hours of rest and recovery for the scaffolding to establish its new normal.

From MRI to Competition in Six Months:
An Athlete Restores Her Slide, Glide, & Stride

Dear Jill,

To answer your question about my baseline change, I no longer squat with pain! I recover. **I actually recover.** I don't work around my dysfunctional tissues. I treat my body so that it works for me in its entirety. Strength gains are made only in a fully functional body.

What I never told you is that I've had chronic pain in my left hip for months but had been hiding my injury for years. I suspected all along that it was stuck fascia (IT band and vastus lateralis were like linoleum and external rotators were locked!) but had an MRI to make sure I didn't have a torn labrum. The results were inconclusive—inflammation in the hip joint?

This past June, I started seeing an amazing manual therapist, Noelle Nieva (who did one of your Therapy Ball Trainings in NYC), and I took to my ALPHA Ball with abandon. The one-two punch of the therapist's help and the ALPHA got me out of pain. I remember walking up the subway steps about four weeks after I began treatment and realized that I had no pain in my hip. I was shocked to not be hurting anymore and knew that I had the tools to keep myself healthy with the Roll Model Balls. It's hard to believe that I put up with that much pain for as long as I did.

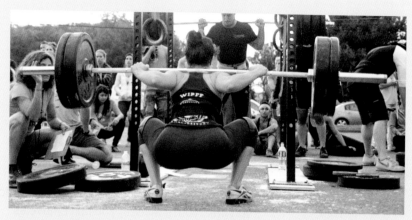

Elizabeth lifted 200 pounds of metal, pain-free, breaking her personal record during a competition.

This squat photo was taken four months after I started to treat my injury, at The Beast of the East in Connecticut in October 2013. I used the balls as my primary warm-up tool since the athlete warm-up area was chaotic and intimidating. The balls got my tissues ready to play, but working with the balls also soothed me and allowed me to relax and focus in the middle of the madness. With very little effort, I achieved things that weekend that I never thought possible. Up to that day I had never PR'ed [broken a personal record] in competition because my nerves took me out of my body. On this weekend I PR'ed in almost every event with confidence and calm.

The event in the picture was a team workout that required each of the four team members to find an eight-repetition maximum back squat in 20 minutes. My goal for the day was 185 pounds. I hit that number with ease and then went on to 195 pounds. With about 90 seconds left I loaded the bar to 200 pounds and squatted that eight times. At 41 years old and weighing 140 pounds, I moved 4,640 pounds in less than 20 minutes and walked away without pain.

From the MRI to the competition was about six months.

My confidence in my body returned, and I now coach and compete better than ever. I feel like I have the magic "rubber bullets" that can annihilate my fears of competition and the pains that I was hiding from you, from myself, and from my students.

Best,
Elizabeth

Elizabeth Wipff, 41

*Lead Coach and Director,
CrossFit Virtuosity
Coaching Program*

Brooklyn, New York

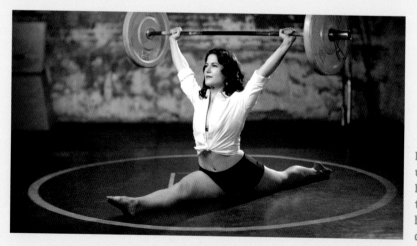

Elizabeth has been using the Roll Model Balls for more than three years and lifting heavy things for dozens.

Proprioception:
Your EmbodyMap

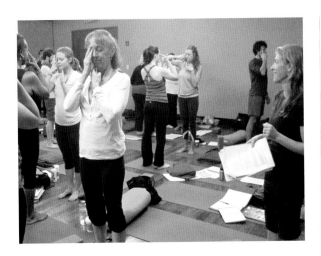

One of my favorite quizzes that we use in my anatomy trainings is the Anatomical Sobriety Test. Trainees close their eyes, and then I call out different body parts, and they have to locate them. This is a great way to define what you know and don't know about your anatomy.

I firmly believe that one of the greatest causes of musculoskeletal disease is a lack of total body awareness. Most bodies are littered with blind spots–areas of overuse, underuse, and misuse. These body blind spots cause dis-coordination and movement confusion. Have you ever noticed that when you're injured, you don't move as gracefully? Your brain relies on feedback from your sensory nerves to move your body through space. Your brain's ability to collect and understand this information is called *proprioception*. Proprioception is trainable, and improving it is an important factor in your long-term health.

PROPRIOCEPTION: *Your body's sense of itself; your inner GPS system. The ability to sense the position, location, orientation, and movement of your body and its parts.**

* Jaap C. van der Wal, "Proprioception, mechanoreception and the anatomy of fascia," in *Fascia: The Tensional Network of the Human Body* (Elsevier, 2012): 81.

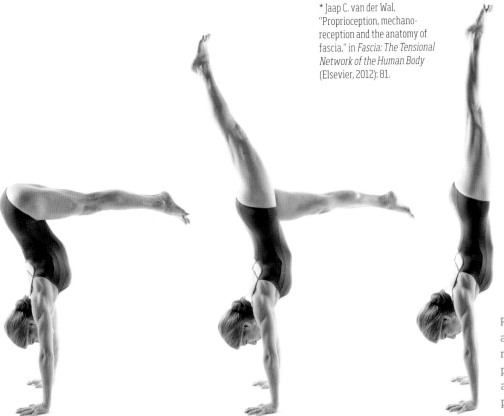

Progress in acrobatics requires knowing precisely where all your body parts are in space.

Think of a gymnast on a balance beam, a circus performer on a tightrope, or a yogini performing a gravity-defying pose. These athletes move with unflappable precision in order to get from point A to point B. Every cell is unified in intent and purpose. The process of training your nervous system to be more physically self-aware comes with repetition, concentration, and discipline in attempting to improve the way you perform whether in still positions or in motion. It is the ultimate embodiment of yourself. My term for this is *EmbodyMap*.

> **EMBODYMAP:** *Your constant positional sense of the interrelation of all your body parts in stillness or in motion. Your keen self-perception of your inner proprioceptive landscape.*

Unfortunately, many people rush into fitness fads without a good sense of their own EmbodyMap. They last a few weeks and then get injured. Systematically preparing your body for movement by using the Roll Model Balls will improve your proprioception for any endeavor you choose. But if you continue to walk into activities blind to your body blind spots, you will continue to tread the same patterns that take you out of the game.

The balls stimulate the nerves that provide positional feedback to your brain; consequently, you can sense whether you are in or out of alignment. You are able to make better choices about your position in space as it relates to your activities. Your EmbodyMap becomes more nuanced, detailed, and adaptable to whatever you choose to do. You become the most durable and agile version of yourself.

Remember this motto whenever you work out:

Exercise with great posture to get great posture!

To become a skilled Roll Model, you must master the mapping of your own body. You are a pioneer armed with rubber scalpels to do nonsurgical surgery on yourself. Become the cartographer of your own EmbodyMap to create your own proprioceptive awakening.

The easy way to become aware of your EmbodyMap is to practice deep palpation with the balls and then attempt to incorporate your awareness of that deep level of touch in all the actions you perform throughout your day. You earn this skill set through practice; you cannot gain it just by reading about it. Practice self-soothing and self-locating daily. Once you have mastered the sequences outlined in chapter 8 and have absorbed the locations and nuances of your own anatomy, you will feel comfortable improvising on yourself and will confidently create new ways of using the balls for healing and relaxation.

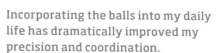

Incorporating the balls into my daily life has dramatically improved my precision and coordination.

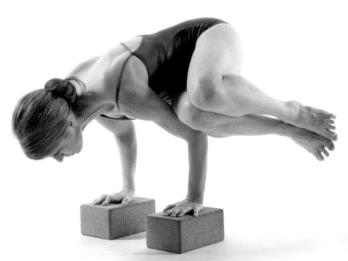

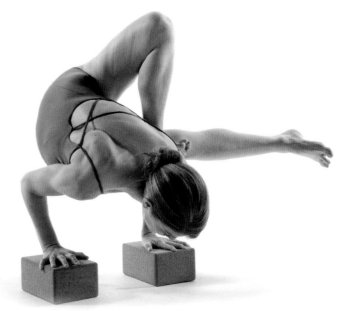

ANATOMY LIVES IN YOUR BODY, NOT IN YOUR HEAD: THE PROCESS OF EMBODIMENT

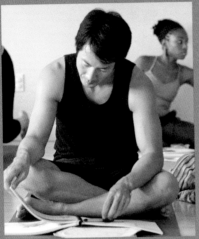

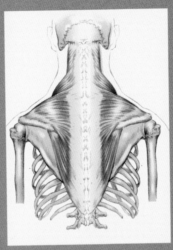

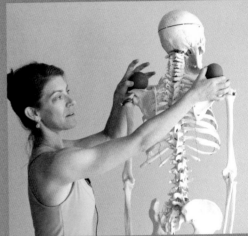

To help with the embodiment process at live trainings, we first look at an image of the myofascial structure we're locating. Our target here is the upper trapezius.

Then I demonstrate where the balls are placed on a "bony" model.

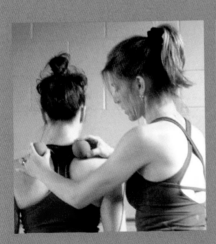

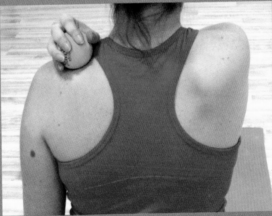

Then I demonstrate on a human model (far left).

Then the students try to locate the spot on themselves with their fingers (near left).

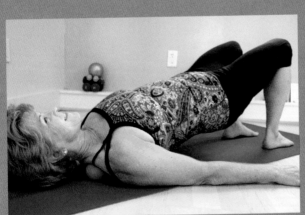

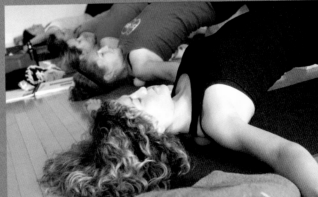

Then the students get down and roll on the balls.

YOUR INNER COMPASS
Developing an EmbodyMap involves sharpening your kinesthetic awareness (an all-encompassing sense of touch) and proprioceptive sense (the ability to sense where your body is without seeing it). The Roll Model empowers you by increasing your ability to internally sense and *correctly* activate (or deactivate) your tissues in every movement so that you are aligned properly and move efficiently according to the natural design of your physique. Cultivating a well-defined EmbodyMap allows you to reduce uneven wear on your joints and tissues, increasing their health and longevity while preventing and diminishing pain.

The Science of Touch: Sensory Nerve Endings

Awakening your EmbodyMap and learning to decipher it may seem as daunting a task as decoding the Rosetta Stone. It's actually quite easy to heighten your body's sense of itself by using the Roll Model Method. Your body is a festival of nerve endings longing for stimuli and novelty. The balls give them just the right kind of rub to help your tissues get a better sense of themselves. Your discipline in regularly stimulating your tissues will make your nerve conductivity more accurate and help the nerves themselves maintain balance and function. The balls will tumble across all sorts of nerves. Some larger ones, such as your sciatic nerve, can be quite uncomfortable and should be avoided, but the smaller nerve endings thrive on therapeutic contact.

The sensory nerve endings that are of particular interest are those associated with proprioception. These nerve endings that contribute touch- and pressure-sensitive information to your proprioceptive sense are called *mechanoreceptors*. And because it's inevitable that some of the sensations created by ball-rolling will be genuinely unpleasant and at times a bit painful, you'll want to distinguish the feeling of painful *nociceptors*. These are the nerve endings that relay noxious information where true hurt exists.

All these nerve endings are laced throughout your fascias within your body's nerve network and are accessed at different depths and through

MECHANORECEPTORS: *The nerve endings that relay specific touch and pressure-sensing information to the central nervous system.*

NOCICEPTORS: *Sensory nerve endings that relay pain perception to the brain.*

different modes of touch. You will constantly roll over them and tease them with the Therapy Balls.

1. **Muscle spindles:** These stretch sensors are located within the fascial tissues of your muscles, specifically within the wrapping around groups of muscle fibers called perimysium (see page 106). When stimulated with sustained tolerable pressure, they facilitate local lengthening and reduction of sympathetic arousal in the contacted tissues. *In other words, relaxing these sensors reduces muscle bracing and helps the myofascia lengthen.*

2. **Golgi tendon organs:** These stretch sensors are located within tendons of all types, including myotendinous junctions, aponeurosis attachments, ligaments of peripheral joints, and joint capsules. Stimulating these proprioceptors affects the tone of their associated muscles as well as neighboring Golgi tendon organs. *In other words, relaxing these sensors reduces tendon tension at joint junctions and tougher soft-tissue seams.*

3. **Pacinian corpuscles:** Located in spinal ligaments, facet joints, deeper joint capsules, muscular tissues, and myotendinous junctions, these sensors respond to rapid pressure changes and vibration and help heighten the body's sense of movement and position. *In other words, massaging these sensors reduces local tension and improves proprioception.*

4. **Ruffini endings:** These nerve endings are found in the ligaments of peripheral joints, outer capsular layers, and dura mater and also are prevalent in the deepest layers of superficial fascia and abundant in the loose membranous layer of fascia that comprises the sliding surface between superficial and deep fascias. They are specifically aroused by stretching and being contacted through slow, deep pressure at oblique angles. This approach can globally inhibit the sympathetic tone in the central nervous system.* *In other words, massaging these sensors reduces whole-body tension and improves proprioception.*

5. **Interstitial fibers:** Unmyelinated (uncoated) free nerve endings that relay information about touch and pain.** These nerve endings are found all over the body, with extra-high density in the periosteum (dense layer surrounding bones). They respond to rapid pressure changes as well as sustained pressure. When stimulated, they create changes within blood vessels, also known as *vasodilation.* Massaging these sensors relays different types of touch, including pain. It also affects blood flow and fluid circulation. *In other words, massaging this complex set of nerve fibers might generate competing sensations of pleasure and discomfort.*

Did you know that there are 20,000 muscle spindles in your body, and the highest concentration of them is located in the back of your neck?*

* Robert Schleip et al, *Fascia: The Tensional Network of the Body* (Elsevier, 2012).

** Excerpted in part from Schleip's article "Fascial plasticity - a neurobiological explanation" in *Journal of Bodywork and Movement Therapies* 7, no. 1 (2003): 11-19 and 7, no. 2 (2003): 104-16.

*** Jonathan Cole, *Pride and a Daily Marathon* (Bradford Books, 1995): 26.

HERE'S THE BIG-PICTURE TAKE-AWAY FROM THIS TOPIC:

One biological fact of utmost importance for all Roll Models is this: there is a mutually inhibiting relationship between pain (nociception) and proprioception (body sense).

Increasing fascial proprioception diminishes your perception of pain. Conversely, an increase in pain diminishes your ability to propriocept.****

IN OTHER WORDS:

The more pain you have, the less coordinated and more prone to injury you are. The balls erase pain while they increase your coordination and body sense.

**** "Proprioceptive signaling tends to inhibit potential myofascial nociception, particularly if accompanied by a state of mindfulness." Robert Schleip and Amanda Baker, *Fascia in Sport and Movement* (Handspring Publishing, 2015).

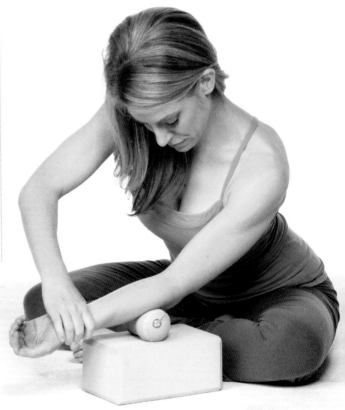

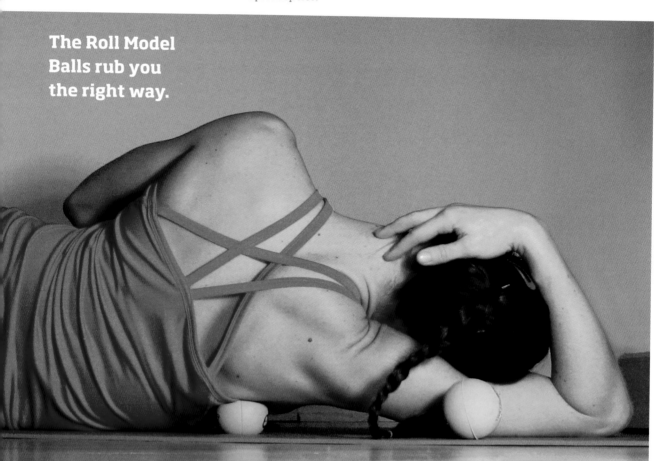

The Roll Model Balls rub you the right way.

The balls are super-grippy and pliable so that they can stimulate these wonderful nerve endings and give them a chance to be heard by your brain. Pain is loud and can dominate the concentration of your brain. But using the grippy, springy balls can flip the sensory-nerve communication switch so that you flood your brain with positional sense that increases your chances of moving better with postural correctness. Over time, this changes your pain portrait.

MORE ON PROPRIOCEPTION

There is a slightly larger picture to the faculty of proprioception than I am able to cover in this book. Your body's sense of seeing itself on the inside also includes your vestibular system, the balance controls located in your inner ear. This system plays a key role in your overall coordination to minimize slips and falls. The methods in this book don't explicitly access this system in depth, as it concentrates on arousing the touch receptors nestled within your fascial and myofascial tissues. The head/neck and jaw sequences will impact your vestibular sense in part. Refer to www.tuneupfitness.com for exercise-based courses that enlarge the scope of proprioception-based training.

In Summary:
Sensory Nerves and Fascia

You have six times as many sensory neurons loaded in your fascias as in any other tissue of your body, except for your skin.* Your fascia is your secondary sensing organ. So much of what you feel physically is relayed by the well-functioning nerve endings laced throughout your soft-tissue scaffolding.

Your nerves, like all your other tissues, depend on proper motion, nutrition, and a balanced, fluid environment in order to signal correctly. When these nerve endings are underfed or squashed together because of tissue tension or dehydration, they are not apt to communicate sensation or location as clearly. So many of these nerve endings are devoted to providing location and position information to your brain (see page 110 on EmbodyMap). Location and position translate to coordination. Improve your fascial environment by lubricating these tissues with the Roll Model Balls, and you'll gain better coordination and grace. You'll become a *BALLerina!*

It's interesting to note that the zones in your body that have the most slide & glide also have an abundance of sensory neurons called *Ruffini endings.* These Ruffini endings are the most prevalent proprioceptors that live inside the membranous layers of loose fascia. To access this transitional layer between your superficial fascia and your deep fascia, simply grab a big pinch of your skin and its underlying fatty layer and then shift it as far as it will move over the stiffer underlying deep fascia. Then attempt to twist or wring that pinch. Well done! You've just mobilized your membranous layer and all the Ruffini endings within it!

When you arouse this transition zone with its thicket of Ruffini endings, those Ruffini endings have two specific messages for your central nervous system:

1. They increase body awareness, or proprioception, in the stimulated area.

2. They tamp down sympathetic outflow, sedating your entire nervous system and reducing global tension in your body. (See chapter 9 for more on the sympathetic nervous system and relaxation.)

Historically, fascia has not received the kind of attention that other body systems have enjoyed, but if this is the first time you've read about it, I *guarantee* that it will not be the last. More and more research is being done on the ties that bind you, and you will be doing your own embodied research every time you use the Roll Model Balls. It's really not that exotic; whole-body movements, specific positioning, and deep listening all enhance your awareness of your fascia. Your soft-tissue scaffolding has been moving with you all along, but certain angles, vectors, and palpation approaches can highlight perception in the seams of your body's inner wetsuit. The sequences presented in chapter 8 will help you gain this proprioceptive insight.

* Robert Schleip, *Terra Rosa* e-magazine (December 2012): 12). Accessed via https://issuu.com/terrarosa/docs/terrarosa_emag11

Flipping the Switch on Pain and Proprioception

Eric Johnson, 47
Estate Manager
Toluca Lake, California

When I met Eric, he was 41. He wore ankle and lower-leg braces, carried 60 extra pounds, and had the slumpiest C-shaped posture I've ever seen. His wrists and hands were so weak that he was unable to button his own shirt. In fact, his whole body was so weak and pain-filled that he could not roll over in bed, and the clothing on his body caused him nonstop irritation. He came to me at the suggestion of his psychiatrist, with complaints of unbearable chronic pain, an inability to relax, and massive anxiety. Eric was on the highest dose of prescription pain medication allowed by law, 100 milligrams of fentanyl. It is 100 times more powerful than morphine and hundreds of times more potent than street heroin. He said to me:

> **//** I am under the care of a set of doctors and medical specialists, and I am right now in intensive psychotherapy. I need to learn how to both relax and create exercise opportunities. I have, it seems, remained in a perpetual 'fight or flight' state for about 35 years. The weakest parts of my body are my wrists and ankles, due to the atrophy of the musculature. The atrophy is due to lack of enervation, or neurological communication with the muscles. They are there; I just can't talk to them. **//**

Eric has a genetic neuropathology called Charcot-Marie-Tooth disease (also known as hereditary-sensory motor neuropathy), which withers the neural messaging into and from the peripheral appendages of the body. The nerve conduction from his brain to his body and back to his brain is deeply damaged and continues to worsen. There is no cure. Those who suffer from Charcot-Marie-Tooth lose control over the mechanics of their ankles, feet, wrists, and hands, and their limbs progressively weaken and wither. The nerves within them lose their myelin sheath, the protective coating that helps nerves do their jobs. Without their myelin layer, the nerve endings become dysfunctional and quite often act as nociceptors, which are signalers of pain. Nerves that were once muscle-firing motor neurons now have no capacity to conduct motion. Nerves that were once sensory neurons, proprioceptors, and mechanoreceptors no longer sense motion, position, temperature, or touch. Most of Eric's nerves had become pain nerves. When I first met him, he also had total numbness in his feet and could not move his toes.

Fentanyl was only one of the many medications Eric was taking when I started teaching him in 2008. He was taking Oxycontin, Wellbutrin, gabapentin, nortriptyline, cannabis, and clonazepam, all to help with his pain and mood. He was also taking Flomax and Prilosec for urinary incontinence and acid reflux. His doctors told him that there was really nothing he could do other than to live with the progression of the disease and remain on pain medications for the rest of his life. He was also discouraged from exercising, as it inflamed many of his conditions, which he likened to "being tortured." He was told that he'd never be able to articulate his ankles or have fully functioning opposable thumbs, among other messages that we have since disproved.

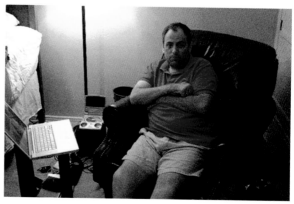

Eric when he and I first met.

Eric felt unable to operate or even sense his own body. His proprioception failed him constantly, and he frequently suffered from falls and knee dislocations. He felt trapped inside his body, held hostage by pain, with no long-term relief in sight. His body was inescapable, and his pain was a daily terror. During my first session with him, I tried to figure out which moves I could teach him that would reduce his pain rather than increase it.

First, I taught him to breathe while lying down. When I walked toward him to adjust his feet, he violently recoiled and shrieked, "You can't touch me! I was sexually assaulted as a child, I can't be touched!" His trauma pierced me like a shotgun. His wounds were not just physical, but deeply linked to his sense of self and his soul. On top of his physical challenges, he shared that as a boy he'd been the object of a sick adult's fantasy, and was sexually abused repeatedly from age 7 to age 12. He was the one who couldn't run away. And given his strict religious faith, he was afraid to let his family or elders know about it.

I calmly breathed through my startle and responded, "No problem, I won't touch you. Instead, I'd like to give you these," and I handed him two well-worn Roll Model Balls. "You'll learn to use them to touch yourself." He placed the balls along his upper back and allowed them to nuzzle into decades of braced tension. I taught him to breathe directly into the pressure and to relax in spite of the initial discomfort. Eric finished that first twenty-minute spinal self-massage with ecstatic relief. He had no idea that he could feel so good. And he did it all by himself, with my guidance. Then I taught him different stretches and strengtheners to help his hips, finishing up with meditation at the end of the hour. I maintained our strict no-touch boundary and have never found it awkward other than that initial moment of shock.

Eric emailed me the day after the session to tell me that he could not remember having a deeper sleep in years. We began a diligent regimen of twice-weekly sessions for the next several years. Over time, I gained his trust. We both knew that we were literally rolling into uncharted territory. Here was a man who could not allow therapeutic touch to his body. Here was a body that had been neglected for decades and transferred from one doctor to the next, dismissed as unfixable and on a course of progressive degeneration. I did not look at Eric as a disease or a symptom, but as the whole person he is. The interconnectedness of his physical, emotional, and relational pains was constantly influencing his ability to concentrate, move, and develop new, supportive habits.

I recognized early on that his medical team's messages had become internalized beliefs about weakness, helplessness, and hopelessness. Sadly, this gifted man's self-esteem had taken a tumble as a result. Given the progress we were making, we decided that we were not going to believe any preconceived notions about what he could or couldn't do.

I approached Eric with new eyes each time we met. Sometimes he would have an unthinkable episode of pain, and other times he had robust energy. No matter how he showed up, he walked out with better posture, completely coordinated, and rid of, or with significantly less of, whichever symptoms he'd walked in with that day. And this was all done simply by our one-hour session of Therapy Ball rolling and Yoga Tune Up corrective exercise (see chapter 11). None of his doctors could have predicted the changes in his weight, body, mind, or confidence or the steady reduction in pain medication that took place over the next five years.

Two years into working with me, Eric declared that he'd like to fly across the country and attend my advanced Core Immersion training. By this time, he had eradicated his urinary incontinence and acid reflux, which I attribute to the deep core training, Coregeous Ball work, and diaphragm strengthening I had taught him. I said to him, "In my trainings, there is a lot of partner work, and a lot of contact and touching. Will you be okay with that?" "I'm ready," he said. He was so ready, in fact, that he leapt at the chance to volunteer in several of my hands-on demonstrations.

Then, about two and a half years into working with me, he said that he wanted to start wearing tennis shoes again and stop wearing his corrective ankle/leg braces. The next session, he walked in holding a box of new sneakers.

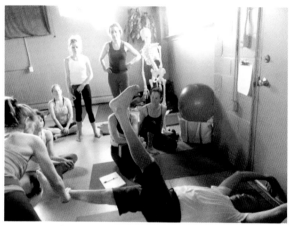

Eric is the class demo. This is the first time I ever touched him.

I watched him lace them up himself with fingers his doctors had told him would never be able to pick up a penny, let alone lace shoes. A new Eric was born.

The Roll Model techniques I used to awaken his proprioceptors are exactly what I use with all my students. But Eric is unlike most people I have met, in that he is ravenous to know himself and un-cover all the layers that have held him captive for so long. His appetite for self-massage, motion, and meditation surpasses those of any student I have ever met. His will to change his life motivated him to create new habits of self-care healthcare. He did his homework and dedicated space in his house to roll and exercise. His new daily dosage of self-care provided unimaginable benefits. Over the past six years, he has awakened a proprioceptive gift

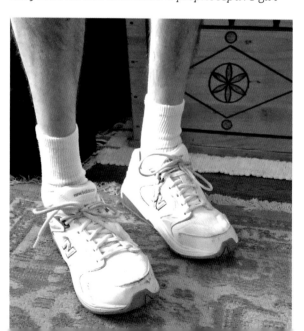

that has enabled him to feel powerful inside his own skin for the first time in his life. He routinely moves his mind into his (new) muscles and relishes the experience with a passion that brings tears to my eyes.

One day three and a half years into his diligent studentship, I went with Eric to see his pain doctor. He had slowly been reducing his pain medications, losing weight, improving in all his reflexes, and gaining muscle mass. His physician wanted to meet me, as he'd never seen this kind of reversal of the disease. Dr. Avrom Gart, the Director of Pain Management and Rehabilitation Medical Director at Cedars-Sinai Spine Center in Los Angeles, encouraged us to get Eric off of pain medication completely, and we all agreed that it would be our next goal.

Weaning off of highly addictive narcotic pain-killers is not a gentle proposition. Withdrawal is ugly. The body responds like a hunted beast; the mind offers up torturous messages and images that are mental agony. One tactic for breaking through addiction is to transfer the dependency onto something else. Eric had the Roll Model Balls. He'd been using them for years with me and at home to self-treat his pain and to prevent more pain from entering his life. But it would be a gamble to find out if he could help his innate chemistry kick in and resolve his pain. Would he have the fortitude and presence of mind to turn to his tools, or would the drive to medicate domi-nate his life forever?

In year 4, Eric was able to successfully wean himself off of fentanyl. Both of us and the rest of his medical team will admit that it was not an easy process, nor without its setbacks. But he did it. He was able to do the medically unthinkable. He stopped Charcot-Marie-Tooth in its tracks and transformed his life from depression, regression, and degeneration into progression, optimism, and regeneration.

Eric reclaimed fine motor skills that most of us take for granted; in addition to tying his shoe-laces, he no longer had to pay others to trim his nails. His larger movement patterns gained coordination and clarity as well; he could roll over in bed with ease and do squats and long-held planks. Subsequently, he lost 60 pounds of excess weight. And he could now walk across his parents' mole-ridden lawn barefoot without falling. He had physiological breakthroughs such as eradicating acid reflux and urinary incontinence. His chronic high blood pressure dropped from 140/90 to 120/70 and has remained steady. And he even lost the bald patch on his head! (Spontaneous dark hair regrowth is one of his proudest accomplishments.)

As Eric gained muscle mass, his neglected body awoke from a slumber of underuse and abandonment that had damaged his psyche for decades. The ultimate result of this inside-out transformation is that toward the end of our third year together, he had so changed himself that he was finally able to allow therapeutic and relational touch back into his life, and he entered into a relationship with a loving girlfriend.

Eric is an astonishing Roll Model for others living with his disease. I presented his journey as a case study at the International Symposium on Yoga Therapy in 2011 and at the International Fascia Research Congress in Vancouver in 2012. Eric is a poster boy for how improving proprioception diminishes pain in the body. He is a walking billboard for how improving coordination minimizes accidents, injuries, and further pain. He did it all with the ultimate deck of cards stacked against him. Using the Roll Model tools and other Yoga Tune Up exercises, Eric unraveled bound and inefficient connective tissues, heightened his global proprioceptive ability, awakened new strength, and massively decreased his stress. His life is forever changed.

This is what Eric taught his doctor, Avrom Gart of the Cedars-Sinai Spine Center:

> "Eric has shown outstanding progress. I have seen firsthand how pain and neuromuscular dysfunction can be drastically improved with Yoga Tune Up. The method sensitively accommodates each individual's personal needs. This is not a cookie cutter approach, but an incredibly intelligent rehabilitative format."

This is what Eric taught me:

> Our neurons are not dead ends… they can be revived.

And this is what Eric taught himself:

> "I am enough. I have enough. All is well."

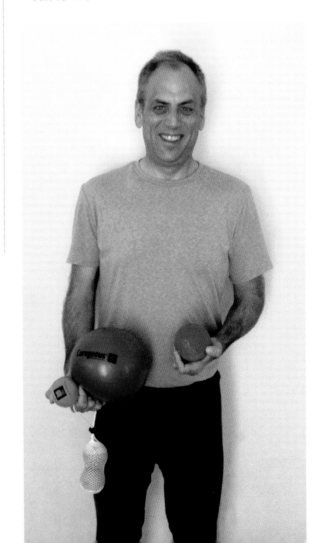

5 Know Your Body Better: An Embodied Orientation to Bones and Muscles

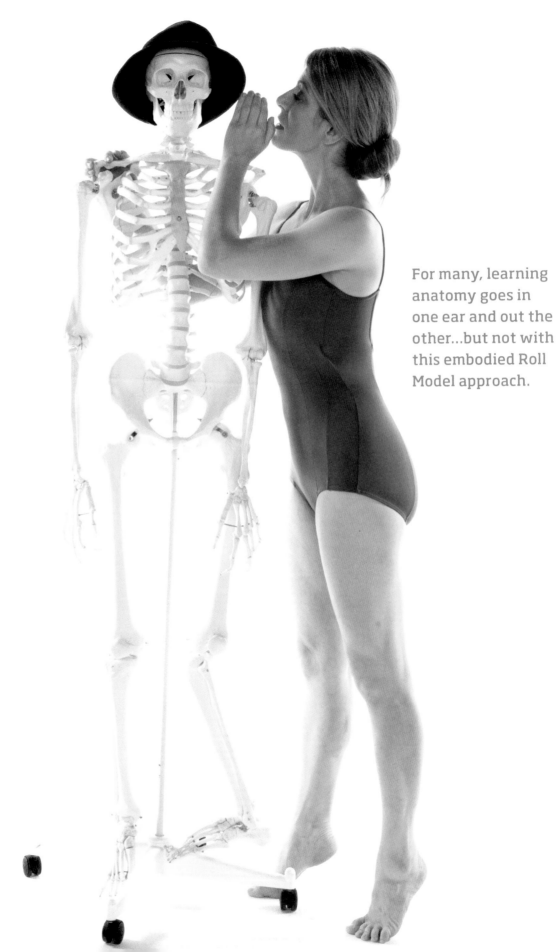

For many, learning anatomy goes in one ear and out the other...but not with this embodied Roll Model approach.

While I personally find learning the names of my body parts enriching and gratifying, it is by no means a precursor to erasing your pain. You don't need a PhD in anatomy or a clinical license to rub out your aches. I believe that you were born equipped to heal yourself, and you have the right to tackle your tight spots whether you are anatomically fluent or use the intuitive skills of a cat. Therefore, you can skip this chapter and review it later if you'd prefer to start rolling now. Whenever you choose to probe the specifics of this chapter, it will deepen your understanding of how and why the Roll Model Balls make a difference.

I share the following information with you out of my own insatiable need to explain why the Roll Model Method has been so helpful. So much wisdom about the human body has been kept behind closed doors, and I want you to know it. Based on my years of teaching these techniques and the questions that typically arise, I have distilled some essentials that I feel will illuminate the potential of these "magic balls"; they are not just another gimmick or widget, but valuable self-care tools that need to be in every hospital, medicine cabinet, car, and gym bag.

Learning the names of your body parts will only enhance and empower your exploration, especially when you are discussing your tissue issues with doctors or therapists, should the need arise. It also gives you a basic vocabulary to understand terms that doctors may use in describing treatments to you, and you will be better able to discern the best course of action for you. Knowledge is power.

To know your anatomical structures is to feel them. To be able to feel them is to be able to propriocept them. The more aware you are of your body at rest and in motion, the easier it will be for you to intelligently roll out your knots and kinks.

36 Knead-to-Know Bony Landmarks

Your bony landmarks give you a veritable living grid of nooks, crannies, buttes, hilltops, and spires that you can identify as guideposts as you perform self-massage with the Roll Model Balls. Often these landmarks are obscured by clothing, body position, or thick superficial fascia, so you must develop a keen sense of them on yourself in order to become accurate with your ball placement.

Alexandra Ellis wears her ink proudly. Here she displays her scapulae prominently, highlighting her medial borders, inferior angles, and spine of scapulae. (For more, see page 130.)

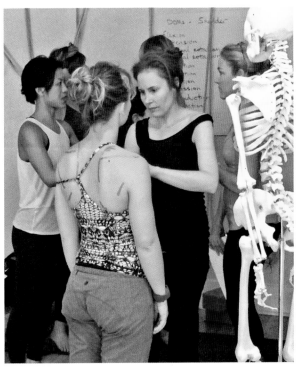

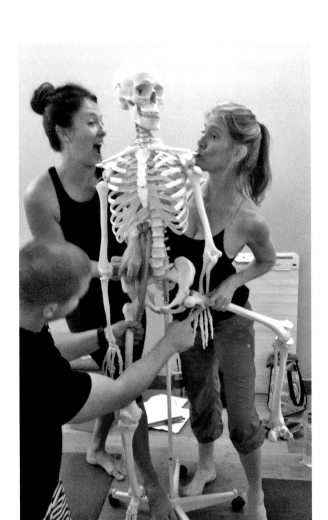

Learning anatomy is mandatory fun in my classroom.

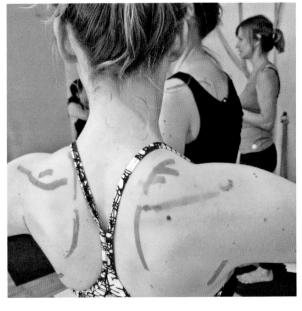

The following are "knead-to-know" bony landmarks that anchor key myofascial structures. Train yourself to sense and see these landmarks, as they will help you visualize your postural integrity.

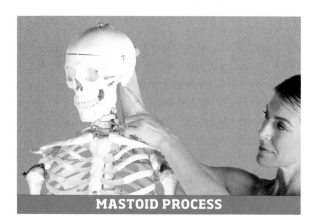

MASTOID PROCESS

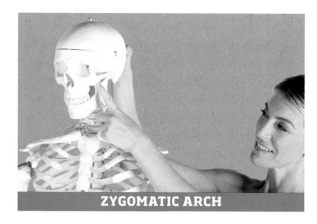

ZYGOMATIC ARCH

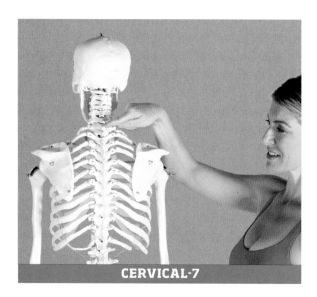

CERVICAL-7

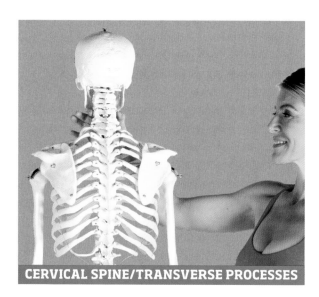

CERVICAL SPINE/TRANSVERSE PROCESSES

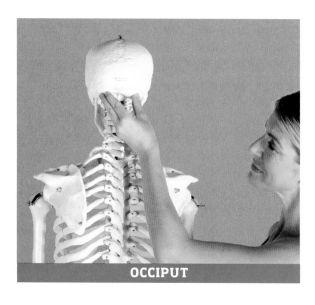

OCCIPUT

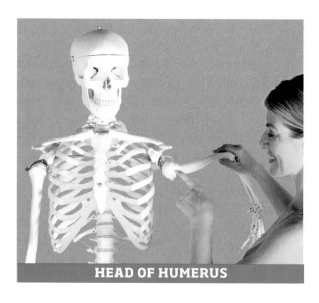

HEAD OF HUMERUS

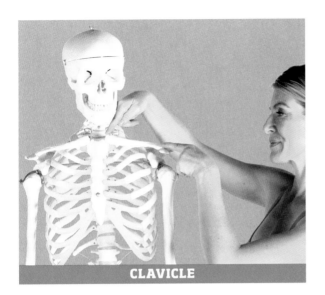

CLAVICLE

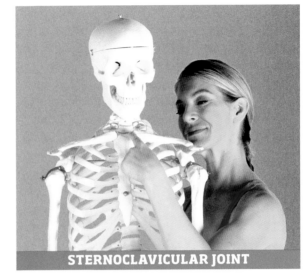

STERNOCLAVICULAR JOINT

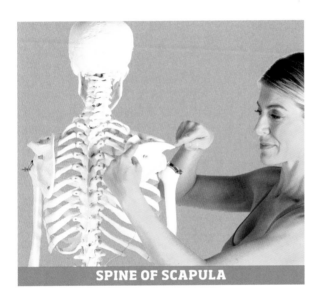

SPINE OF SCAPULA

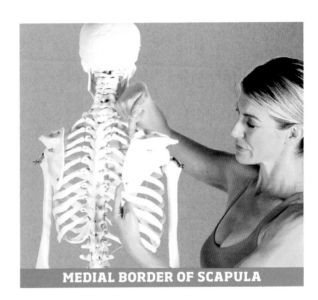

MEDIAL BORDER OF SCAPULA

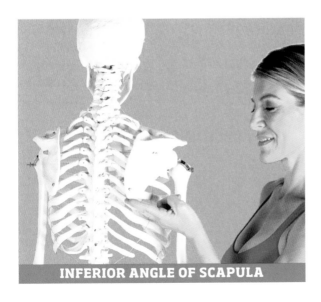

INFERIOR ANGLE OF SCAPULA

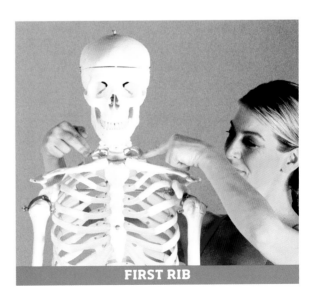

FIRST RIB

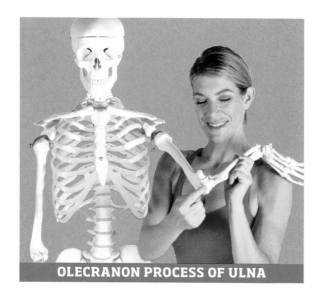

OLECRANON PROCESS OF ULNA

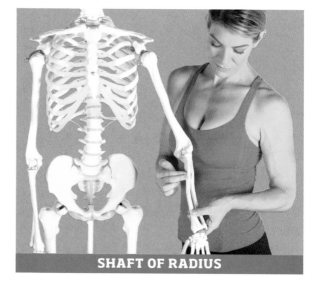

SHAFT OF RADIUS

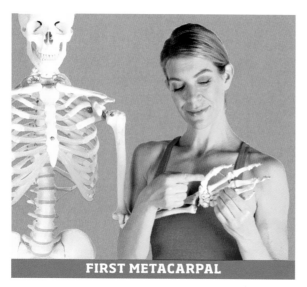

FIRST METACARPAL

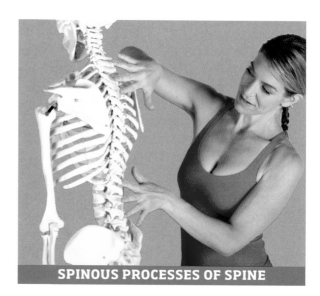

SPINOUS PROCESSES OF SPINE

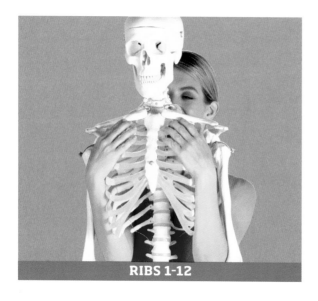

RIBS 1-12

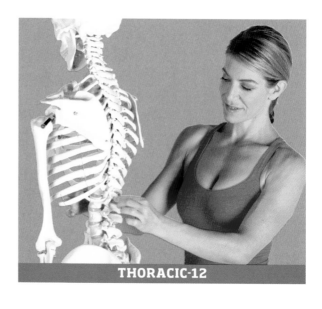

THORACIC-12

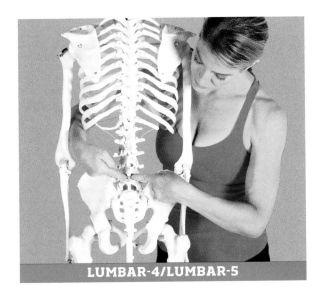

LUMBAR-4/LUMBAR-5

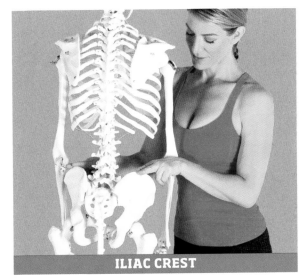

ILIAC CREST

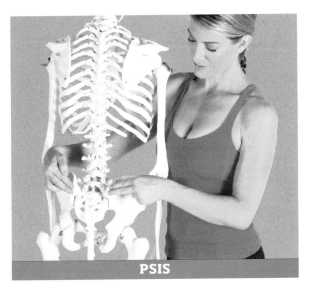

PSIS

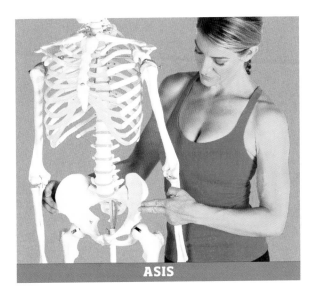

ASIS

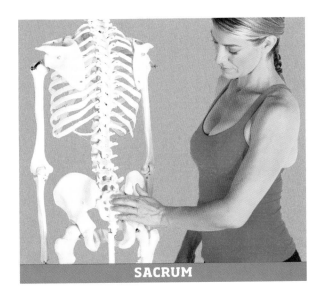

SACRUM

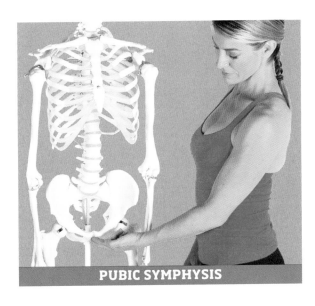

PUBIC SYMPHYSIS

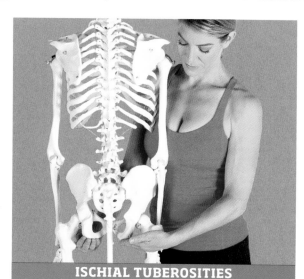

ISCHIAL TUBEROSITIES

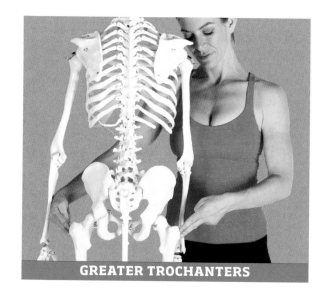

GREATER TROCHANTERS

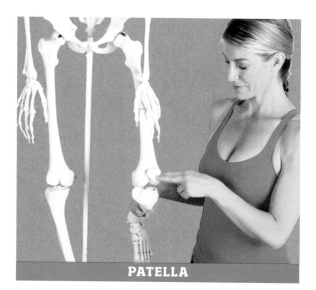

PATELLA

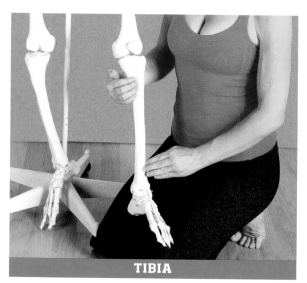

TIBIA

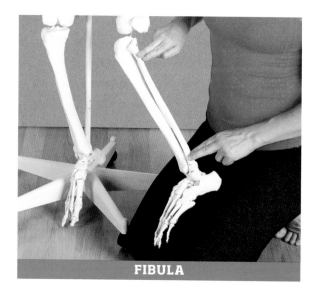

FIBULA

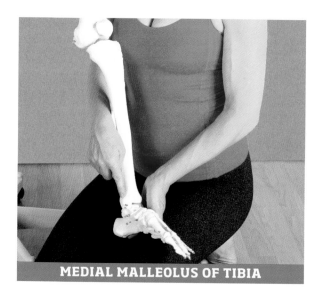

MEDIAL MALLEOLUS OF TIBIA

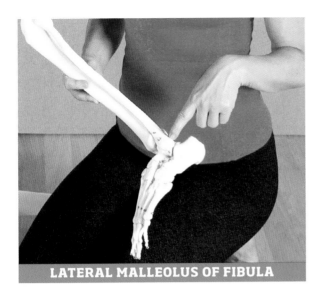

LATERAL MALLEOLUS OF FIBULA

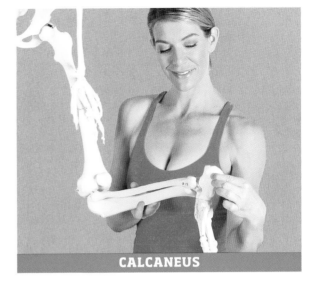

CALCANEUS

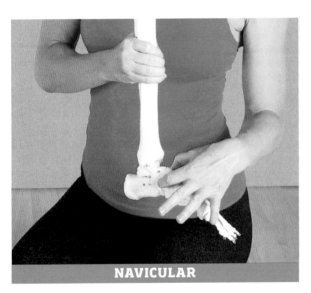

NAVICULAR

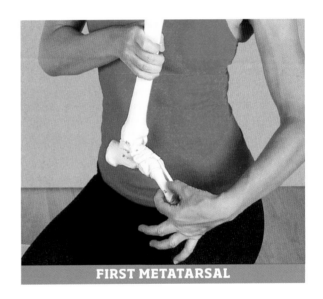

FIRST METATARSAL

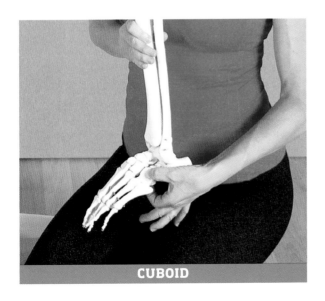

CUBOID

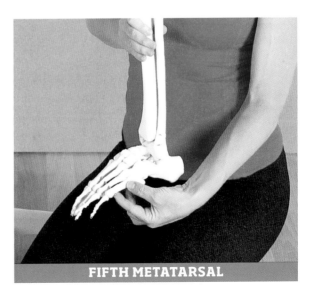

FIFTH METATARSAL

In my Roll Model Therapy Ball trainings worldwide, I have my students draw these bony landmarks on one another so that they learn to feel them on themselves and others, and also to train their eyes to see differences from person to person and from one side of the body to the other. Learning these landmarks is an incredibly useful tool. If you are working your way through this book with a friend, invest in some nontoxic washable markers and use one another as canvases to improve your ability to see your own structure and the structures of others. Think of it as war paint to get you out of war with your pain.

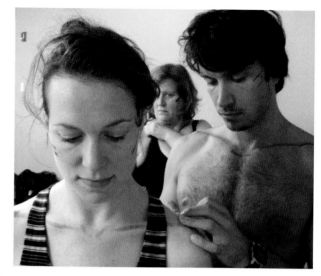

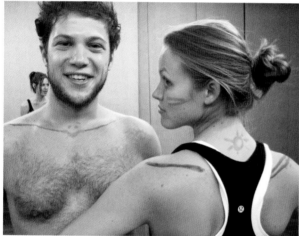

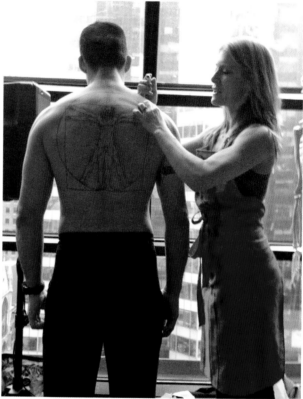

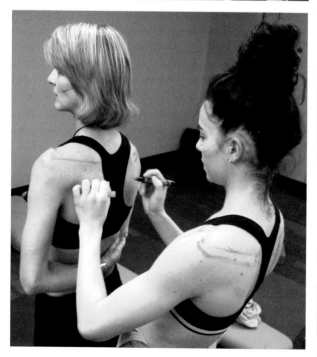

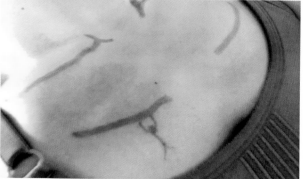

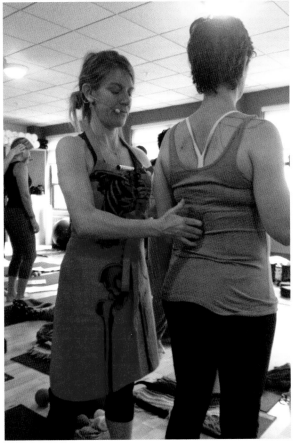

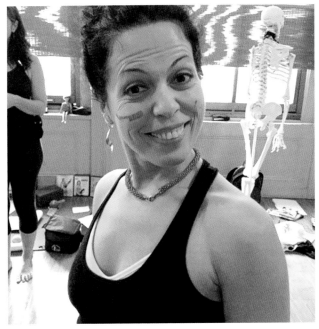

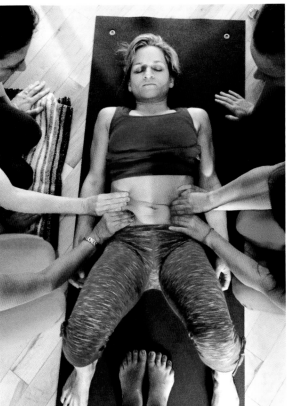

Follow these suggestions for making the abstract concept of bone locations an embodied, integrated experience:

1. **Feel each landmark.** Use the Roll Model Balls to "tour" and "site-see" all these bony locations. Notice where you have easy access, get curious about the surrounding tissues, and investigate these landmarks with their unique soft-tissue attachments.

2. **Memorize these locations on yourself by reviewing images in anatomy books or online.** Repeat their names aloud, and then start investigating them on partners, family members, and friends (or even your students if you're a fitness professional). Try scanning crowds of people and look for variations of these landmarks as they model themselves around you. Develop an eye for seeing these structures anywhere and everywhere.

3. **Learn the major and minor muscles that attach to each of these landmarks.** Doing so will increase your workable map of the human body.

44 Knead-to-Know Muscles

There are more than 700 named muscles (myofascial structures) in the human body. You will contact almost all of them directly or indirectly by using the Roll Model Balls. I am sharing 44 muscles with you here as a starting point–a mere 6 percent of your myofascial structures.

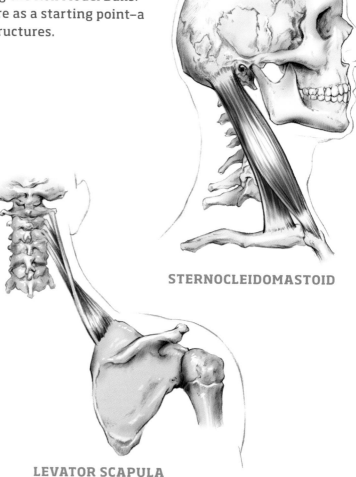

STERNOCLEIDOMASTOID

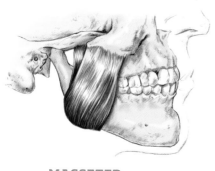

MASSETER

LEVATOR SCAPULA

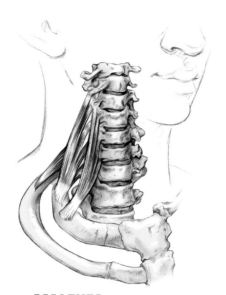

SCALENES

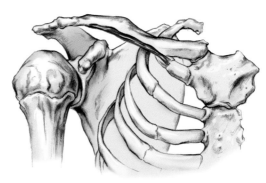

SUBCLAVIUS

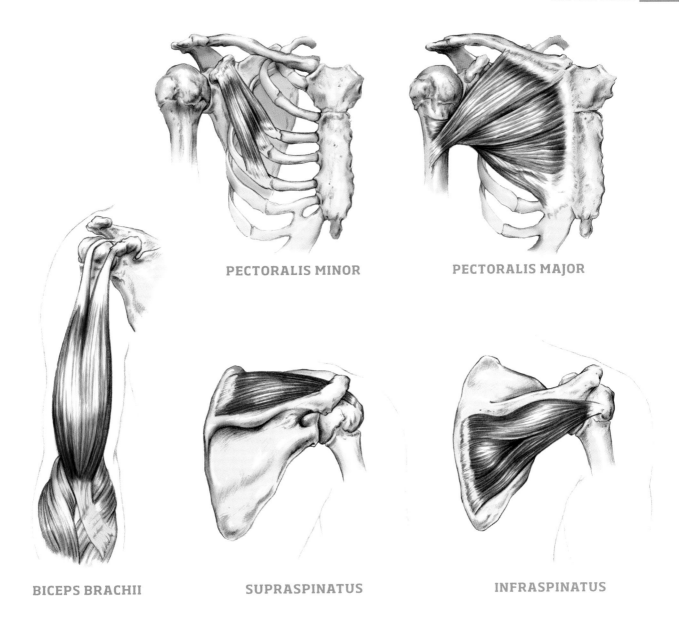

PECTORALIS MINOR

PECTORALIS MAJOR

BICEPS BRACHII

SUPRASPINATUS

INFRASPINATUS

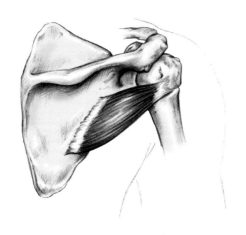

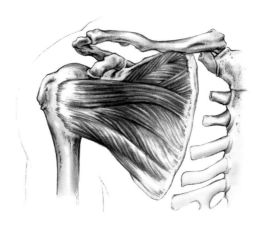

TERES MINOR

SUBSCAPULARIS

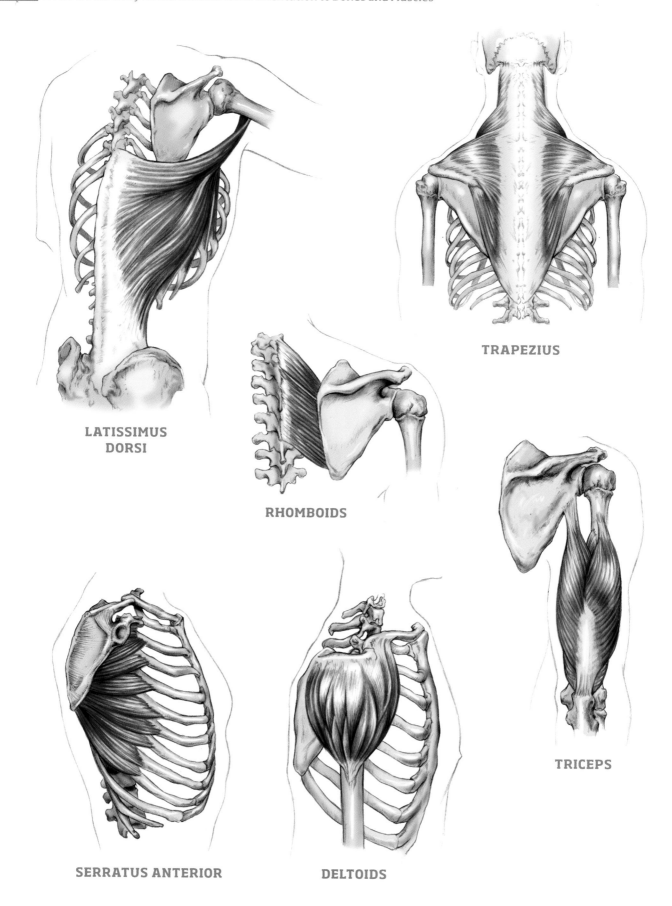

**LATISSIMUS
DORSI**

TRAPEZIUS

RHOMBOIDS

TRICEPS

SERRATUS ANTERIOR

DELTOIDS

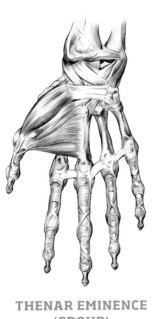

**THENAR EMINENCE
(GROUP)**

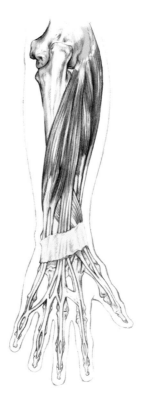

**EXTENSOR
DIGITORUM**

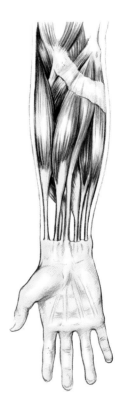

**FLEXOR DIGITORUM
SUPERFICIALIS**

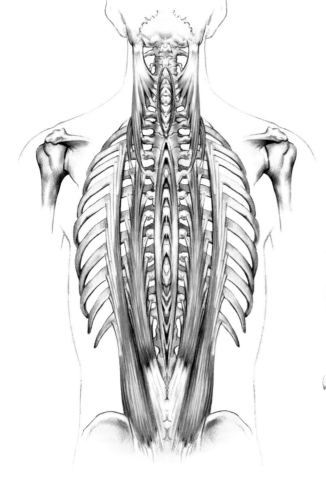

ERECTOR SPINAE

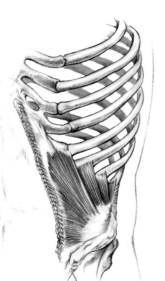

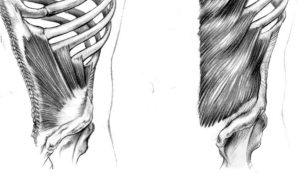

**EXTERNAL AND INTERNAL ABDOMINAL
OBLIQUES**

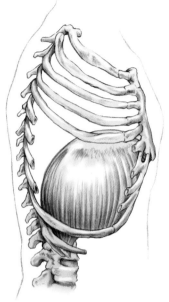

**RESPIRATORY
DIAPHRAGM** (side view)

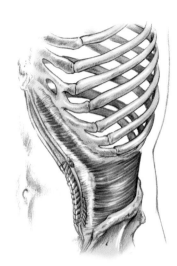

**TRANSVERSUS
ABDOMINIS**

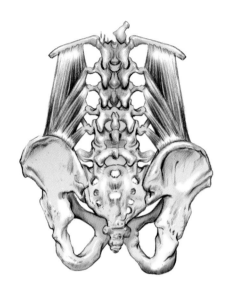

**QUADRATUS
LUMBORUM**

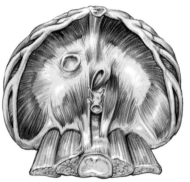

RESPIRATORY DIAPHRAGM
(inferior view)

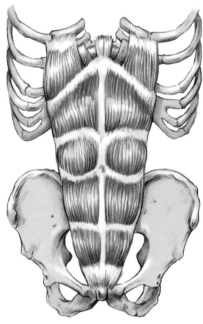

**RECTUS
ABDOMINIS**

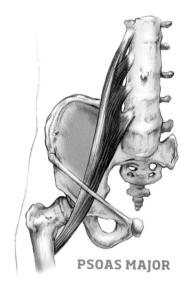

PSOAS MAJOR

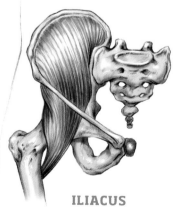

ILIACUS

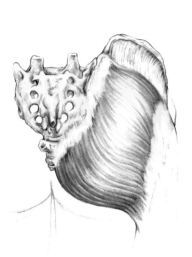

GLUTEUS MAXIMUS, MEDIUS, MINIMUS

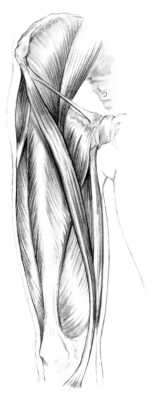

SARTORIUS

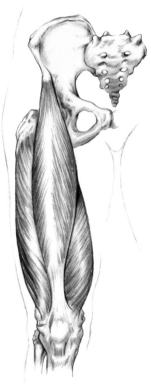

RECTUS FEMORIS OF QUADRICEPS GROUP

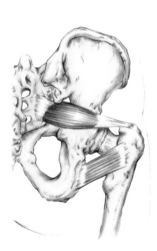

PIRIFORMIS AND QUADRATUS FEMORIS

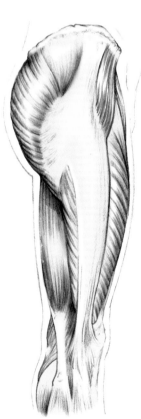

TENSOR FASCIA LATAE

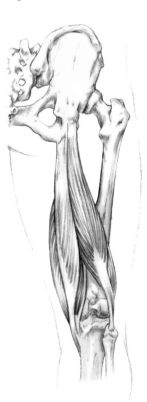

HAMSTRINGS–BICEPS FEMORIS, SEMIMEMBRANOSUS, SEMITENDINOSUS

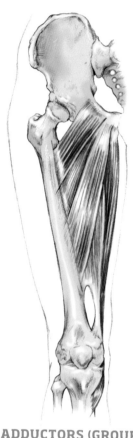

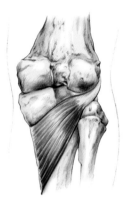

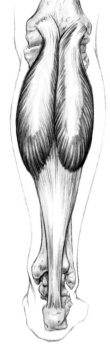

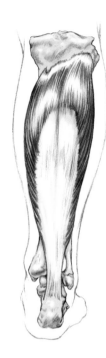

POPLITEUS

GASTROCNEMIUS

SOLEUS

**ADDUCTORS (GROUP
INCLUDES GRACILIS)**

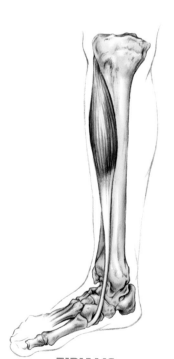

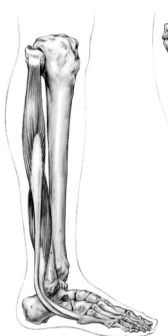

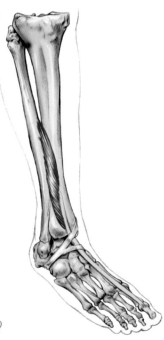

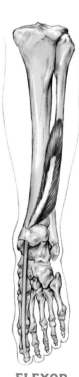

**TIBIALIS
ANTERIOR**

**PERONEUS
LONGUS
(AKA FIBULARIS)**

**EXTENSOR
HALLUCIS
LONGUS**

**FLEXOR
HALLUCIS
LONGUS**

Your aches and pains may not be located in any of these muscles, but thankfully, they are fascially interconnected to everything else in your body. At a minimum, familiarizing yourself with the muscles on this list will help orient you as you probe into neighboring tissues. Get to know these major muscles through self-palpation, by reviewing anatomy books or websites, and by using the Roll Model Balls. Doing so will give you an accessible soft-tissue grid to trace through the issues in your tissues and begin to make lasting change.

As you study these myofascial structures, take a close look at the way the striations (stripes) are drawn. The angle of these lines is known as their *line of pull* and represents how the muscle pulls on neighboring structures, especially joints. Identifying the lines of pull of your muscles helps you tailor your strokes accordingly. For example, the erector spinae run up and down your back, so you roll the balls up and down to *Strip* them, you

roll from side to side to *CrossFiber* them, and you arch and relax your back in order to *contract/relax* them. (See chapter 6 for much more on the nine key rolling techniques.)

It's also helpful to recognize where a muscle "begins" (known as its *origin*) and "ends" (its *insertion*). Learning the origins and insertions of your muscles will help you refine your ball positioning, which is very helpful when you are treating injuries. It will also enhance your awareness of how each myofascial structure interconnects to its neighboring structures. But in truth, these myofascial tissues are 100 percent connected and attached along every surface. Each tissue is in constant contact with the fascias that surround it. (Traditional "origin and insertion" locations may seem obsolete when you recognize that your tissues are infinitely originating and inserting themselves into the inter- and intramuscular fascias.) These fascial encasements are soft-tissue envelopes that affect the position, function, and physiological health of the myofascias they surround and interpenetrate.

Additionally, because your body is a layered structure, when you target one specific muscle with the Roll Model Balls, you will likely be rolling the myofascias that are on top of and below it.

> **LINE OF PULL:** *The vector of motion according to the organization of muscle fibers and fascia relative to their origin and insertion.*
>
> **MUSCLE ORIGIN:** *The portion of a muscle that moves less during a contraction (often more proximal/closer to the midline).*
>
> **MUSCLE INSERTION:** *The portion of a muscle that moves more during a contraction (often more distal/farther from the midline).*

Identifying a few muscles will stir your curiosity to probe, palpate, and investigate every nook and cranny of your body. I don't know about you, but I'd rather do this exploration on myself with rubber balls than have a surgeon's scalpel dig into me further down the road.

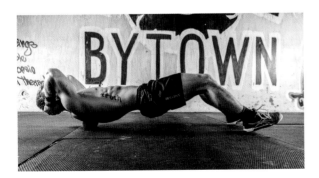

6 The Nine Essential Roll Model Ball Techniques

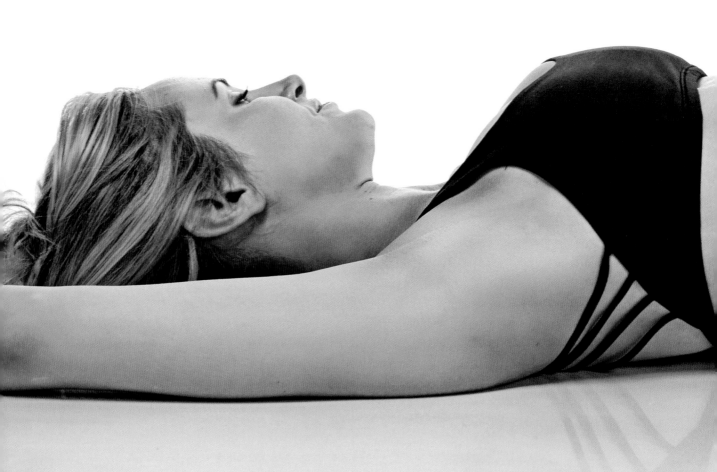

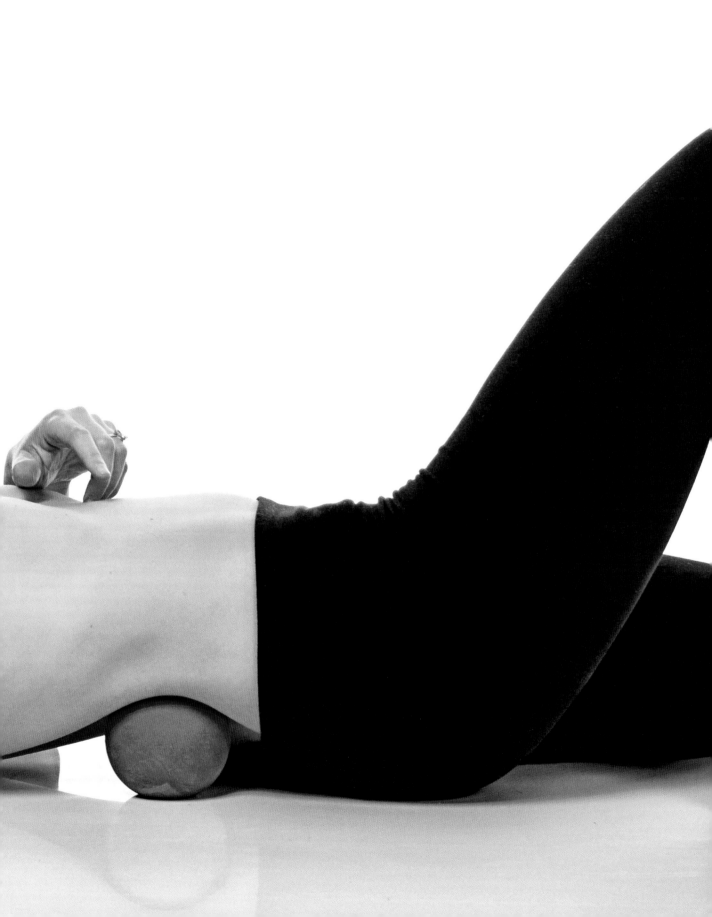

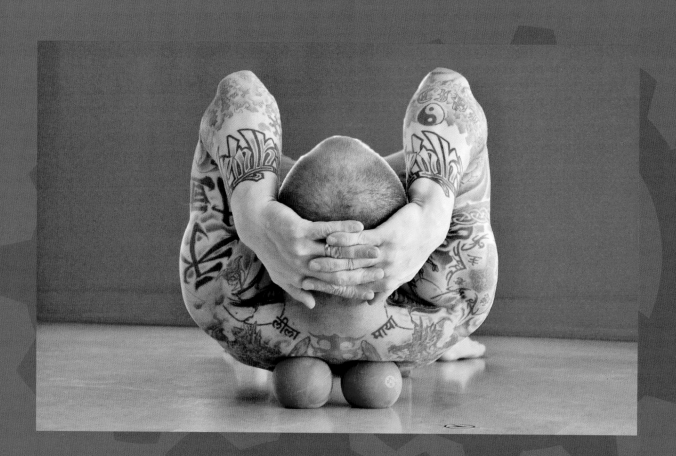

There are many strategies and techniques for working out your kinks with the Roll Model Balls. This chapter details the nine key ways to experiment on different areas of your body. You know your body best, and certain techniques may make a big impact in one area but hardly affect you in another. Interchange the techniques and different-sized balls to find your own deep relief.

These nine techniques will also help you become aware of your body blind spots, tension patterns, and imbalances. You will likely be surprised that one technique may gloss over a knot, while another finds the mother lode of tension that is buried in the exact same spot. Be patient and inquisitive, and be willing to tinker and play to find resolution to your unique discomfort.

These moves are at the heart of the Roll Model sequences detailed in chapter 8. Refer to this chapter often to refine your understanding of each technique.* Let your own tissue stiffness guide you, and feel free to swap techniques within the sequences to soothe yourself. This is the key to erasing your pain.

* For a video review of all Roll Model Method techniques used throughout the sequences, visit www.tuneupfitness.com/roll-model-videos

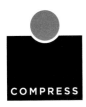

1. Sustained Compression

COMPRESS

For **sustained compression,** use a Roll Model Ball to find the "epicenter" (there may be more than one!) of an adhesion, trigger point, or area of tense tissue and apply consistent pressure straight into it. (The direction of the pressure depends on your angle of approach.) Allow the ball to sink into your tissue like warm quicksand and make a soft-tissue indentation, and hold the position for 90 to 120 seconds.

What's happening physiologically: Steady, constant pressure combined with deep breathing helps the muscle spindles (the stretch sensors/ proprioceptors within muscles) get the message to stop contracting. The constant pressure should be at the edge of what you consider "tolerable discomfort" in order to help the muscle spindles unlock their habit of contraction. The associated fascias will also lengthen to accommodate the pressure of the ball.

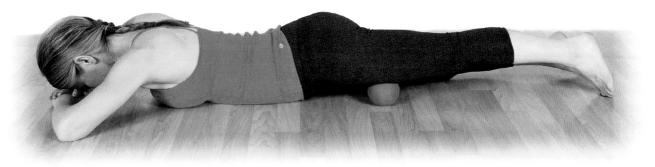

HOW: Allow the ball(s) to sink into your tissue like warm quicksand and make a soft-tissue indentation.

2. Skin-Rolling/Shear

SKIN ROLL

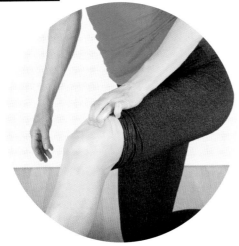
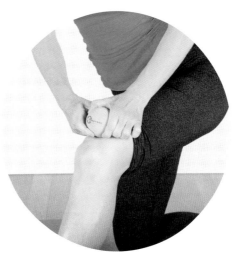

HOW: Use the ball(s) to pull, twist, and wring the skin and its underlying tissues away from your body.

Skin-rolling, also known as **shear,** is fascial stretching in which you use a Roll Model Ball to gently pinch your skin while you pull, twist, and wring the skin and its underlying tissues away from your body. The goal of this technique is to create a moving transition of the skin and its underlying fatty layer (superficial fascia) over the deep fascia and myofascia. The ball acts on the skin and the spongy layer underneath to crimp, fold, and pile your superficial tissues at a faster pace than the deeper underlayers of myofascia. This is similar to a car's rubber tires skidding on a muddy road: the tire catches the slimy surface mud and scrapes it away from the drier, more solid mud beneath. The effect is that these tissues become warmer and more pliable and feel "fluffy," just like a flat pillow that you've fluffed to bring it back to life. The balls skin-roll most effectively against exposed skin, although their grip is powerful enough to effect skin-rolling through a layer of fabric. Multiple layers of fabric, however, will interfere with their ability to create shear.

What's happening physiologically: The grip of the balls takes hold of the skin and its underlying superficial fascia. This grip, coupled with tractioning the ball along the skin, creates a shearing force that transitions the superficial fatty layer several degrees beyond its "normal resting range" atop the deep fascia. Mobilizing the fatty layer away from the underlying deep fascia stimulates the production of hyaluronic acid to enhance local tissue hydration. It also stimulates the Ruffini endings (proprioceptors within the superficial and deep fascia), which has two major effects:

1. It enhances proprioception, or body sense, in the area being rolled.

2. It turns down sympathetic nervous system arousal and turns up parasympathetic nervous system arousal (see page 363 for more on the nervous system). In other words, skin-rolling/shear acts as a global sedative.

> **HYALURONIC ACID:** *A lubricating fluid produced by fascial tissues throughout the body. This fluid permits slide & glide among the multiple layers of soft tissue.*

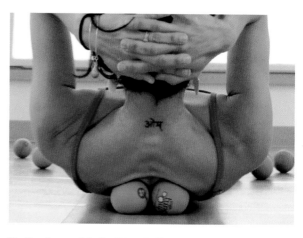

Notice how this Roll Model's skin buckles ahead of the pressure of the balls? This is the shear effect of the grippy pressure of the balls shifting her skin and underlying fascia.

STRIP

3. Stripping

HOW: Slide the ball(s) from one end of the muscle to the other, like combing conditioner through tangled hair. The ball(s) act like a rubber rake through the length of the myofascia.

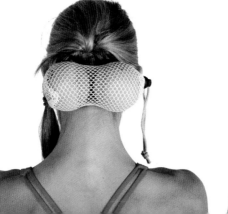

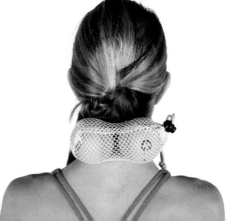

To **strip** is to maneuver a Roll Model Ball along the "grain" of a muscle. (All the fibers/cells in a muscle line up in the same direction, like a brand-new box of spaghetti.) In order to strip a muscle, it is essential to learn the origin and insertion points of the muscle so that the ball can follow its line of pull. For example, to strip your erector spinae muscles (the group of muscles running up and down your back), you roll the ball up and down along your spine. To strip the anterior tibialis (the muscles on the front of your shin), you roll the ball up and down your shin bone. See pages 132–139 for a list of Knead-to-Know muscles and to view their lines of pull.

What's happening physiologically: The ball rolls to lengthen the myofascia from end to end, much like combing out fine knots in tangled hair. This re-establishes the resting length of the muscle. (See the "Stripping and CrossFiber" box on the next page.)

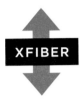

4. CrossFiber

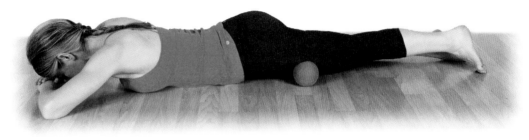

HOW: Move the ball across the muscle fibers, as if prying apart stuck spaghetti noodles.

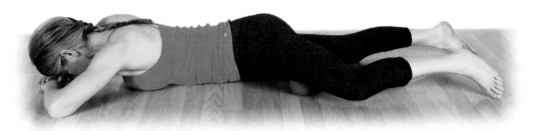

To **CrossFiber** is to move, slide, or drag a Roll Model Ball against the "grain" of a muscle, or across the muscle. CrossFiber can also be performed at various oblique angles, as long as you roll *across* the line of pull of the muscle. In order to CrossFiber a muscle, it is essential to learn the classical origin and insertion points of muscles so that the ball can crisscross that myofascia. For example, to CrossFiber your quadriceps, you track the ball from side to side across your thigh. To CrossFiber your quadratus lumborum, you scroll the ball from side to side across your lower back. See pages 132–139 for a list of Knead-to-Know muscles and to view their lines of pull.

What's happening physiologically: One of the most effective techniques for addressing fascial stiffness, CrossFiber teases apart stuck or dehydrated adhesions and stimulates fibroblasts to produce collagen in the direction of the cross, thus re-establishing the crimpy wave-form of healthy fascia.

STRIPPING AND CROSSFIBER: THE LONG AND SHORT OF IT

Many muscles cause pain because they are locked in an overstretched position ("locked long"). For example, your neck muscles may be full of knots and trigger points because they are sustaining long-held contractions to hold your heavy head while it slumps forward at your desk or bows over a texting device like a tuna at the end of a fishing pole. Trigger points form within those long neck muscles as local hyper-contracted bands of muscle tissue try to prevent your head from falling farther forward. For every inch forward your head travels, an additional 10 pounds of stress and strain is added to the muscles holding your head.* Your neck muscles fatigue and ache as a result.

Stripping will only further elongate myofascias that are already "at the end of their rope." In the case of a muscle that is locked long (overstretched), you want to try to shorten the myofascia by using a CrossFiber technique.

Conversely, many muscles cause pain because they are locked in a tightened position due to injury, overuse, or poor habits. In the case of a muscle that is "locked short," resetting the myofascia's pliability from end to end through stripping resolves its claustrophobia. It can then help neighboring soft-tissue seams and joints resolve their range-of-motion restrictions.

For example, in our deskbound culture, the accumulated stress of sitting creates extra-tight hip flexors that are locked short (while the buttock muscles opposite the hip flexors are locked long). Stripping the Roll Model Balls along the grain of the short hypertonic hip flexor myofascias can help restore a more optimal, healthy tone. CrossFibering these adaptively shortened hip flexors will not necessarily resolve their tension, but the gluteal muscles opposing the hip flexors might benefit from CrossFiber since they are "locked long."**

If you are unsure whether a muscle is locked long or short, don't let it prevent you from getting on the ball. These are helpful guidelines, but they are not laws. Because the majority of your myofascias are interconnected, your technique stroke (no matter which you choose) will likely help some unhappy tissue in that region.

* http://erikdalton.com/forward-heads-funky-necks/

**Explore this concept further in Thomas W. Myers' book, *Anatomy Trains* (Churchill, Livingstone, 2014)

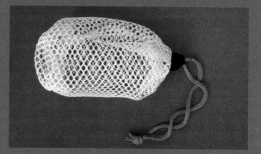

This empty Snug-Grip Tote represents normal myofascia. Notice that the "cells" have a diamond shape.

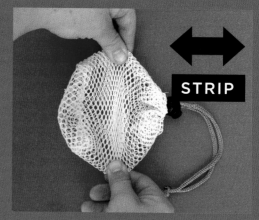

STRIP

Here the tote is stiffened into a "locked short" shape. Stripping resets the tension in overtightened fascias and returns them to their balanced diamond shape.

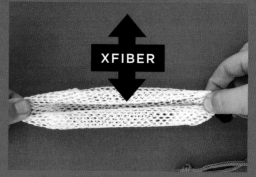

XFIBER

Here the tote is stiffened into a "locked long" shape. CrossFiber resets the tension in overstretched fascias and returns them to their balanced diamond shape.

In short, you strip muscles that are locked short, and you CrossFiber muscles that are locked long.

5. Pin & Stretch

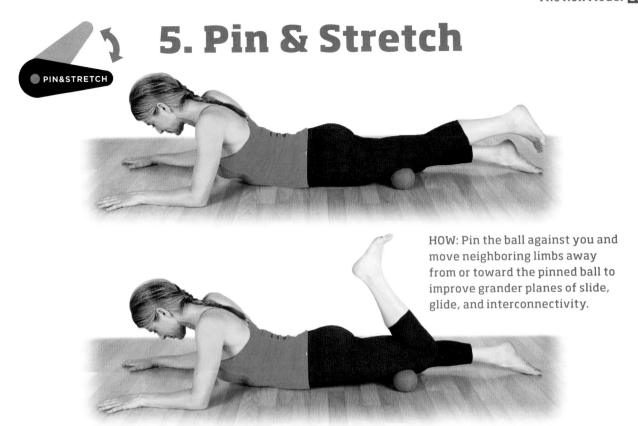

● PIN&STRETCH

HOW: Pin the ball against you and move neighboring limbs away from or toward the pinned ball to improve grander planes of slide, glide, and interconnectivity.

To perform the **pin & stretch** technique, find a location along a muscle that feels tender, tight, knotty, or guitar string-like and lodge your ball into it. Use your body pressure to create a "ball sandwich" between your target and the floor, wall, or other surface against which you are rolling. Now move any appendage that is close to the pinned area in any possible direction. In other words, move the "uptown joint" or "downtown joint" while you keep the ball locked in place (like a grippy hinge) at the tender point. As the ball tacks down the tissue there, your nearby joint movements will pry apart and loosen the myofascial fibers that are under the ball.

What's happening physiologically: This technique is extremely effective at eradicating trigger points and building body awareness.

1. The pressure into the pinned location on your muscle combined with the stretch across the rest of the muscle (the muscle's "belly") returns the fascia to an elastic state and restores full contractile ability to those muscle fibers. Over time, using this technique

deactivates trigger points and can train the muscle itself to regain its optimal length and functionality.

2. Pin & stretch helps you identify the direct relationship of a knotty area (which is pinned under the ball) to its surrounding tissues (the areas being moved and stretched). You may also notice referral sensations into distant fascial attachment sites.

With that knowledge, you will be able to isolate the degree of restriction along the line of pull between the moving part and the pinned tissue. This will make you more aware of how your movement or non-movement pattern defines the balance of motion between these parts. While moving, you are stretching body parts away from or toward the pinned spot. This encourages the fascial connections and muscle fibers in between to become more supple, hydrated, "conscious," and relieved.

When performing pin & stretch, you will notice the distinct fibrous "threads" within the greater "weave" of your fascia. This awareness truly helps improve your proprioception and your perception of your body as an interconnected organism.

CONTRACT
RELAX

6. Contract/Relax
(Proprioceptive Neuromuscular Facilitation)

Contract/relax, also known as **propriocep-tive neuromuscular facilitation (PNF),** techniques request that the tissue being targeted by the ball actively contract as the ball is either pinned on the tissue or within movement-based strokes. In other words, you stiffen the tissue where the ball is placed, hold for seven to thirty seconds, and then relax that tissue.

What's happening physiologically: Both contracting and relaxing target the Golgi tendon organ (GTO)–the proprioceptive stretch receptors located in tendons and fascial junctions (myoten-dinous aponeuroses; see page 109 for more on proprioception). When the targeted tissue is con-tracted, the GTO is stimulated and communicates a quick reflex loop with the spinal cord. When the targeted tissue is relaxed, the entire muscle and its associated connective tissues slacken and re-lease. This allows the muscle and its internal and external fascias to become more pliable and thus helps the ball dig deeper with less resistance to eradicate trigger points. (The terms *contract/relax* and *PNF* can be used interchangeably.)

HOW: Dock the ball onto a tight spot and contract the spot pinned by the ball, then relax it. Contract/relax is the fastest way to reduce muscle bracing.

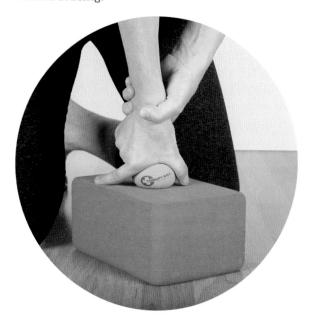

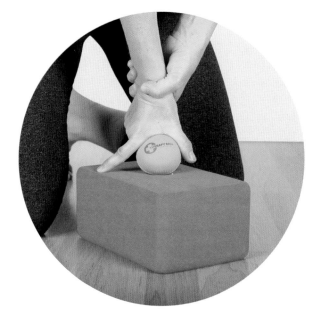

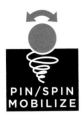

7. Pin/Spin & Mobilize

PIN/SPIN MOBILIZE

Pin/Spin & mobilize combines multiple techniques. It is the ultimate quick fix to facilitate as much tissue turbulence as possible. You place a ball on your target area, lean your body weight into the ball, and use a hand to spin and wring the ball deeper into your tissues. While it burrows and screws its way deeper into that target, you mobilize a neighboring joint in multiple directions, and you will clearly feel the interconnectedness of the fascia. Alternatively, you can lock the ball in place and then spin your body on top of the ball to create the same wind-up effect, and then mobilize the neighboring joint. For maximum effect, spin in only one direction while gathering as much tissue as possible, then mobilize, increase the tension on the spin, and mobilize again. After 90 to 120 seconds, wind the tissue in the opposite direction.

What's happening physiologically: The spinning of the ball into your tissues dramatically increases the skin-rolling/shearing effect on those tissues. Pin & spin finds the interrelated tensions that connect soft-tissue motility with joint mobility. As in the pin & stretch technique, you will clearly identify the relationships of fascias to their neighbors. The goal is to create as much piling and pinching of multiple fascias at once in the vortex of the twisting ball. This frees up inter- and intrafascial motion, stimulates the flow of fluids, and creates warmth. This technique, more than any other, might make you acutely aware of how fluid you are. Pin/Spin & mobilize makes a soft-tissue slurry out of your inner body.

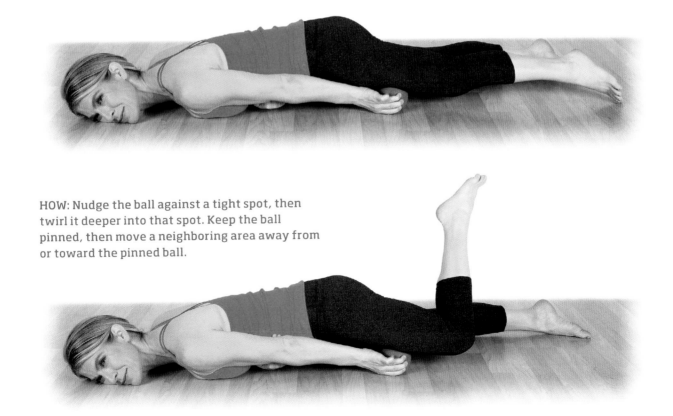

HOW: Nudge the ball against a tight spot, then twirl it deeper into that spot. Keep the ball pinned, then move a neighboring area away from or toward the pinned ball.

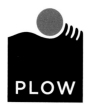

8. Ball Plow

The **ball plow** technique takes full advantage of the body's seam structure. It is especially lovely for enhancing slide & glide among deep fascial layers. This is the ultimate technique for mobilizing and transitioning large layers of superficial fascia over deeper fascias. It utilizes one ball (or multiple balls in close proximity) to act as a "squeegee" in an attempt to create a grand sliding motion within entire sheets of myofascia at once. The ball plow technique seeks out a fascial partition where one muscle converges into another. The ball acts like a plow to create massive tissue transition and shift in only one direction, much like a snowplow clearing snow.

Unlike stripping or CrossFiber, where the balls move and sometimes bump across tissues, the intention of the ball plow technique is to gather as much of the soft tissue as possible and move it as a mass in one direction. For the greatest effect, plow in one direction, lightly reset the balls in the original position, and then plow the same area in the same direction for several more strokes. Sometimes you may want to ball plow in only one

direction and then move to another area or technique. Other times you may want to plow that tissue from every conceivable direction.

This technique works best across broad planes of tissue, such as the trapezius, latissimus, gluteus maximus, and quadriceps. Unlike skin-rolling, which applies primarily to shallow and superficial layers, the ball plow is a deep technique that targets deep fascial layers. Ball plow aims to scoop the deep fascial relationships and sweep them along in motion. Naturally, any superficial fascias and tissues connected on top of the tissues being plowed will also come along for the ride.

What's happening physiologically: The one-directional deep shearing motion enhances intramyofascial motion among the planes of tissue being mobilized. This hastens the hydration of the tissues being plowed, resulting in deep warmth and relaxation. Think of the ball plow as maximum perfusion for large sheets of tissue. It will make your tissues feel extra pliable–what I call "petting zoo soft."

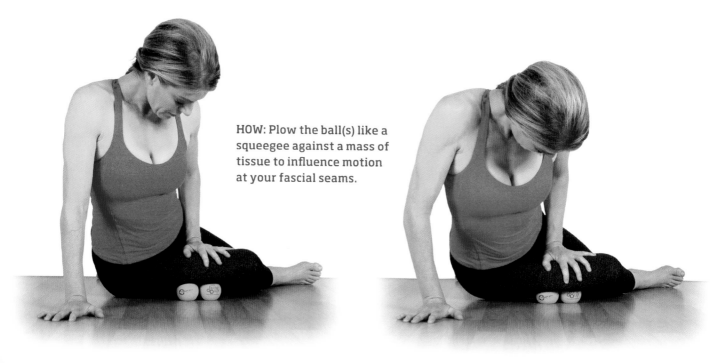

HOW: Plow the ball(s) like a squeegee against a mass of tissue to influence motion at your fascial seams.

9. Ball Stack

STACK

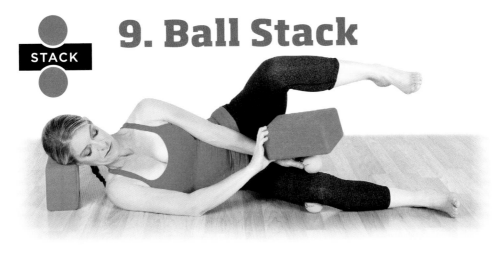

HOW: Stack the balls like a soft-tissue vise grip to unglue stuck masses of tissue–a great way to clear tensions "down to the bone."

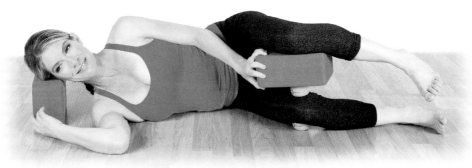

The **ball stack** technique attempts to apply loads of compression and squeezing to the targeted tissue. It feels as if a giant rubber vise grip or C-clamp is pinching large chunks of myofascia to stretch, pry, and partition the tissue away from its bones. Ball stacking is most useful on limbs, or even on the skull and face. It involves multiple balls, sometimes of the same size and sometimes of different sizes. Place one ball(s) underneath the tissue you want to address, place another ball(s) on the opposite side of that tissue, and then apply pressure to both sides simultaneously to compress the tissue between the balls. In some cases, you may need to use your hand, arm, or leg or an object like a book or yoga block to help you apply pressure for an optimal stack.

Once you have learned to stack, you can combine it with other techniques, such as pin & stretch or contract/relax. I find the most relief by seeking out the deep fascia interfaces–the seams between muscles. For example, in the Quad Kabob pictured above (see page 221), one ball nuzzles onto the outer thigh by landing in the partition between the outer quadriceps and the outer hamstrings (vastus lateralis and biceps femoris), while the ball on the inner thigh partitions the seam between the innermost quadriceps and the inside of the upper thigh (vastus medialis and gracilis).

What's happening physiologically: Stacking adds pressure to larger myofascial continuities and addresses fascias that may be hard to reach with just one ball. This "two-handed" approach applies concise vectors of pressure toward fascial attachments in deep fascial compartments. You may even feel a sense of your myofascias lifting or peeling away from your bones. The dual-sided approach also quickly addresses tensions in all the tissues associated with the stack: a great way to clear tensions "down to the bone."

7 Breath Reset

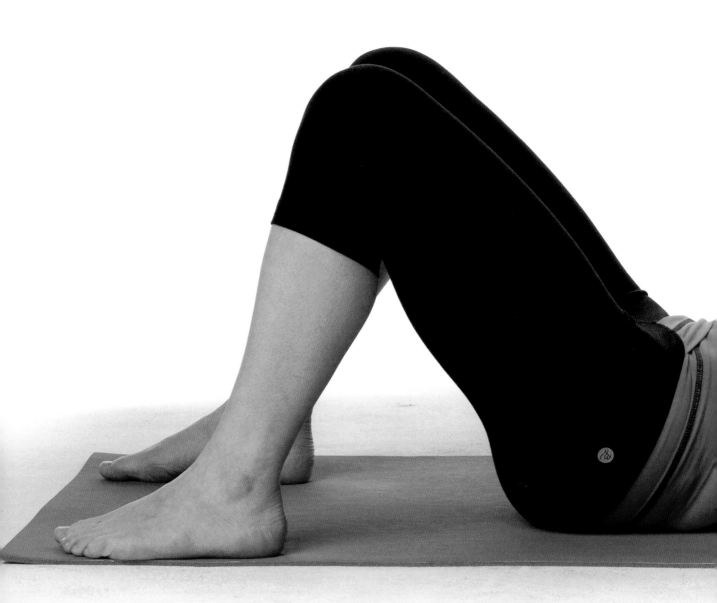

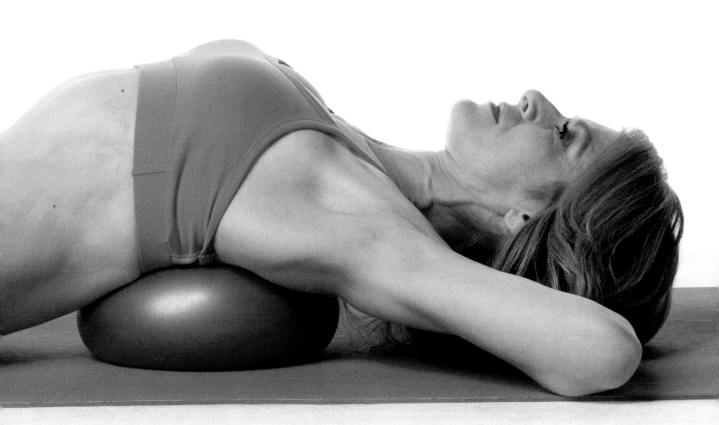

"Most people breathe enough to not die."
–Esther Gokhale,
author of *8 Steps to a Pain-Free Back*

Your breath is a primal life impulse. Its rhythm is a chief barometer of your well-being. In order to breathe skillfully in the most embodied way, it's helpful to understand a bit about the muscles, fascial tissues, bones, joints, and nerves associated with breathing. This chapter peers into the depths of your breath. You'll discover how its health and suppleness are *mandatory* for optimizing your personal Roll Model program.

Your breath muscles are plentiful, especially throughout your torso. The deepest of these muscles line the innermost surfaces of the bony canister of your ribcage, spine, and pelvis. Any muscle of the torso can arguably be a muscle of respiration, since the tissues are either stabilizing or mobilizing to promote breathing. If your muscles are tight and rigid from the inside out or the outside in, they create a stressful type of physical, emotional, and physiological body armor. To unglue and remodel these tissues, perform "non-surgical" surgery on yourself with the Roll Model Balls.

Think of your body's breathing muscles as the inner lining of a suit that you can re-tailor so that your "suit lining" fits you better. Here's the analogy: if you buy an off-the-rack designer knockoff suit, one of the giveaways is that the lining does not line up well with the outer fabric. The stitching is haphazard, and the suit does not move well with you. But if you buy a suit that is custom-tailored to your body, every stitch of the fabric moves effortlessly and efficiently, and it looks beautiful to boot! Most of us have been walking around wearing "knockoffs" instead of custom-fit cores. Now is your chance to custom-fit your physique the way nature intended!

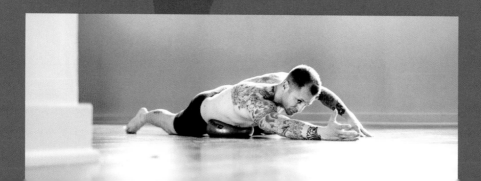

The Respiratory Diaphragm

Your diaphragm is the "heart" of your respiratory system. While the diaphragm muscle is less popular than the core muscles that surround it or the heart that sits on top of it, it is arguably the most important muscle in your body. If it ceases to function, you will expire. Its dome shape serves as a partition dividing your lungs and heart from your other organs. Its attachments are sewn to the insides of your lower six ribs and along the front of your lumbar spine. When it contracts (during an inhale), its plunger-like downward action draws oxygenated air into your lungs. When it relaxes (upon exhale), the plunger flies back up, which pushes carbon dioxide-rich air out.

Most people are unaware of the diaphragm until they have the hiccups, which are spasms in that muscle. It is difficult to perceive the diaphragm working because it is so deeply hidden and has very few sensory neurons. The simplest way to recognize its movement is to notice the motion of the structures that surround it. During an inhale, the diaphragm contracts, descending upon the soft tissue layers below it and the organs wrapped inside them. These myofascias surrounding your organs are seamed together with the diaphragm at their fascial interfaces. (Gil Hedley playfully describes the diaphragm as a "stocking cap" on top of the "abdominal sack.") A healthy abdomen swells like a balloon in all directions. (This is different from the way your gut protrudes when you forcefully bear down or try to push your belly out.) During an exhale, the diaphragm relaxes and returns upward, which relieves pressure on the ballooning abdomen. The abdomen becomes soft again. This abdominal motion is evidence of the layers' interconnectivity. Said simply: with each inhale the abdomen rises, and with each exhale it falls.

It's an unusual muscle because it is regulated by both somatic and autonomic nerves, meaning that you have both voluntary and involuntary control over it (it will soldier on whether you control it or not). This positions the diaphragm to be a portal for any mind that wishes to change its own behavior. Yoga and many Eastern arts, like Qigong and other martial forms, have developed strategies to play around with breath techniques in order to access the nervous system and control states of mind. These breath exercises deeply condition the diaphragm, along with all the associated respiratory muscles. These include all "core" muscles (transversus abdominis, obliques, rectus abdominis), back muscles (latissimus dorsi, erector spinae, multifidi, quadratus lumborum, and more), intercostals, pectoralis, rhomboids, trapezius, and truly all torso tissues! Consciously mobilizing the diaphragm through repeated contractions and relaxations impacts the muscle spindles and Golgi tendon organs (somatic proprioceptors–see chapter 4) within the diaphragm as it changes in texture and mobility. This persistent controlled activity will undoubtedly alter your consciousness and affect your alertness or sedation. Deep breathing also improves your lung capacity and blood chemistry. Each of these elements factors into the volitional modulation of your nervous system.

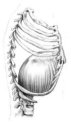

Diaphragm (side view)

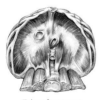

Diaphragm (inferior view)

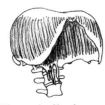

Thoracic diaphragm

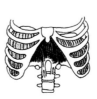

Attaches to ribs and lumbar spine

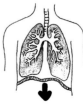

Diaphragm moves downward on inhalation

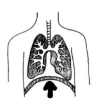

Diaphragm moves upward on exhalation

Images by Harijot Khalsa and Ismael Pinteño

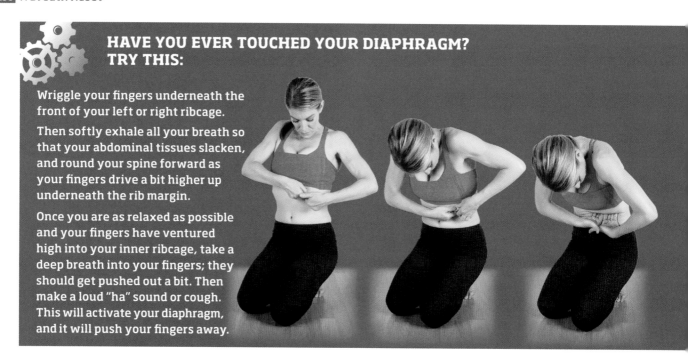

The Stress Response

If your torso and breath myofascias are stiff, immobile, and conditioned toward tension, you will have a hard time taking deep breaths that cool and relax your nervous system. All that body armor renders you stressed out and up-regulated, placing you in a state of sympathetic dominance, or perpetual fight-or-flight. *The goal of using the balls on your respiratory tissues is to help them perform their proper function.* All that detangling and resetting of your breath tissues to help them normalize quells stress and serves as a natural relaxant. You will enter into states of down-regulation ruled by the parasympathetic portion of your nervous system. It's akin to taking a sedative, but with no nasty side effects. (See chapter 9 on the "roll" of relaxation.)

The more time you spend in states of anxiety, the weaker your body becomes. Shallow, rapid breathing is associated with the fear response and higher levels of cortisol. Over time, living in states of fear, trauma, exhaustion, and overload affects your performance on every level. Most illnesses can be traced to a weakened immune system due to stress. The key to healing is to spend more time in the parasympathetic realms of rest and relaxation, which is easily induced with deep abdominal breathing. During this "quiet time" for your body, growth hormone is released and permeates injured tissues to help repair them and bring your body back to balance. Deep breathing is an age-old secret that reverts the body to soothing parasympathetic dominance.

SYMPATHETIC: *The portion of the autonomic nervous system that prepares the body for arousal, action, and defense. It is catabolic, meaning that it tears the body down, using the body's energy for fuel and activation. You access it through shallow clavicular breathing.*

PARASYMPATHETIC: *The portion of the autonomic nervous system that governs rest, digestion, and regeneration. It is anabolic, meaning that it builds up and repairs the body. You access it through deep abdominal breathing.*

The Three Abodes of Breath

In addition to the diaphragm, there are many other muscles that contribute to breathing. These secondary muscles of respiration cluster in three distinct areas of the body. Each type of breathing affects the nervous system, and subsequently your muscles' resting tone, in different ways.

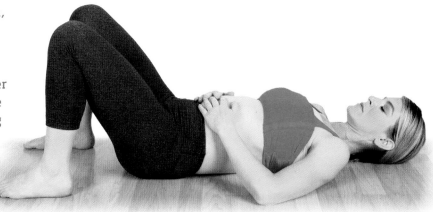

1. **Abdominal breathing**, or belly breathing, uses the diaphragm and the transversus abdominis, a cummerbund-style muscle that wraps horizontally around your waist from front to back. It attaches to the lower spinal vertebrae via a broad plane of connective tissue called the thoracolumbar fascia, and in front to a similar plane called the abdominal aponeurosis (a deep fascia of many layers that wraps around the rectus abdominis, or rectus sheath). This style of breathing is the most calming and triggers parasympathetic dominance. Think of a sleeping baby's belly inflating and deflating. This is the ideal breath for much of the Roll Model Therapy Ball work, as it helps the parasympathetic nervous system induce relaxation into the myofascias that the balls are targeting.

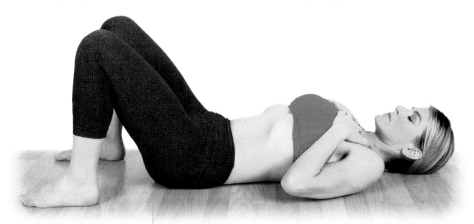

2. **Thoracic breathing**, or chest/ribcage breathing, recruits the diaphragm, intercostals, pectoralis major and minor, and rhomboids. It is used to increase the saturation of the lung sacs with oxygen and to increase total lung capacity. In thoracic breathing, the transversus abdominis is held in a state of tension in order to stabilize the lower-back bones while restricting the downward contraction of the diaphragm. Thoracic breathing is often maligned for not being as restful as abdominal breathing, but it is an absolutely vital area in which to have full facility; otherwise the dozens of joints that connect the ribs to

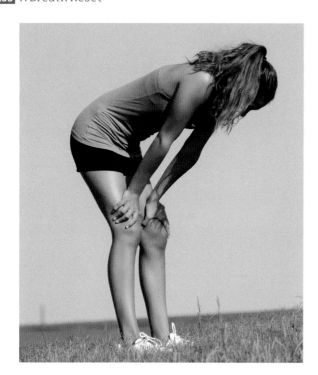

the thoracic spine will stiffen from lack of use. Thoracic breathing does have negative consequences if it is overused or used exclusively, however, as it begins to trigger the fight-or-flight response in the body.

>**//** *Habitual chest breathing not only reflects physical and mental problems, it creates them. It mildly but chronically over-stimulates the sympathetic nervous system, keeping the heart rate and blood pressure too high, precipitating difficulties with digestion and elimination, and causing cold and clammy hands and feet.* **//**
>
>–David Coulter,
>*The Anatomy of Hatha Yoga*

3. **Clavicular breathing**, or stress breathing, practically eliminates the diaphragm, recruiting the deeper pectoralis minor, upper trapezius, levator scapulae, sternocleidomastoid, scalene, and subclavicular muscles. This is the freaked-out panic breath that your body defaults to in emergencies. For example, as you startle at the sound of a gunshot, your shoulders fly up toward your ears, and air rushes into the highest point in your lungs. Another example of clavicular breathing is runners hunched over at the end of a race, their shoulders hiked up to their ears and their hands perched on their upper thighs as their heads fold forward, straining to gulp in a breath.

Asthmatics are all too familiar with this type of breathing and often have tension in the neck and shoulders as a result. But so many of us have Teflon-like stiffness and imbalances in these muscles from poor positioning at computers or texting devices. This buildup of tension is your body mimicking the most stressful arrangement for your breath muscles. Help turn off these stress muscles of respiration by using the Roll Model Balls frequently throughout your workday. I guarantee that it will make you more focused and productive, like pressing your internal reset button. (If the above describes you, make Sequence 14: Neck Gnar and Sequence 10: Ribcage Rinse & Respire a regular part of your daily maintenance.)

Everyone benefits from enhancing their connection to abdominal breathing and learning to intelligently intermix thoracic breathing as well. The Abdominal-Thoracic Breath provides a wonderful combination of relaxed alertness as you practice ball-rolling. But in order to achieve this balancing breath, you must detangle the tissues that obstruct your diaphragm and intercostals from moving fully.

Abdominal and Thoracic Breathing Primer

Try these techniques to get to know your breath before digging deeper with the smaller, firmer balls.

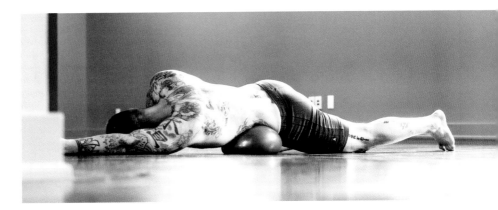

1. **Abdominal Breathing with Hands on Abdomen:** Place your relaxed hands on your abdomen near your navel. Inhale and attempt to balloon your gut so that your abdomen and hands rise. On the exhale, allow your hands to fall back into your belly toward the floor. Do this for 10 breaths without straining or "bearing down." Then move onto step 2.

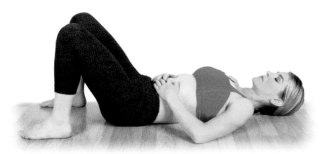

2. **Abdominal Breathing with Coregeous Ball:** Place the Coregeous Ball directly over your navel and lie on top of it for 3 minutes. Practice abdominal breathing. As you inhale, your abdomen will bulge into the ball. As you exhale, your abdomen will passively hollow as the ball burrows into your belly.

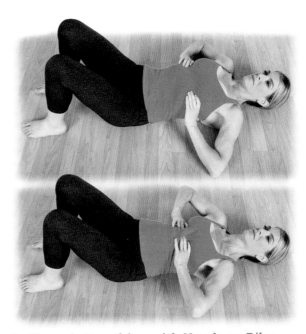

3. **Thoracic Breathing with Hands on Ribs:** While reclining, sitting, or standing, place your hands on either side of your ribcage, your thumbs wrapping around toward your back and your fingers spread wide. Firmly clamp your hands around your ribs to make a "finger cage" surrounding your ribs. Without letting go of your hand tension, breathe into your ribs 8 times, and feel the action of the intercostals attempting to pry your ribs (and fingers) apart.

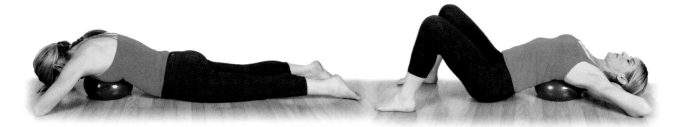

4. **Thoracic Breathing with Coregeous Ball:** Place the Coregeous Ball on your sternum and lie on top of it for 3 minutes. As you rest, practice thoracic breathing. As you inhale, your ribcage will bulge into the ball. As you exhale, your ribcage will seem to become flatter and shallower.

These simple exercises help you gain awareness of your breath patterns and discover different breathing strategies for ball work.

5. **Thoracic Breathing from Your Back with Coregeous Ball:** Place the Coregeous Ball behind your ribs and allow your torso to drape over it. If your back lacks the ability to arch easily, place a pillow, a blanket, your hands, or a book behind your skull so that you can relax into the shape. Breathe to expand your ribcage in all directions. Attempt to feel your chest and back simultaneously growing larger with each inhale and smaller with each exhale. Spend 3 minutes with the ballooning pressure of your ribcage breath.

THE IMMUNE RESPONSE AND GUT MASSAGE

Lying on and breathing into the Coregeous Ball may seem like an awkward way to fight a cold, but lodging that large, pliable ball into your core just might be better than your mom's chicken soup.

The gut area is the most abundant site in your body for lymph. Your lymphatic system (which is a fluid connective tissue) stores the majority of your disease-fighting cells. Your lymphatic ducts and tubing are an odd one-way highway; there is no upward movement out of the ducts and tubes other than being pressed and squeezed through motion, position, palpation, or muscular contractions. Motion around your lymph ducts helps propel those disease-fighting cells into your bloodstream, where they can fight off infection.

Your abdominal lymph is loaded with immune-rich cells. The white blood cells within it have been highly sensitized by the gut's bacterial environment and thus are the superheroes of your lymphatic system. Helping your gut lymph move north into the larger blood vessels is not the easiest proposition. You can do so by inverting your body or doing intense abdominal contractions and mobilizations, or you can use the Coregeous Ball for self-massage.

Lisa Hodge shared her breakthrough studies on rats* at the 2012 International Fascia Research Congress. She infected rats with lung cancers and then created a seven-day protocol of rhythmic massage on their bellies for four minutes at a time, with a break between rounds. She found that the rats that received the abdominal massage saw a decrease in the size of their lung tumors and contracted far fewer pneumonias.

Deep, deliberate abdominal breathing while lying belly-down on top of the Coregeous Ball, coupled with movement, is quite similar to the actions Dr. Hodge induced on the rats' bellies. She claims that myofascial release, or traction and release of the diaphragm, helps remove restrictions to lymphatic vessels. The mobilization of white blood cells was done through deliberate motion and made a massive difference in these animals.

Luckily, your lymphatics are all over your body, and their immune-boosting flow is easily stimulated wherever the balls tumble. The next time you feel under the weather, consider giving your belly a rub.

* Lisa M. Hodge, PhD, "Osteopathic lymphatic pump techniques to enhance immunity and treat pneumonia," *International Journal of Osteopathic Medicine* 15, no. 1 (2012): 13-21.

Breathing Strategies with the Balls

Throughout the Roll Model sequences, you will be instructed to breathe in the following ways. Once you're comfortable with the sequences, you can explore interchanging breath strategies and note their different effects.

1. **Abdominal Breathing:** Swell your abdomen like a balloon on the inhale, and let it deflate on the exhale. Abdominal breathing is the most relaxing and establishes a precondition for deep relaxation.

2. **Thoracic Breathing:** Swell your ribcage like a bony balloon on the inhale, and allow it to deflate on the exhale. Thoracic breathing is not as relaxing as abdominal breathing because it prevents the diaphragm from moving fully through its range of motion, but it is helpful to awaken the intercostals and mobilize your ribs.

3. **Abdominal-Thoracic Breathing:** Generate an inhale that swells your abdomen and then transitions into your ribcage. On your exhale, allow all those areas to relax and deflate. This maximizes the use of all your respiratory muscles and progressively increases your lung volume.

Practice Abdominal-Thoracic Breathing by placing one hand on your abdomen and the other on your chest. Feel your belly expand first, like a giant soft-tissue balloon, then your ribcage, like a bony balloon, followed by both areas emptying. Your hands will rise and fall with each inflation and deflation.

4. **Contract/Relax Breathing:** This can occur in any of the first three strategies. To contract/relax breathe, inhale fully into your abdomen, ribcage, or both, then hold that breath for 5 to 10 seconds. While holding your breath, stiffen your muscles of respiration, then exhale and relax all of your breath muscles. Begin another round once you feel normalized. Contract/relax breathing should not be done with extreme force and should not make your eyes bloodshot or your face beet red; use just enough tension to lock in the held breath. This type of breathing can help speed up the pliability of your muscles of respiration in a very short time.

Whichever strategy you use*, remain aware of your breath. Your mindfulness while breathing will magnify the relaxation induced by the Roll Model Balls. I often tell my students, "Your breath is your safe word. If you cannot stay connected to your breath when you hit a potent body blind spot, you need to modify." Breath training is mental training. Your biology provides you this free tool to help you face seemingly insurmountable emotional and physical stresses. Deep breathing is always at your disposal; just let it *inspire* you.

* For a video review of all breathing strategies used throughout the sequences, visit www.tuneupfitness.com/roll-model-videos

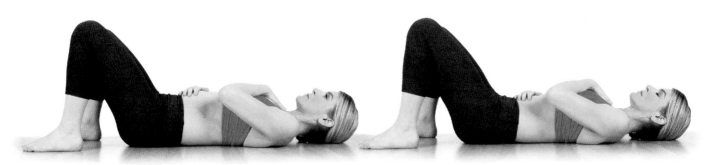

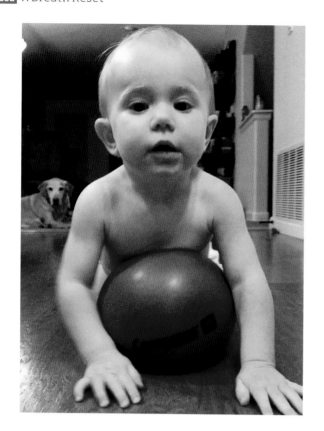

Baby's Breath: Babies haven't piled on years of stress and bad habits, and their breath practices are full of the ease that naturally follows the body's design. As we mature, we tend to get in our own breath's way. This baby climbed on top of her mom's Coregeous Ball one day after she'd seen her mama using it for her own Breath Reset.

Hold Your Breath: A Blow-by-Blow on Beating Asthma

Kelly Starrett, DPT, 40
Physical Therapist and
Human Function Specialist
San Francisco

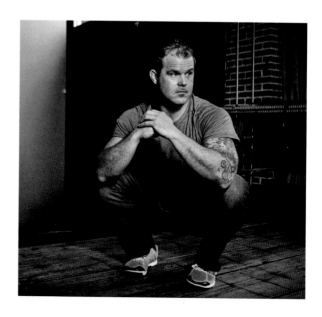

Kelly Starrett is a megastar in the worlds of strength and conditioning, professional sports, human performance, and CrossFit. His popular YouTube channel features hundreds of his self-made MobilityWOD videos that teach people how to fix themselves. At last count, it had more than 18 million views. Kelly is a superior athlete, having competed and won in slalom canoe and white-water kayak for the U.S. national team. His first book, Becoming a Supple Leopard, *is a* New York Times *and a* Wall Street Journal *bestseller and a runaway hit on Amazon. (Full disclosure: we share the same exceptional publisher, Victory Belt.) He is magnanimous, provocative, electrifying to be around, and one of the funniest human beings I've ever met. He makes me laugh until I hurt.*

I first met Kelly face-to-face a few years ago at his treatment clinic, housed in a tiny portable shelter in a small corner of his San Francisco CrossFit "box" (CrossFit gyms are known as boxes) in a chilly, windy parking lot less than a mile from the Golden Gate Bridge. Our mutual friend Keith Wittenstein had introduced us via email in early 2011. Kelly and I emailed a few times after I watched dozens of his MobilityWOD videos and recognized that we share a similar worldview on self-care healthcare. I was headed to lead a teacher training in the area and swung by to show him some self-care strategies for better breath function, something I thought was missing from his catalog of brilliant videos.

Within fifteen minutes of meeting, talking, and sharing some of my ideas, he handed his cell phone to his friend Jesse Burdick, and we shot three videos covering some of my approach. Those three spontaneous MobilityWOD videos tackled diaphragm mechanics, the psoas, and the interplay of the nervous system, breath, and performance. As we filmed, Kelly revealed something that he had kept secret for years: he had been a severe asthmatic.

Twenty-two million Americans have asthma*, a disease that affects the movement of air into and out of the lungs. In an asthma attack, the airways narrow in three ways:

1. Muscular tightening around all of the soft-tissue tubing within the lungs

2. Internal swelling of the air passages

3. Extra mucus production

All these reactions reduce the surface area of the lungs, so fresh oxygenated air cannot get into the bloodstream and carbon dioxide cannot get out. When you have an asthma attack, you feel as if you are simultaneously choking, being suffocated, and drowning.

As a child, I grew up watching my mother suffer from daily asthma attacks that were triggered by allergens, emotional stress, and physical activity. This experience was terrifying for me, as there is very little a bystander can do to help someone in the throes of an attack. When an asthmatic is stricken, she will often hike her shoulders up toward her ears, gasping for air as if she's been running for her life. The terror in the body is real:

suffocation is life-or-death to the nervous system. The muscles of the upper back, shoulders, neck, and chest over-engage to try to suck air in and expel carbon dioxide. This overuse and compensatory use leaves many asthmatics with specific muscular pain in these areas. The majority of asthmatics take pills or inhalants to prevent or tame attacks. (The most "effective" of these are steroids, which have long-term side effects.) Asthma causes more than 500,000 hospitalizations in the U.S. each year and is one of the five most expensive diseases to our healthcare system.**

In our first five-minute video, entitled Jill Miller Fixes Your T-spine and Breathing, Kelly and I explain some of the diaphragm's connections to other tissues in the body. I also share the Rib Rock move with the Roll Model Balls (see page 290). In our second video, with its expressively long title Jill Miller Smashes Your Guts! (and psoas, and tacked down viscera, and matted down abdominals), I teach him how to use the Coregeous Ball to create global shear and slide & glide among all the layers of the abdomen. He deadpans to the camera, "I just did this, this is wretched, this is disgusting, this thing makes me vomit in my mouth a little bit. This is my goat." He also goes on to say for the

* www.aafa.org/display.cfm?ID=5&Sub=105&Cont=725

** www.healthcaresouth.com/pages/asthmadef.htm

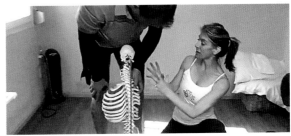

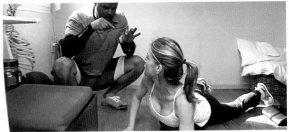

From our first MobilityWOD collaborations.

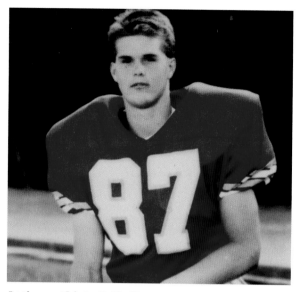

Asthma athlete Kelly Starrett at age 16.

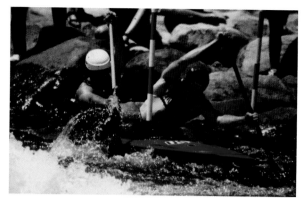

At his kayak peak.

first time to his millions of viewers, "I have always felt tacked down in the area of the diaphragm. I was a bad breather as a kid. I had asthma."

During high school, in 1989, Kelly recognized that something was very wrong with his breathing. His father, a physician, was the first to diagnose him with severe athletic-induced asthma. Later, Kelly realized that his asthma was also triggered by allergens and the environment. He was soon puffing an albuterol inhaler sixteen to twenty times a day to get through practices and competitions. In spite of the threat of passing out (or worse), he charged on in his pursuit of athletic excellence.

Kelly was an "asthma athlete," which meant that he received a grant to attend the University of Colorado at Boulder. To prove his eligibility, he was required to run on a treadmill to induce an attack and then test his breath capacity, which was 40 percent of normal. The lab technicians were shocked that he was still alive after the test and that he was performing "so well" with such a terrible score. Over the next ten asthma-ridden years, Kelly's body made up its own rules to help him get by. He remembers feeling crushed, buried alive when attacks flared. "I had so many inhalers everywhere—I always had an inhaler with me," he says. He remembers registering his inhaler with the National Olympic Committee when he made the slalom canoe team in 1998. He could count on an attack every time he trained, but still he persisted.

His worst attacks came on with his favorite recreational sport, skiing. The cold air was a massive irritant, and Kelly had to be vigilant about having an inhaler on the slopes. He discovered that coffee had a similar effect as his inhalers, and he became a "user" of strong hot coffee to help his lungs. He was never hospitalized; he was able to stave off the worst attacks with his inhalers, gallons of coffee, and occasionally over-the-counter Primatene Mist. Specialists prescribed seven different drugs, but Kelly admits that he was willfully "not good" on a pill regimen. Instead, he continued to rely on inhalers, sometimes twice an hour to survive and win in competition. And win he did, becoming a national champion in slalom and whitewater canoeing and representing the United States at the World Whitewater Championships in 2000, where he met his future wife, Juliet, also a two-time world-champion whitewater paddler.

At that same time, his paddling career ended, not directly due to asthma but because of severe nerve pain in his wrist that frequently caused his hand to go numb. Treatments for his wrist were not working to get him back into competition. It took years for Kelly to recognize that his default asthma breath pattern was intricately involved in the nerve pain. Those overused neck muscles had essentially sutured the nerves down to his thumb, and he was unable to fix this issue without changing his breathing behavior. "I'm convinced that part of that was my asthma breathing pattern, a passive-accessory breathing pattern. It's not an accident that my neck muscles and my scalenes clamped down really hard on some of my nerves," he says. In retrospect, Kelly can see that the way *he was training his body, mind, and nervous system were choppy waters that no top athlete could overcome:*

1. *He engaged in paddling sports for years, twice a day, 300 days a year, which meant a wet and cold environment and extreme upper-body exertion (typically in one direction, depending on which side of the canoe he was on).*

2. *He was not coached into any formal strength, conditioning, or mobilization program to help with his musculoskeletal imbalances.*

3. *His asthma-associated stress-breathing pattern constantly reinforced his asymmetries.*

Each time he practiced, he added more brokenness to his inefficiencies. His friend Gray Cook, DPT, calls it "pressing Save on your Word document, every time."

The nerve pain forced Kelly to change his entire life. He married Juliet, moved to San Francisco, and discovered CrossFit in 2003, diving into the creative hotbed of this human performance cross-training system close to its inception. He also adopted an anti-inflammation diet. He noticed that his asthma symptoms started to diminish the more he ate clean, minimized insulin spikes, reduced his exposure to allergens, and trained his aerobic threshold (maximum body exertion without tipping into a state of lactic acid buildup). In the meantime, he and Juliet opened San Francisco CrossFit. His larger coaching and teaching mission to serve mobility to the masses began to take shape.

With this new goal, Kelly entered physical therapy school and earned a doctorate degree from Samuel Merritt in 2007. He remembers asthma being mentioned in PT school, but no hands-on protocols for helping clients were taught. Kelly thought through his own asthma and wrist pain issues in typical maverick style, recognizing that all systems of the body are interdependent. It was around this time that he figured out the connection between his nerve pain and his neck stiffness: his bad breathing habits from asthma were contributing to his hand pain. So he began to reprogram his breath pattern.

By the time I met Kelly in June 2012, he had made more than 300 videos. His asthma symptoms had disappeared, but there were a few blind spots in his approach to self-treatment, and my decades of yoga practice, meditation, gut massage, and down-regulation training were the yin to his yang, the jelly to his peanut butter. What Kelly had not yet cleared up were the decades of soft-tissue stiffness in the relationships between his neck muscles, intercostals, diaphragm, psoas, and quadratus lumborum—what he refers to as "matted down tight tissues." His "Word document" needed to go through a shredder. There were areas in and around his torso that had zero slide & glide, and the grippy, pliable Roll Model tools I brought, coupled with my method of application, finally uncorked the tension that had been built up from a long-standing bad breath pattern. Back when he was training, he says, "I had a breathing pattern that was not diaphragmatic in nature, but was passive-accessory. And one of the key concepts to healing this is accessing the parasympathetic nervous system through the diaphragm. The Coregeous Ball gives you the immediate feedback that you're breathing right or breathing wrong."

Kelly started to use the Coregeous Ball on his abdomen religiously and taught his athletes and coaches to detangle their own knotty messes of overtightened abdominals. He also began to program self-massage of the psoas, diaphragm, or quadratus lumborum every ten to fourteen days in his classroom and Daily Rx videos. He has recommended these techniques for those who have had hernia surgeries; for rehab of abdominal tissues from carrying babies, Cesarean sections, and pelvic floor dysfunction; for all kinds of breathing issues; and much more. He also shares with his students and coaches that even the fiercest athlete is not immune to the effect that emotional stress plays on these sensitive tissues.

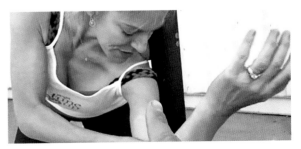

From November 2012, *Jill Miller and Your Dys-Supple Neck.*

Months later, I went back to visit Kelly and shared another fix, dubbed Jill Miller and Your Dys-Supple Neck, also known by the goofball shorthand title of Neck Gnar (the Neck Gnar rolling sequence begins on page 327). This fix uses an Original Yoga Tune Up Therapy Ball to massage the scalenes and other passive-accessory "stress muscles" of respiration, all while mobilizing the first rib. Kelly found this area to be the last vestige of his wrist pain, the Vulcan death grip that had impinged the nerves all the way down his arm. Though I had focused our original collaborations on this stress-breath pattern and all of its body consequences, Kelly and I received feedback from hundreds of people who used the videos for other chronic pain syndromes that were not directly related to breath. As he says, "Your body is a system of systems," and clearing up an issue in one specific area will have a positive ripple effect into many other areas.

Kelly loves that when you lie belly-down on the Coregeous Ball, it gives you tactile feedback of exactly how and where to breathe. "Breathing into the ball can cue you how to breathe properly; otherwise, it's really difficult to figure out. Any parent reading this who has a kid with asthma needs to get them the Coregeous Ball and get them to breathe into their belly as part of their treatment." He also champions this self-belly rub for eliminating back pain: "What's nice is that it gives people access to their diaphragm and breathing mechanics, which is also going to improve their spinal positioning while undoing the stiffness from asthma or other poor breath patterns."

The diaphragm piece is a natural highway into the parasympathetic nervous system: the relaxation response, recovery, and the importance of down-regulation. None of this response is possible when your breath muscles are armored and working against you. In June 2012, we expanded these concepts into a 26-minute video titled Down Regulation, Heart Rate Variability, Adaptation, Stress, and Turning Off.

Kelly says about asthma, "If we look at the neural mechanics of this thing, you're in an adrenal 'freakout'–an overblown sympathetic response that becomes your default because you've trained yourself to breathe incorrectly under extreme stress. It's easy to feel out of control, but what can you do about it physically? You can have correct breathing patterns, you can address the tissue dysfunction, and you can address the inefficient pattern that results from it. Take five minutes a day on the Coregeous Ball, or use the smaller balls for Neck Gnar. The soft-tissue component is the other 50 percent of asthma. If you can get ahead of it and stay ahead, you're fine, but once you're behind, it's hard to shut it down."

Kelly Starrett is a Roll Model for so many reasons. He's been one of the biggest catalysts for my own thinking, health, and programming. He proves

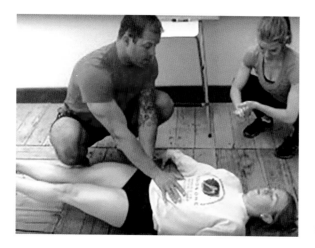

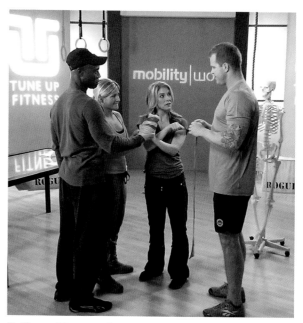

Kelly and I on set for *Treat While You Train* with Roll Model Greg Reid and cover model Sarah Kusch.

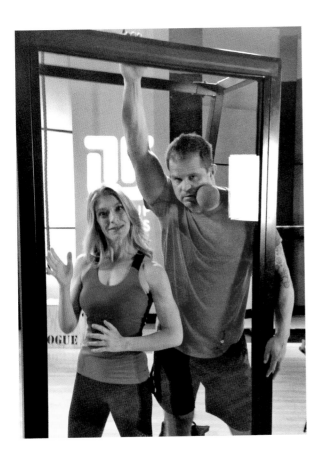

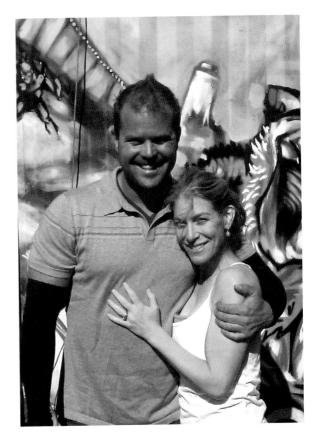

that with dedication to lifestyle, including soft-tissue self-care, you can stifle the progression of asthma and eliminate it from your life altogether. Kelly and I share a wish that if you have asthma, you will spend a few minutes a day trying these techniques for your long-term health.

Kelly says:

// People intuitively want to wean off of their medication, and for me it happened organically. Don't be afraid to pay attention, notice how you're feeling, and track your needs to use your inhaler. In an emergency breathing situation, these muscles are always gonna be tight, so deal with them. Asthma is something I have, but I can control it. There's no need to get beat down by it. **//**

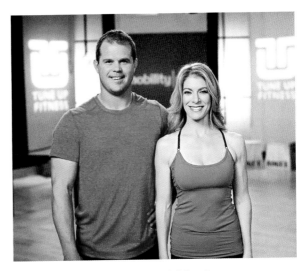

Out-of-the-box thinkers and friends.

Don't let asthma suck the life out of you. Take control with the Roll Model Therapy Balls.

8 The Sequences That Reset Your Body

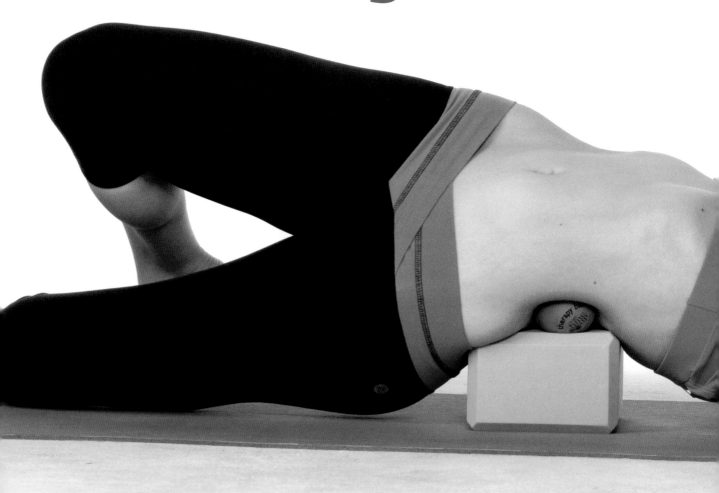

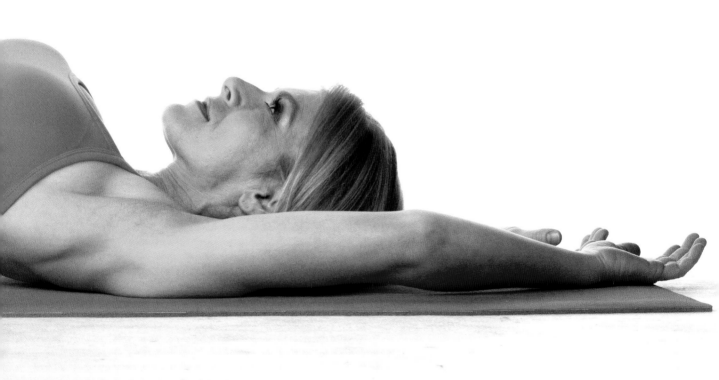

You have reached the heart of this book—the collected practices that have helped hundreds of thousands of people "take life by the balls" to eliminate medications, avoid surgeries, erase pain, maximize movement potential, and perform better than ever.

Drill into the body parts that seem relevant to your aches, but also remain open to exploring other areas. You may be surprised by your results! Because your fascial seam system is constantly interconnected (see chapter 4), tweaks may manifest in one area due to imbalance in another. For example, if you suffer from back pain, simply doing the back sequences will not necessarily address the full scope of the issue. With back pain, it is prudent to address your abdomen and hips also, since they are often the origin of back pain; at a minimum, these neighboring body areas are most certainly pulled into the soft-tissue tension that back pain creates.

Welcome to your inner sanctum. Here are your keys. It's time to enlighten your body to its own interconnectedness.

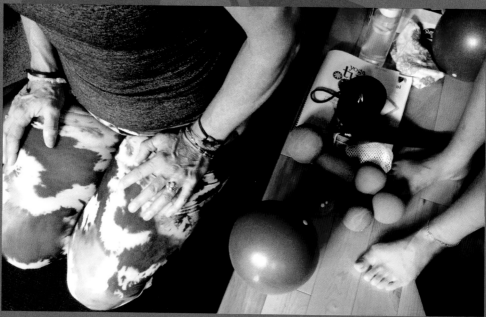

Your new movement medicine cabinet full of "rubber pills."

What Are the Roll Model Therapy Ball Sequences, and How Do You Use Them?

The Roll Model Therapy Ball sequences are carefully crafted deep-tissue self-massage explorations of different regions of your body. Each sequence targets specific muscles, connective tissues, and joints and attempts to induce compression, friction, penetration, motion, circulation, relaxation, and length into muscles and fascia all over your body. The balls are used in novel and unexpected ways to mimic the educated touch of a skilled massage therapist.

These sequences have been road-tested on hundreds of thousands of students worldwide in classes, in private training sessions, and via DVDs and online videos. They by no means exhaust all of the possibilities for any of the body parts listed, but this book gives you a fantastic array of sequences to keep your body happy, humming, and moving better than ever before. As you familiarize yourself with the sequences, begin to incorporate the nine key Roll Model Ball techniques outlined in chapter 6. Intermix those techniques and find moves that soothe you. Refining your knowledge of the bony landmarks and muscles (see chapter 5) will help you continue to raise the bar on your self-care healthcare.

As you begin doing the sequences, be sure to do the Check In and ReCheck suggested at the beginning and end of each sequence. These moves test whether your efforts elicited change. You'll be amazed at the immediate results you'll see! (Find more detail on Check Ins and ReChecks on page 175.)

Think of these sequences as your new movement medicine cabinet—a medicine cabinet full of rubber "pills" with only beneficial side effects. Alternate the different-sized balls to find just the right amount of pressure, grip, or penetration depending on where you are rolling and how you are feeling. Take your daily dose for routine maintenance, or increase the time you spend rolling in order to tackle specific aches and pains.

I suffer from a bad back and bad knees. Usually when I start feeling pain in my lower back, I pull out my Roll Model Balls. Just the other day, I was helping my family push our car into our driveway, and I started getting that sharp pain in my lower back. Once we were done, I pulled out my Therapy Balls and started rubbing the pain away. It literally felt like I was slowly pushing the pain away, down each vertebra. And the next day I had no aches or pain in my lower back. The Roll Model Balls are my pain reliever, and I'm glad I came across them.

–Jeslene Moore, Vallejo, California

Each sequence takes between ten and twenty minutes to roll through. If you have time, do the complete sequence; if you are short on time, choose a few points from within a sequence or mix and match moves from different sequences. The time you spend on the balls each day will begin to add up, and the Roll Model Method will uncover and erase pains that were previously hiding in plain sight. You'll also remodel your body into a supple fortress that pain cannot penetrate.

Here's an at-a-glance menu of the body areas you'll be rolling:

GLOBAL SHEAR TECHNIQUES FOR CORE/TORSO

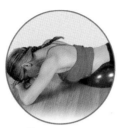

Sequence 1:
Global Shear Warm-up

LOWER-BODY SEQUENCES

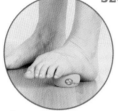

Sequence 2: Feet:
Save Your Sole

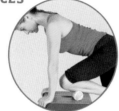

Sequence 3: Ankle &
Lower-Leg Treat

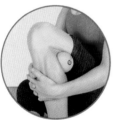

KNEE & ITS NEIGHBORS

Sequence 4:
Kneed to Knead

Sequence 5:
Pliable Thighs

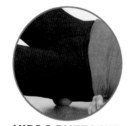

HIPS & BUTTOCKS

Sequence 6: Healthy Hips
& Fluffy Buttocks

Sequence 7:
Pelvic Funnel

BONUS: Pelvic Floor

SPINE SEQUENCES

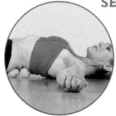

Sequence 8:
Lower Back

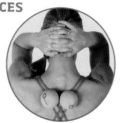

UPPER BACK

Sequence 9:
Upper-Back Unwind

Sequence 10: Ribcage
Rinse & Respire

SEQUENCES FOR SHOULDERS TO FINGERS

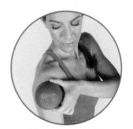

Sequence 11:
Shoulder – Rotator Cuff

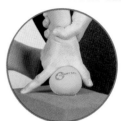

Sequence 12:
Shoulder – Elbow

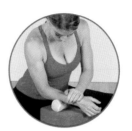

Sequence 13:
Forearms, Fingers,
Hands, & Wrists

NECK AND HEAD SEQUENCES

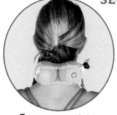

Sequence 14:
Neck Gnar

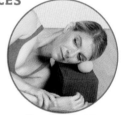

Sequence 15:
Head, Face, & Jaw

FREESTYLE EXPLORATION SEQUENCES

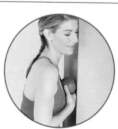

Sequence 16:
Front Seam

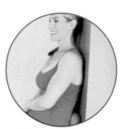

Sequence 17:
Back Seam

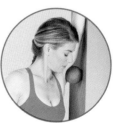

Sequence 18:
Side Seam

Your Movement Medicine Chest: Tools for the Sequences

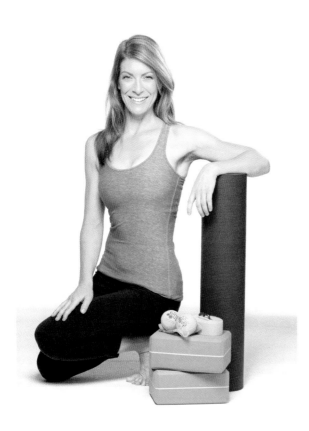

A full set of Roll Model Balls plus a few extra props are all you need to proceed with the sequences. You can easily substitute your favorite balls or tools if you don't have all of this equipment; I've made a few suggestions below. The props can easily be found at most sporting goods stores or online. You'll also find the Roll Model Balls and stretch strap at www.tuneupfitness.com.

The Roll Model Balls

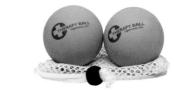

ORIGINAL YOGA TUNE UP BALLS

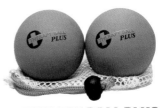

THERAPY BALL PLUS

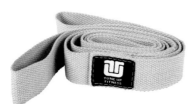

STRETCH STRAP SUBSTITUTIONS: LONG BELT OR SCARF

For the Roll Model Balls, substitute tennis balls or racquetballs. For the Coregeous Ball, you can use a rolled-up soft blanket or an extra-soft children's ball.

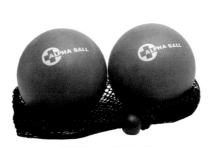

ALPHA BALLS

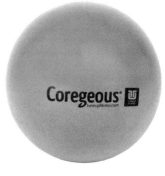

COREGEOUS BALL

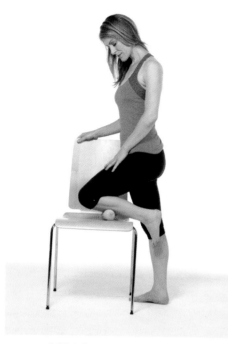

LOW STOOL OR CHAIR

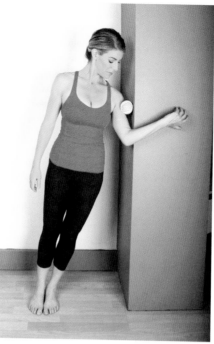

WALL CORNER OR DOORWAY

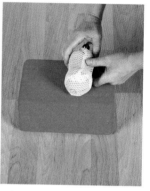

1 OR 2 BLOCKS SUBSTITUTIONS: LARGE BOOKS OR THICK, FIRM PILLOWS

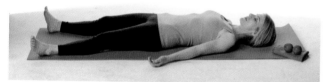

MAT (IF YOU ARE ON ITCHY CARPETING)

As you practice the sequences, you will naturally find your own best setup for each series. You will also inevitably innovate and discover new ways of untangling your own specific aches and pains, and you may introduce new tools or remove some of the ones listed above.

QUICK MODIFICATION RECAP: What to Do if the Pressure Is Intolerable

1. Take your balls to the wall (or a bed or sofa).

2. Use a larger ball on that area, or use two balls instead of one.

3. Move the balls uptown (higher), downtown (lower), or across town (to the right or left).

4. Stay on the surface with skin-rolling or shear.

5. Contract/relax until you achieve change or stop making change.

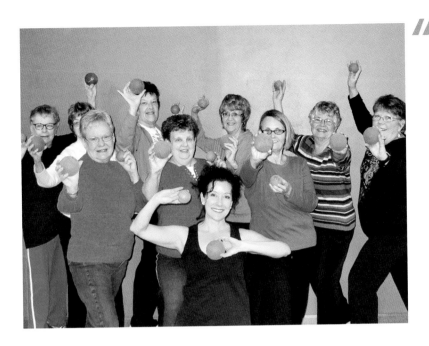

This picture was taken at my studio with our Seniors Yoga Class—possibly the biggest fans of Roll Model Balls EVER! Every one of these ladies owns her own balls or multiples, and I'm constantly getting testimonials on how Yoga Tune Up poses and the work with the Therapy Balls has alleviated pain for them and allowed them to do the things they want to do with more zest and joy! They are showing their balls to their doctors, chiropractors, friends, gardening club, you name it. They love it!

–Cathy Favelle,
Wautoma, Wisconsin

Check In/ReCheck

After you finish any of the sequences laid out in this chapter, you will likely feel different. Whatever your goal may have been before you rolled, whether it's relief, better movement, relaxation, or awareness, rolling will effect some kind of change. In the clinical space, this before-and-after scenario is called Test/Retest. I call it Check In/ReCheck. Basically, it means to do the following:

1. Bring some embodied awareness to the area that you are targeting *before* you roll, and **Check In** with the following:
   - pain
   - range of motion
   - stress level
   - breath
   - awareness

2. Then, *after* you roll, **ReCheck** those same elements. Sometimes you'll check just one, and other times you'll check several.

I have provided a simple Check In move for each of the sequences in this chapter.* Practice them before and after rolling and feel your movement changing. As you start to experiment, feel free to invent your own Check In stretches or moves, always ReChecking them afterward to find out whether the routine you created was helpful.

* For a video review of all Check In/ReCheck moves used throughout the sequences, visit www.tuneupfitness.com/roll-model-videos

For example, when doing the Neck and Jaw sequence, you can Check In by moving your neck in any of the many ways your neck moves:

1. Side bend
2. Forward bend (flexion; not pictured)
3. Backward bend (extension; not pictured)
4. Rotation
5. Rotation with forward bend (flexion)

Then do the sequence, and check one or all of these same ranges afterward.

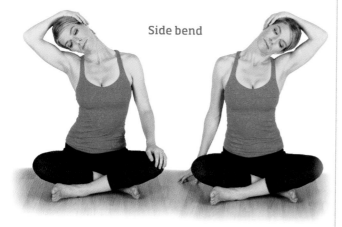

Side bend

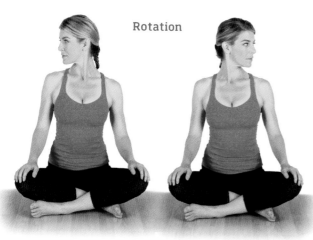

Rotation

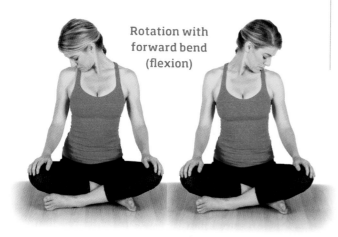

Rotation with forward bend (flexion)

The goal of the Check In/ReCheck is to give you a chance to see change and improvement. If you are familiar with each of your joints' directions of movement, you will be able to craft some very methodical Check Ins. A kinesiology textbook* or an Internet search on *kinesiology* will show you the many ways your joints can move and enhance your exploration. These gross movements of your joints will recruit the surrounding tissues. Sometimes the moves will feel great, and other times they will take you directly into the source of your pain and discomfort. Moving your body in uncomfortable directions sometimes makes matters worse, but it can also be your embodied clue as to which of your tissues are inflamed and malfunctioning. If you are unable to resolve your issues with the approach laid out in this book, consulting a professional is prudent.

For example, in 2006, I tore one of my rotator cuff muscles, the infraspinatus. I winced with pain when I moved my shoulder in certain directions, but not in others. Through my rehab process, I became educated about the factors causing my injury and which moves and soft tissues were compromised because of the injury. My physical therapist, Sean Hampton, and I would check each range of motion regularly, and with his treatment, my self-treatment, and exercises to strengthen my weaknesses, the tear eventually healed completely.

* My current favorite is *Kinesiology: The Skeletal System and Muscle Function*, 2nd Edition, by Joseph E. Muscolino (Elsevier, 2010).

Here are some of the many Check Ins/ReChecks for shoulder motion from the first teacher training manual that I wrote:

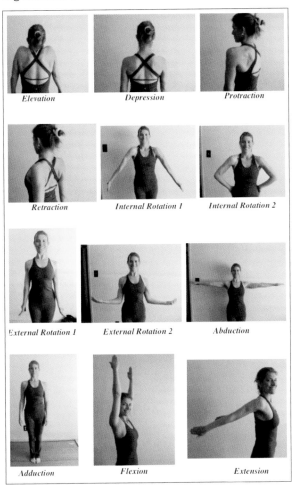

Elevation *Depression* *Protraction*

Retraction *Internal Rotation 1* *Internal Rotation 2*

External Rotation 1 *External Rotation 2* *Abduction*

Adduction *Flexion* *Extension*

This is an incomplete list of the shoulder's directions of movement, but you get the idea. Check In with one or more before you roll your shoulder, then ReCheck with one or any after you roll.

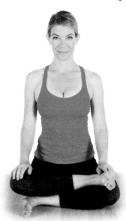

Double Pigeon is the Check In and ReCheck for the Healthy Hips & Fluffy Buttocks sequence.

Check In/ReCheck Options

Use the following list to generate creative Check Ins/ReChecks for yourself:

1. Dynamically move the joint directly associated with the rolled tissue. Check In its range of motion from every possible vector, then ReCheck after rolling. For example, before the Neck and Jaw sequence, Check In with your jaw by opening and closing it. Then open it and move it from side to side, followed by moving it in circles.

2. Create a static stretch of the joint directly associated with the rolled tissue. Design different stretches that you hold for five to ten breaths from every possible vector (choose one per session and repeat for your ReCheck). For example, in the Hips & Buttocks sequence, I suggest Double Pigeon as the Check In (see page 239). With this grand stretch of that buttock area, you will definitely feel a change before and after rolling.

3. Contract the myofascias that you plan to roll, then re-contract them afterward. For example, in that same Hips & Buttocks sequence, you could simply contract your buttocks for your Check In and then contract them again for your ReCheck. You will find that you are able to produce more force, or you will feel more of your buttock myofascias contributing to the contraction.

4. Observe your breathing before and after rolling.

5. Consider your mood before and after rolling.

6. Notice feelings of warmth before and after rolling.

7. Observe the presence or absence of pain before and after rolling.

This book does not offer complete diagnostics for every ache in the human body. I am giving you a general set of things to observe and try, but the book cannot tackle every possible condition of pain. If your befores and afters do not improve over time, please seek professional help.

Global Shear Techniques for Core/Torso

Global shear is perhaps the best way to arouse the greatest number of self-locating proprioceptors at once. It's like lighting up an entire city map instead of just a single street address. This technique quickly heats up and pre-lubricates tissues as a warm-up before you do more specific rubber scalpel work with the smaller balls.

Global shear utilizes the Coregeous Ball as its primary instrument of awakening. You may find that areas such as your back or portions of your side appreciate the ALPHA Ball, too. Interchanging the following four Roll Model Ball techniques (see chapter 6 for details) will give you the best benefits. These techniques naturally evolve from your breath and help reset your breath muscles by de-stiffening the multiple layers of soft and hard torso tissues that impede well-functioning breath.

1. SKIN-ROLLING

SKIN ROLL

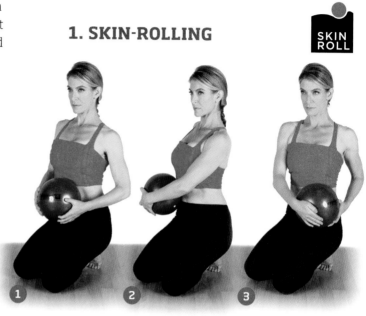

2. CONTRACT/RELAX

CONTRACT
RELAX

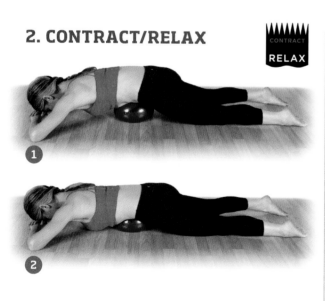

3. BALL PLOW

PLOW

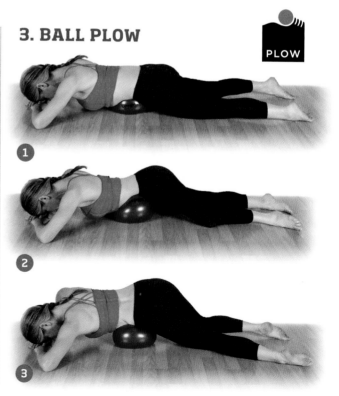

4. PIN/SPIN & MOBILIZE

PIN/SPIN
MOBILIZE

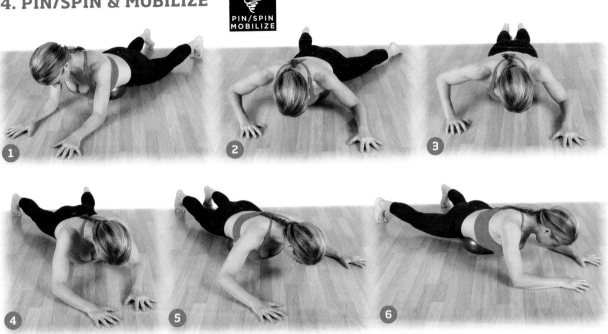

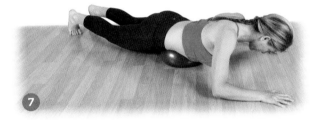

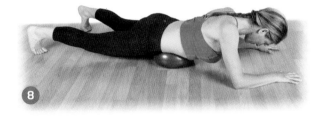

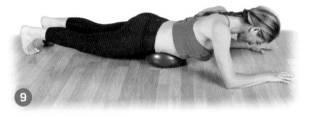

Each of these techniques wrangles the grippy Coregeous Ball into mobilizing the skin and its underlying superficial fascia. This springy top layer is manipulated to shift in multiple ways over the deep fascia to provide maximum slide and glide. To maximize global shear, the sticky rubber should feel like it is taped to your skin (bare skin works best). The ball will conform to your shape and allow your body and bones to sink into it. As you pinch, twist, wring, and reshape the outer layers over the inner layers, you source a wealth of heat and yummy fluidity. You also plow into areas that may feel like they have been stapled and stitched together by tension, time, scars, adhesions, and neglect. Occasionally you will find clumps of adhered tissues, remnants of scars, or poor movement patterns. Other times you will encounter a deep fascial seam or partition called a *septum*, the dividing "line" between one myofascial structure and another. A septum naturally is thicker and stiffer than myofascia, as its job is to maintain the integrity of the connections between structures, yet septa should still be pliable.

The Coregeous Ball treads and transitions the largest sheets of tissue over one another. Its size and malleable rubber allow for massive motion without threatening any delicate connections.

Use the Coregeous Ball to create global shear and preheat all of your torso tissues, and then use the smaller balls to do more precise soft-tissue resculpting.

Sequence 1: Global Shear Warm-up

EmbodyMap

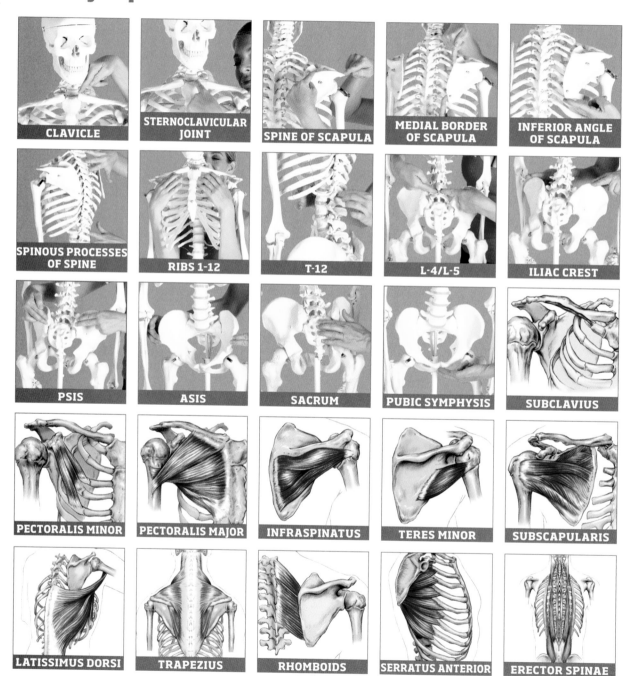

CLAVICLE	STERNOCLAVICULAR JOINT	SPINE OF SCAPULA	MEDIAL BORDER OF SCAPULA	INFERIOR ANGLE OF SCAPULA
SPINOUS PROCESSES OF SPINE	RIBS 1-12	T-12	L-4/L-5	ILIAC CREST
PSIS	ASIS	SACRUM	PUBIC SYMPHYSIS	SUBCLAVIUS
PECTORALIS MINOR	PECTORALIS MAJOR	INFRASPINATUS	TERES MINOR	SUBSCAPULARIS
LATISSIMUS DORSI	TRAPEZIUS	RHOMBOIDS	SERRATUS ANTERIOR	ERECTOR SPINAE

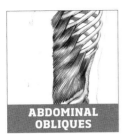
ABDOMINAL OBLIQUES

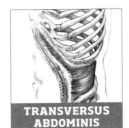
RESPIRATORY DIAPHRAGM

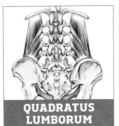
TRANSVERSUS ABDOMINIS

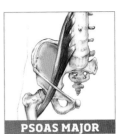
QUADRATUS LUMBORUM

PSOAS MAJOR

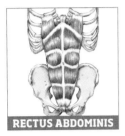
RECTUS ABDOMINIS

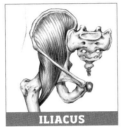
ILIACUS

Basic Ball Stops

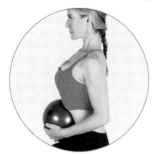
Abdomen

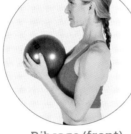
Ribcage (front)

Ribcage (back)

Check In: Abdominal-Thoracic Breath

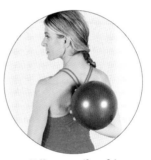

- Practice Abdominal-Thoracic Breathing by placing one hand on your abdomen and the other on your chest. (Once you have mastered sensing that these areas move as you breathe into them, you will no longer need to place your hands on your body; you can leave your arms resting comfortably at your sides.)

- (1) Feel your belly expand first, (2) then your ribcage expand like a giant soft-tissue balloon is making its way from the bottom of your torso to the top, followed by both areas emptying. Your hands will rise and fall with each inflation and deflation.

- Take 5 to 10 complete breaths.

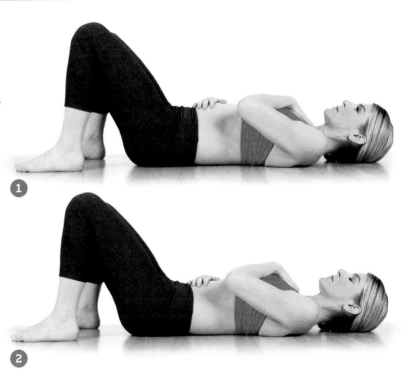

Roll Sequence
ABDOMINAL PEEL

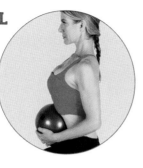

Action 1: Sustained Compression with Abdominal Breathing

Lie facedown with the Coregeous Ball placed on your navel. Take 5 to 10 Abdominal Breaths.

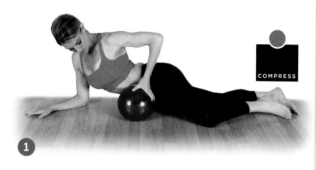

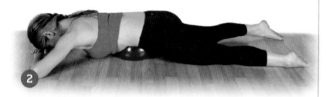

Action 2: Abdominal Breathing with Contract/Relax

- (1) Inhale your abdomen into the ball, tighten your abdomen while holding your breath for 5 to 10 seconds, and (2) then exhale and allow the ball to sink in.
- Repeat for 5 to 10 breaths.

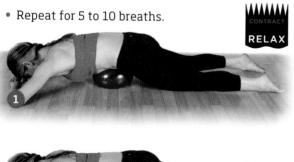

Action 3: CrossFiber the Rectus Abdominis

- Shift your body from side to side, moving the ball across your abdomen. Continue to breathe into your abdomen, and sprinkle in Contract/Relax Breathing as needed for extra-sticky spots.
- Descend the ball below your navel to CrossFiber the lowest abdominals and pelvic bowl.
- Cross back and forth 10 to 20 times. Explore going very slowly and at a brisk pace.

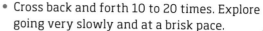

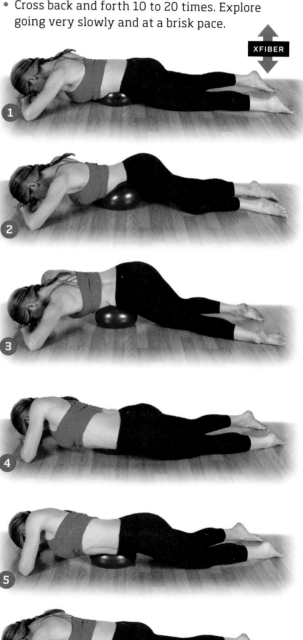

Action 4: Strip the Rectus

- Track the ball in an up-and-down rolling wave along the rectus abdominis from the pubic symphysis to the bottom of your "breastbone" (sternum). Continue to breathe into your abdomen, and sprinkle in Contract/Relax Breathing as needed for extra-sticky spots.
- Do 8 to 10 strips.

Action 5: Core Crawl

- (1) Place the ball on your lower abdomen and (2-3) alternately slide your knees up toward your waist like a crawling baby. Play with a fast or slow pace.
- Do 5 to 10 crawls per side.

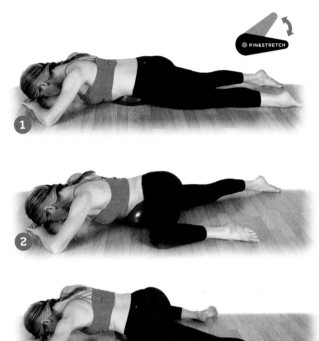

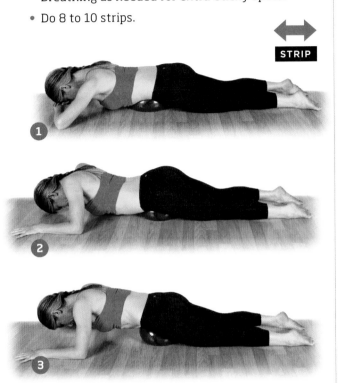

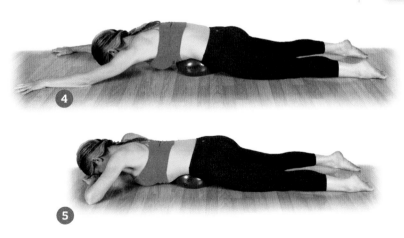

Action 6: Pin/Spin & Mobilize

- **(1)** Place the Coregeous Ball in the center of your abdomen and attempt to lock it in place on bare skin (if possible).

- **(2-4)** Pivot your body as far to the right (or left) as you can, maintaining the original "sticking spot" of the ball.

- **(5-7)** Your body should slowly wind its way around the ball. The ball itself needs to stay in place in order to create maximum wringing and shear.

- **(8-9)** Pivot your body slowly while maintaining deep Abdominal Breaths. You will feel a lot of heat and a sensation of pleasant pinching.

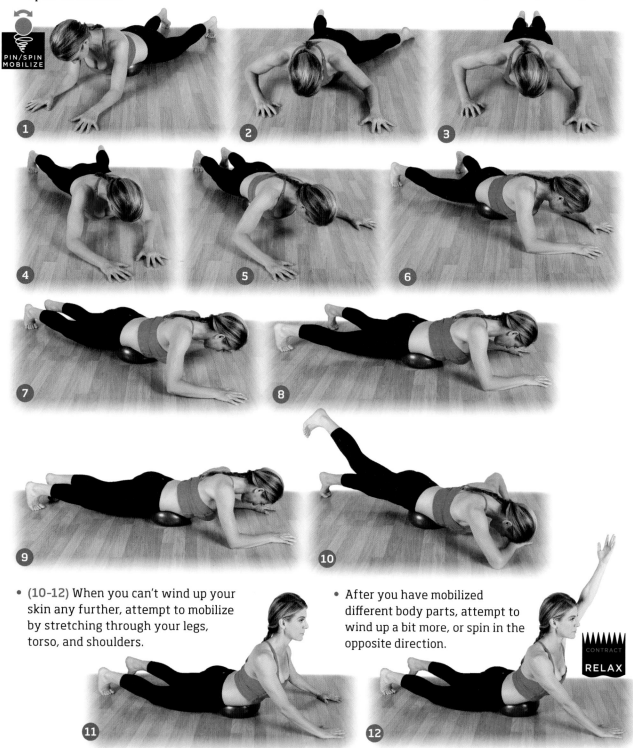

- **(10-12)** When you can't wind up your skin any further, attempt to mobilize by stretching through your legs, torso, and shoulders.

- After you have mobilized different body parts, attempt to wind up a bit more, or spin in the opposite direction.

RIBCAGE REHAB*

Action 1: Thoracic Breathing with Contract/Relax

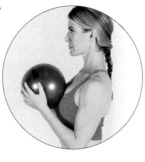

- (1-2) Lie facedown with the Coregeous Ball placed on your sternum. Take 5 to 10 Thoracic Breaths.

- (3-4) Using the pressure of the ball as feedback for your breath capacity, add 5 to 10 breaths with contract/relax: inhale into your ribs, hold your breath for 5 to 10 seconds, then exhale and feel your chest collapse around the ball.

* For more info on breast massage, see "To revert breast cancer cells, give them the squeeze" at www.sciencedaily.com/releases/2012/12/121217140544.htm

Action 2: CrossFiber the Pectoralis

- Slowly slide your torso from side to side and encourage the ball to move across your sternum and chest to find the side of your ribcage.

- Maintain Thoracic Breathing throughout, pausing occasionally to contract/relax in extra-tight spots.

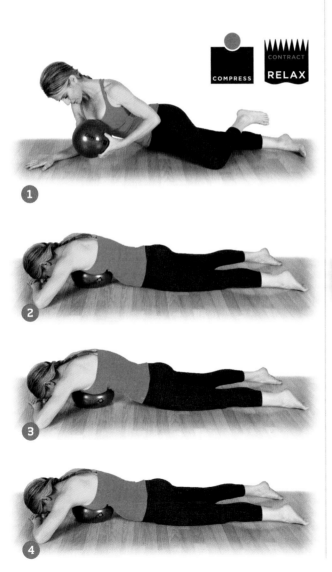

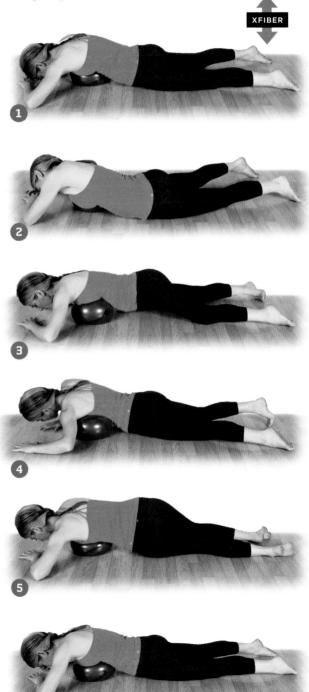

Action 3: Strip the Pectoralis

- Track the ball up and down your sternum and up and down each side of your chest as your sensitivity to pressure on your chest and breasts permits.

- Continue to breathe into your ribcage, and sprinkle in Contract/Relax Breathing as needed for extra-sticky spots.

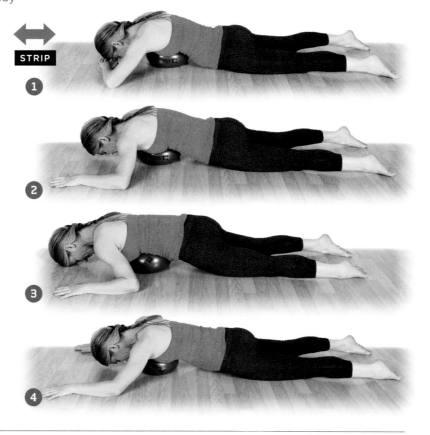

Action 4: Chest Reset with Pin/Spin & Mobilize

- **(1)** Place the Coregeous Ball in the center of your sternum and attempt to lock it in place on bare skin (if possible).

- **(2-3)** Pivot your body as far around to the right (or left) as you can, maintaining the original "sticking spot" of the ball.

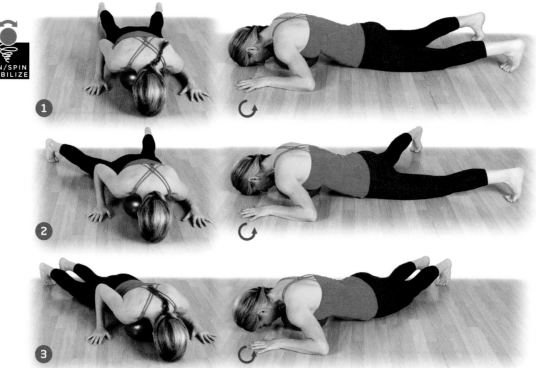

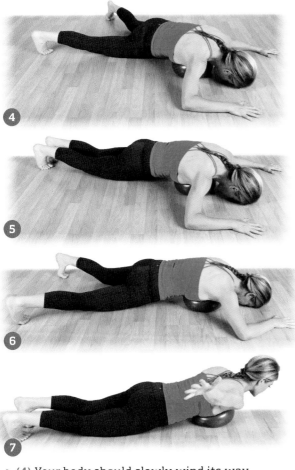

UPPER-BACK SHEAR

Action 1: General Rolling

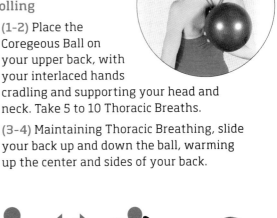

- (1-2) Place the Coregeous Ball on your upper back, with your interlaced hands cradling and supporting your head and neck. Take 5 to 10 Thoracic Breaths.

- (3-4) Maintaining Thoracic Breathing, slide your back up and down the ball, warming up the center and sides of your back.

COMPRESS ⟷ STRIP SKIN ROLL

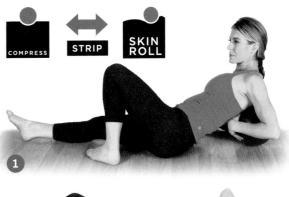

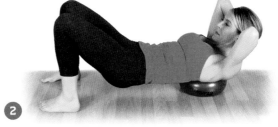

- (4) Your body should slowly wind its way around the ball. The ball needs to stay in place in order to create maximum wringing and shear.

- (5-6) Pivot your body slowly while maintaining deep Thoracic Breaths. You will feel a lot of heat and a large sensation of "pleasant pinching."

- (7-8) When you can't wind up your skin any further, attempt to mobilize by stretching through your shoulders, upper back, and neck.

- After you have mobilized different body parts, attempt to wind up a bit more, or spin in the opposite direction.

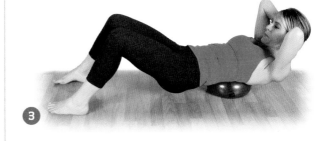

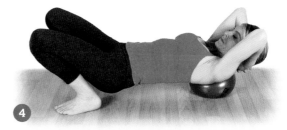

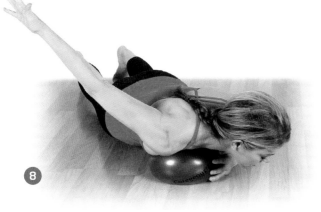

- **(5–7)** Maintaining Thoracic Breathing, slide the ball from side to side across your upper back, rolling from shoulder to shoulder. Explore all areas of your upper back.

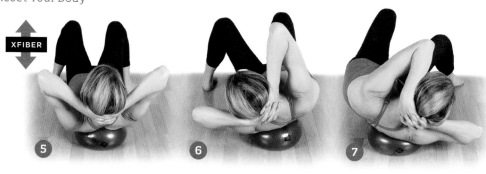

Action 2: Spinal Extension

- Using the Coregeous Ball to help your whole spine backbend, inhale with a Thoracic Breath, then slowly lower your pelvis and skull to the ground.

- Remain there and take 5 to 10 Abdominal Breaths, Thoracic Breaths, or Abdominal-Thoracic Breaths.

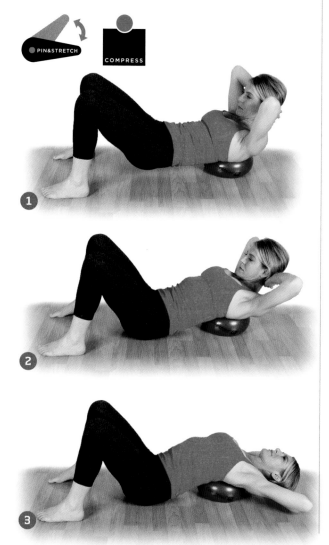

Action 3: Pin/Spin & Mobilize

- **(1)** Lock the ball on your upper back, preferably against bare skin. Support your head with interlaced fingers. Activate your abdominals and buttocks in order to maximize the pressure of your upper back on the ball.

- **(2–13)** Slowly step your feet apart and together (toward the right or the left) in order to "screw" your upper back's skin/fascias/myofascias into the ball's grip.

- **(14–15)** Once your tissues are tightly wound, mobilize by moving your arms/shoulders/back in different directions while breathing deeply.

- Re-spin as needed, then spin in the opposite direction.

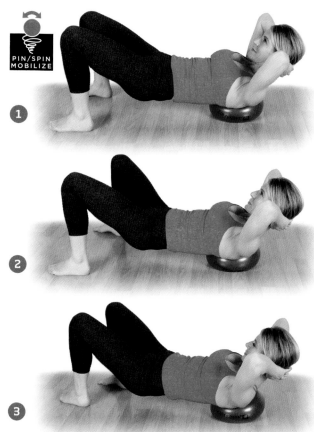

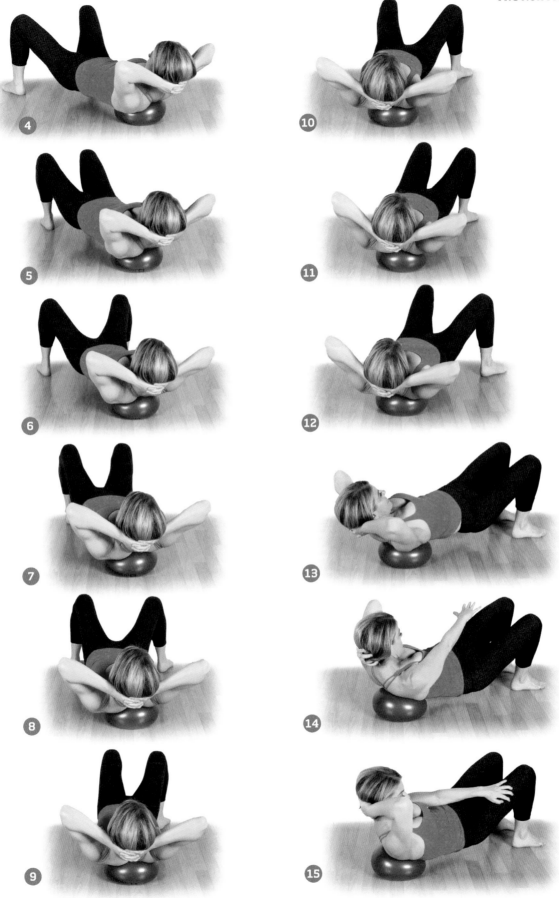

ReCheck:
Abdominal-Thoracic Breath

- Practice Abdominal-Thoracic Breathing by placing one hand on your abdomen and one hand on your chest.
- **(1)** Feel your belly expand first, **(2)** then your ribcage like a giant soft-tissue balloon, followed by both areas emptying.
- Your hands will rise and fall with each inflation and deflation.
- Take 5 to 10 complete breaths.

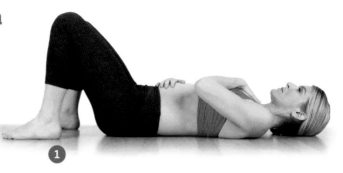

Reflect

1. Are you able to take fuller breaths?
2. Is more of your back in contact with the floor?
3. Finish this statement: I feel _____.

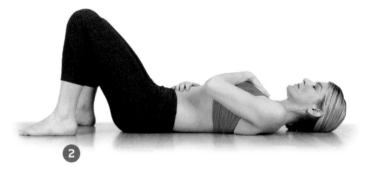

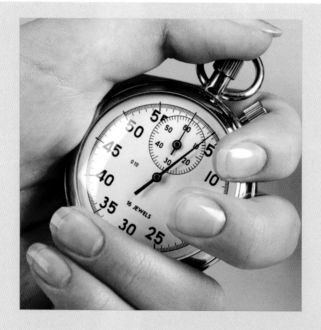

HOW LONG SHOULD YOU DO EACH MOVE?

For some of the moves, I have given you a general time frame or number of repetitions: "5 to 10 breaths" or "roll back and forth 5 to 10 times." There is no time-specific formula that can cater to all readers of this book, and your time on the balls is ultimately quite personal, depending on why you are rolling, how long your aches have been there, and your own time constraints. You will feel that some points and moves are cleared up within seconds or minutes, while others may take weeks of persistent rolling. My favorite "formula" comes from Dr. Kelly Starrett:

> *"Roll 'til you make change,*
> *or 'til you STOP making change."*

In other words, you are the ultimate decider when it comes to how long you roll.

The Wrath of Scar Tissue: An Organ Donor Stitches Herself Back Together

Helen McAvoy, 56
Owner, Balance in Motion
North Windham, Connecticut

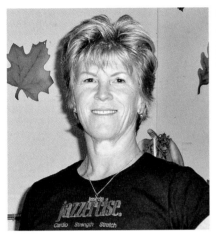

Helen before she donated part of her liver.

Helen McAvoy is a 56-year-old (and growing younger!) mother of two adult sons and the owner of Balance in Motion. She has been a popular Jazzercise instructor for the past 24 years and recently became a Yoga Tune Up teacher. You can find her teaching packed classes at the North Windham Jazzercise Center in Connecticut. She is a firecracker! Her energy levels are off the charts, and her radiant outlook on life make her the type of instructor who inspires others to keep healthy and moving. Lucky for me, over a year ago, she became a student of mine, eager to tackle the aches and pains that were starting to make her miserable.

Helen is a mensch, used to putting others' happiness ahead of her own and following her heart. Twelve years ago, in an incredible act of selflessness, she became an organ donor for one of her studio managers.

"Cindy had Crohn's disease for years and then was diagnosed with PSC (primary sclerosing cholangitis), which affected her bile ducts and caused her to get sick more frequently. As a retired nurse, she recognized the downward spiral of her health and, knowing that there had to be treatment options, she began to pursue a liver transplant. She sought a living donor, did a lot of research, and traveled to various locations in her pursuit. All during her research, which was a few months, I listened and pondered. I said to myself...why can't I donate? I am healthy, and I really felt it was what I was supposed to do at that moment in my life. I never hesitated and still wouldn't if I could again.

"Cindy was a bit upset when I offered, knowing I was a single mom and owned my business. She said no way, and I said yes, way! So that was that. I am type O blood, so it's a no-brainer–universal donor, baby! We began the process in the spring of 2002, going to NYU every few weeks, working with Dr. Teperman, who is amazing, and his three other surgeons. Dr. Teperman wears cowboy boots in the operating room and listens to rock! Love that man! I was tested and had an MRI of my body to check for anything. I also had a long meeting as to the process and what they would do, including removing my gallbladder and outlining details of complications I might have afterward because I would be out for so long. I was also required to undergo an extensive psychological examination with questions like, was I being coerced? do I know I could die? etc.

"So, quick history: I was a single mom with a son in high school and the older one living out in Snowmass, Colorado. I spoke with them both, as

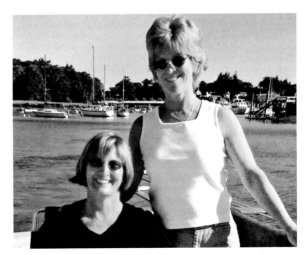

Connected for life, these Roll Models share the same liver.

well as my ex, who remains a friend in my life. I spoke with my family and my sisters were livid, thought I might as well jump off a bridge, but my dad was wonderful. Friends were supportive, and my Jazzercise family was all on board and completely inspirational. Anyway, Cindy and I sat with my staff (at the time I owned a Jazzercise center in Deep River, Connecticut) and explained what was going on. I planned ahead with my will and so forth and my business as to what would happen should something go askew, but truthfully I knew I would be fine. During this whole process I continued to teach eight classes a week, run the business, and handle my teenager.

"The surgery was in September 2002. All went well, ten hours under, I went in first, then a few hours later Cindy in the operating room next to me. Cindy had complications about eight hours afterward and we almost lost her, but she pulled through, thank God.

"When I first woke up I was intubated, argh! Then that came out after a few days, and I had to get a spirometer ball to move up and practice breathing so I could get my lungs back. I couldn't do it at first and it scared the hell out of me. My first thought was, 'Will I be able to teach Jazzercise again?' I couldn't breathe hard. Next came moving out of the bed, eventually to a chair. I have had two 'old-school' C-sections, so abdominal pain is no stranger to me. But 47 staples from my sternum to my right hip was. I was in the hospital for ten days and then came home, still with a drain tube coming out of the bottom of the incision. I had the 47 staples taken off a few weeks later.

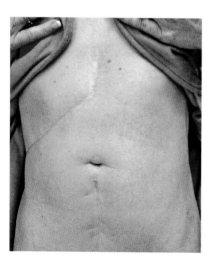

Helen has an 11-inch scar from her liver donation and a 4-inch scar from 2 Cesarean sections.

"So on to my recovery. Boy, do I wish I had had the Yoga Tune Up experience then! But I am very thankful for the knowledge I did have, and a very good friend who was a massage therapist helped me understand the issue of the tissue. Movement is medicine, hoo-rah! And of course Jazzercise! It kept me moving and twisting and dancing...although minimally at first. The liver regrows, and it takes about six weeks. So they took 60 percent of my right lobe, and my left lobe regrew to pretty much fill the spot. My scarring was massive, 11 inches, and I massaged my incision with my own hands and vitamin E oil and slowly got my fanny back on stage by Thanksgiving Day to do a benefit class for the American Liver Foundation, low impact of course!

"How has it affected my body? Jill, just in writing this, I am sitting here realizing all these years I have never really given my body a chance to resynchronize. After the surgery I got right back on my horse and was busy helping everyone else, teaching and being a mom. Jazzercise has been good for the camaraderie and a blessing as it has kept me moving, but I never really addressed all the emotional stuff that has accumulated and intertwined itself within me. So now it begins. I notice if I sit around and don't do any sort of movement, I do experience issues, scar tissue adherence, and knowing what I know now, that darn fascia gets stuck! But thanks to you I can roll out and release. It also affects my elimination if I do not move my body. I had my first colonoscopy a few years ago with Cindy's gastroenterologist. He could not get all the way up, he said probably due to scar tissue adhering, so I had to do a virtual one.

"My alignment has definitely been off, and with your work I am focusing on it more, as I think the surgery has caused me to unconsciously compensate all over my body for years. Fortunately, now that I have the Roll Model Balls, I'll lie on my back and do skin-rolling with the balls on either side of my scar, and this helps to heat up and release that feeling of tightness. The balls are helpful because I can also feel how the scarring in my middle has referred tension to neighboring parts of my body above and below it. I feel it all unwinding, and it feels great.

"There is no denying that the scars have made a lasting impact on my body. There is a sensation of intense resistance and lack of body synchronicity due to the many layers of my body that were cut and sewn back together. And at times, I felt my core was very unconnected to the rest of my body, because it has lost its way from all the surgeries. There was a lot of emotional scar tissue as well that followed into my inner being. I am determined now to revive and re-link to myself on my own terms. I know it might sound corny...but I almost feel as though, even though I was cut open to save someone else, I have been given this incredible opportunity to re-stitch together the fabric of my own life, and it literally starts with me re-knitting my own tissues. It's pretty profound to be fully steering the course of my healing and next chapter. With the Roll Model Balls, I have the tools to do this on my own.

"I use the Coregeous Ball almost daily. I lie face-down on it starting at the sternum and gently roll side to side. Then I remain still with quiet breathing. I continue by moving the ball lower and eventually to the psoas region. I then roll the Coregeous from side to side. When I do the center of my abdominals, I lie stationary and belly breathe with long-held inhales followed by exhales. I also migrate the Coregeous into the obliques, where most of that darn scar is. After using the Coregeous Ball all over, I fall into breathing deeper and yawning. Within the yawn is a second inhalation or yawn as if my body was exuberant at being able to expand more. I feel an amazing stretch among my ribs and intercostal muscles. I've begun to realize that over the years I never fully regained what is true breathing.

"A few months ago I had my annual physical with my doctor, who knows my whole health history and chronic scar tissue discomfort. I explained to her what I had been doing and my recent Yoga Tune Up training and how it was helping to relieve my scar tissue confinement. She said, 'Fantastic, I can see the results it's having, keep on doing what you're doing, it will definitely keep you from having issues with scar tissue adherence.'

"I feel much more empowered to care for my body now than I did a year ago. I still have so much to learn. This last year has been a reawakening for me in so many ways. Yoga Tune Up has been so amazing, it has given me the opportunity

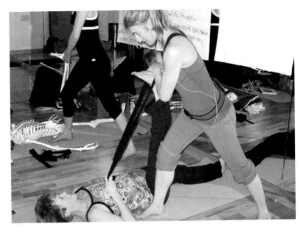

Helen receiving a deep hip stretch from me at a Yoga Tune Up teacher training.

to work on my body, learn about anatomy within my structure, and pass this on to my students."

Helen made the ultimate sacrifice for her friend: she gifted her healthy living body to someone she knows and loves. She willingly opened her body and being to give life to another. And in doing so, she found the nature of who she is and the potential of her body to regrow and heal in a whole new way. She is a true Roll Model.

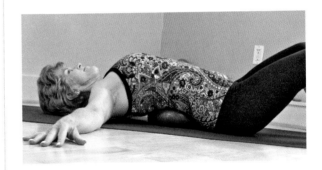

// *A few months ago I had my annual physical with my doctor I explained to her what I had been doing and how it was helping to relieve my scar tissue confinement. She said, 'Fantastic, I can see the results it's having, keep on doing what you're doing, it will definitely keep you from having issues with scar tissue adherence.'* **//**

–Helen McAvoy

Lower-Body Sequences

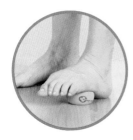

Sequence 2:
Feet: Save Your Sole

Setup

Roll Model Balls:
Original YTU or
PLUS

Chair or wall

EmbodyMap

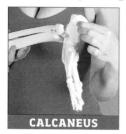

CALCANEUS

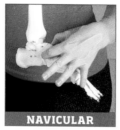

NAVICULAR

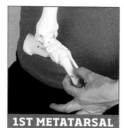

1ST METATARSAL

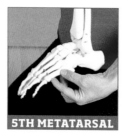

CUBOID

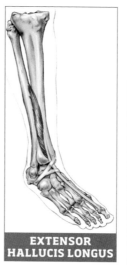

EXTENSOR HALLUCIS LONGUS

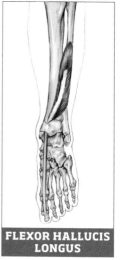

FLEXOR HALLUCIS LONGUS

5TH METATARSAL

Basic Ball Stops

Arch

Inner arch

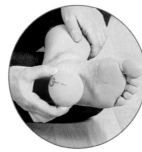

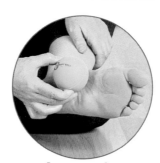

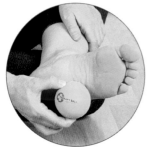

Outer arch

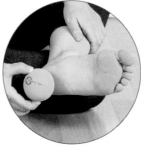

Heel

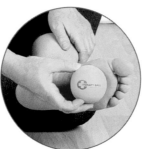

Ball of foot

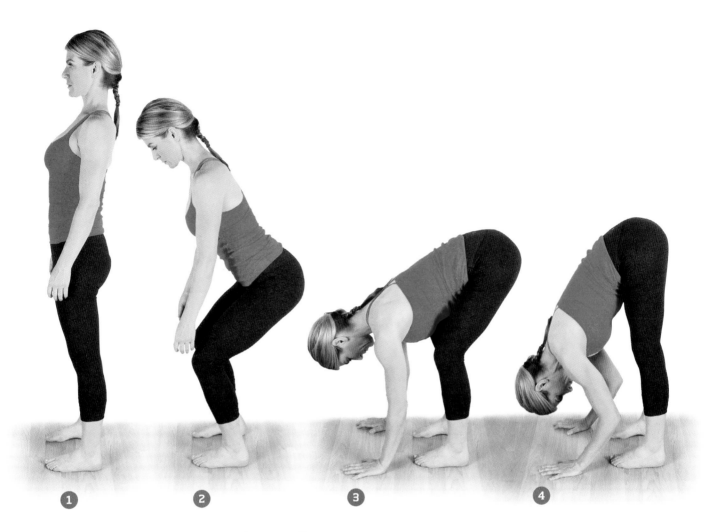

Check In: Forward Bend

- **(1)** Stand with impeccable posture (see page 84).

- **(2)** Brace your core to limit spinal motion, and pivot your forward bend from the hinge of your pelvis rolling over your thigh bones.

- **(3)** Depending on the flexibility of your hamstrings, lock your hands on the floor, a chair, or a wall, attempting to maintain your neutral (non-rounded) spine. (Unfortunately, my spine rounded here; I should have placed my hands on a chair!) **(4)** Then briefly straighten the backs of your knees to feel the sensation of stretch in the backs of your thighs, knees, or calves.

- Hold for 2 or 3 Abdominal-Thoracic Breaths. Notice if you feel more tension behind one thigh than the other. Then return to standing with a flat back.

Roll Sequence

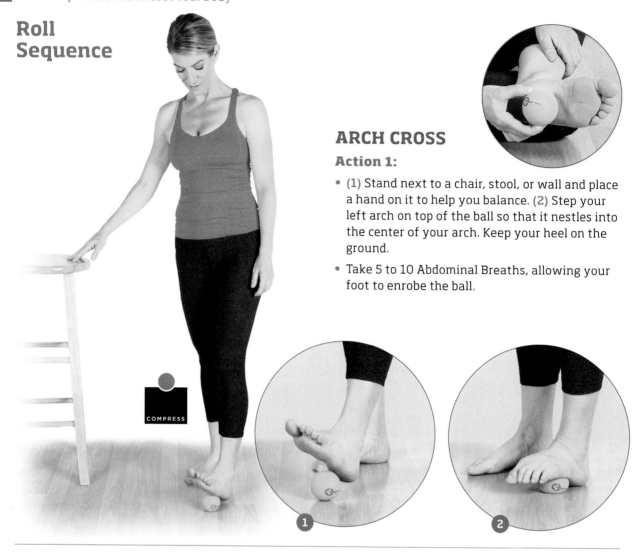

ARCH CROSS

Action 1:

- **(1)** Stand next to a chair, stool, or wall and place a hand on it to help you balance. **(2)** Step your left arch on top of the ball so that it nestles into the center of your arch. Keep your heel on the ground.

- Take 5 to 10 Abdominal Breaths, allowing your foot to enrobe the ball.

COMPRESS

Action 2:

CrossFiber your arch and plantar fascia by pivoting your ankle from side to side (invert and evert your ankle) 10 times. Attempt to smush the ball as you go back and forth.

XFIBER

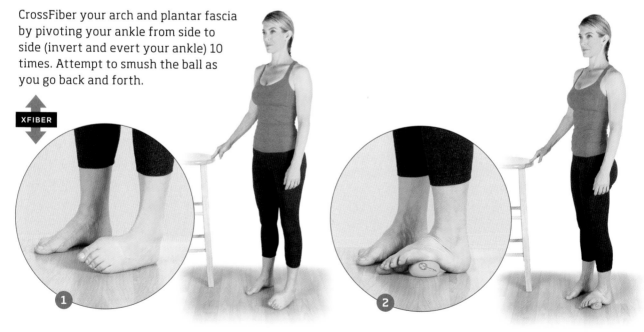

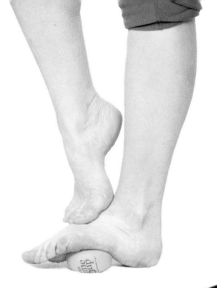

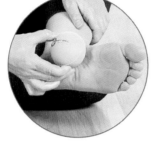

INNER ARCH SUPPORT

- **(1)** Scoot the ball to the inside of your left arch, locking it in place at the highest point on your instep. This is the meeting place of the first metatarsal and the navicular.

- **(2)** Squash the ball with extra compressive pressure, and **(3)** slide your foot to the left so that the ball tacks onto your skin and creates massive shear in your inner arch.

- Reset the ball and repeat this action 2 to 5 more times.

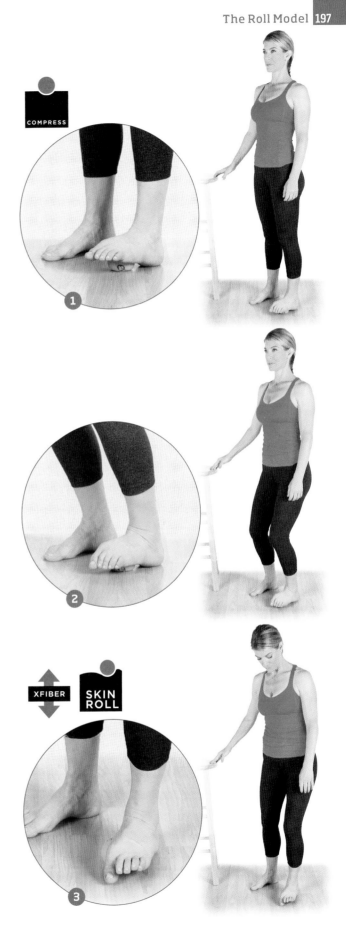

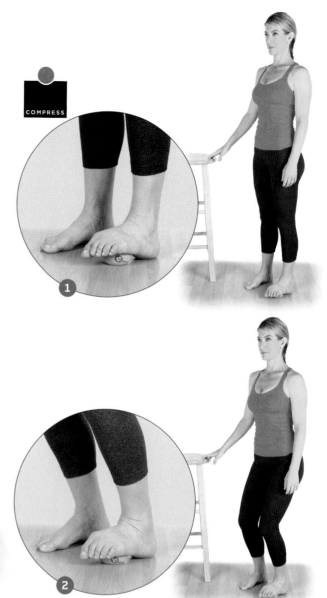

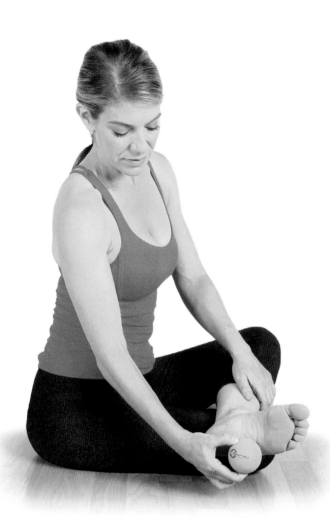

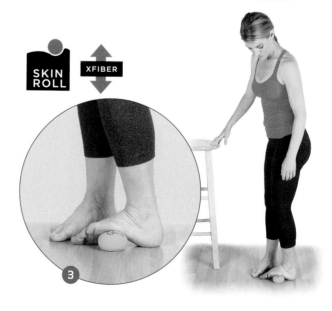

OUTER ARCH SUPPORT

- (1) Move the ball to the outside of your arch and lock it in place. The bony landmarks you are targeting are the fifth metatarsal and cuboid.

- (2) Squash the ball with extra compressive pressure, and (3) slide your foot to the right so that the ball tacks onto your skin and creates massive shear in your outer arch.

- Reset the ball and repeat this action 2 to 5 more times.

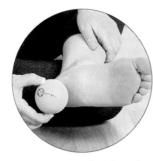

STILETTO TREATMENT

Roll the ball back to the bottom of your heel at the calcaneus, and lock your toes on the ground. Drive your body weight into the ball, then briskly scrub the ball from side to side as if you were trying to scrape gum off the bottom of your foot. Do this brisk motion for approximately 30 seconds.

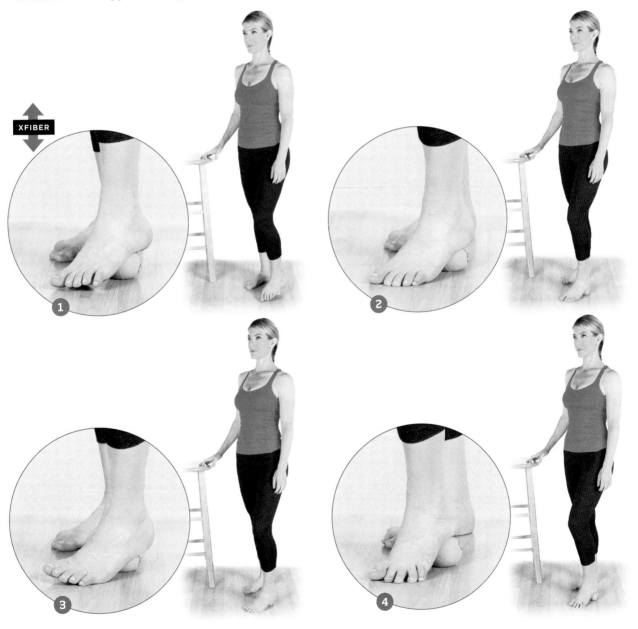

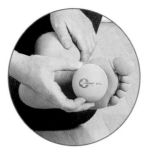

TOE MOTION

Action 1:

(1) Drive the Roll Model Ball into the ball of your foot–this is the transverse arch of your foot. CrossFiber the ball 10 times across the ball of your foot, which will (2) invert and (3) evert your ankle while helping the long bones of your foot spread away from one another.

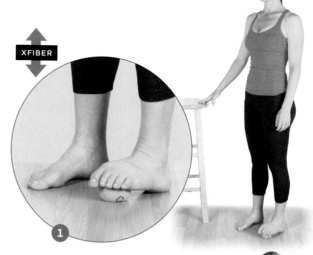

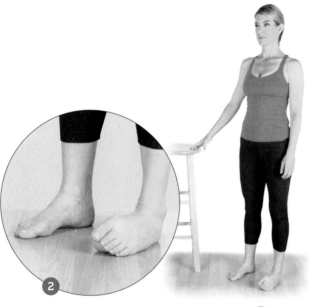

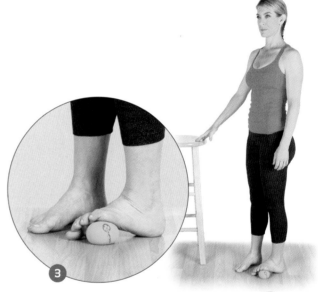

Action 2:

- (2) Squeeze your toes into the ball, making a "foot fist," then (3) spread and lift all 5 toes away from the ball. Do this 5 times.

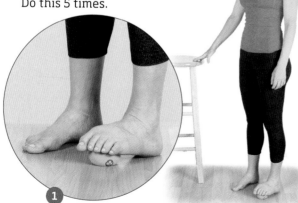

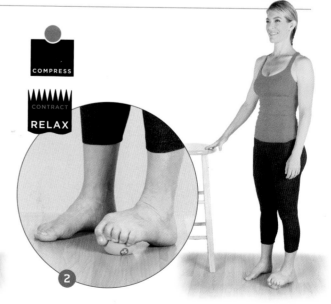

COMPRESS

CONTRACT

RELAX

- (4) Squeeze all of your toes into the ball, then attempt to isolate the motion of your big toe by extending and flexing it without letting your other toes move, going up and down 5 to 10 times.

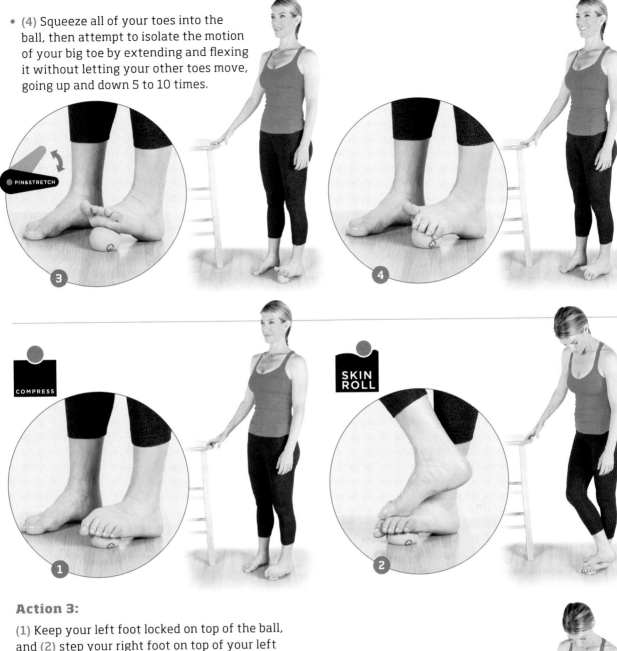

Action 3:

(1) Keep your left foot locked on top of the ball, and (2) step your right foot on top of your left foot. (3) Twist the sole of your right foot into the skin on the top of your left foot to skin-roll and create massive twisting shear, as if you were trying to "remove your pantyhose." Do this until you feel a pleasant heat all over the top of your left foot.

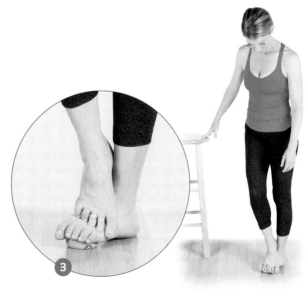

Action 4:

Reset the ball to the middle of your foot and track the ball up and down along the length of your foot several times.

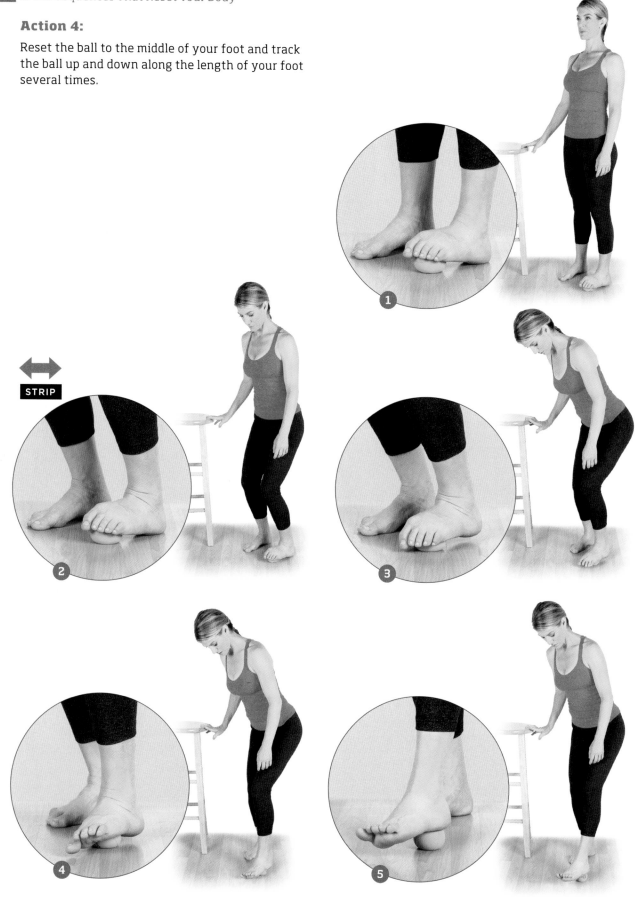

After completing the sequence with one foot, perform your ReCheck.

ReCheck:
Forward Bend

- (1) Stand with impeccable posture (see page 84).
- (2) Brace your core to limit spinal motion, and pivot your forward bend from the hinge of your pelvis rolling over your thigh bones.

- (3) Depending on the flexibility of your hamstrings, lock your hands on the floor, a chair, or a wall, attempting to maintain your neutral (non-rounded) spine. (Unfortunately, my spine rounded here; I should have placed my hands on a chair!) (4) Then briefly straighten the backs of your knees to feel the stretch in the backs of your thighs, knees, or calves.
- Hold for 2 or 3 breaths, and notice if the side you just rolled feels less restricted than the side you did not roll.
- Return to standing with a flat back.
- Repeat the sequence with your other foot.

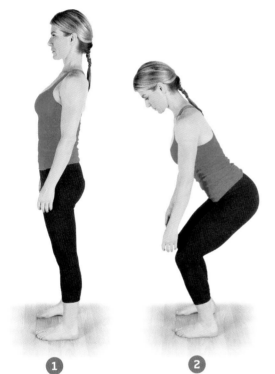
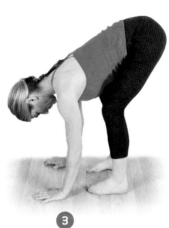
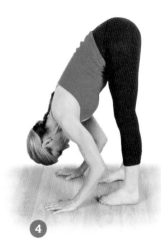

After completing the sequence with your other foot, perform your ReCheck again.

Notice less restriction in the backs of both legs now? This ReCheck helps your body understand the principles of the interconnectedness of your fascias. Your calf, hamstring, buttock, and back muscles are all in a continuity of tissues with the fascias on the bottoms of your feet. They essentially share the same "back seam." When you roll out the local area of the foot, all of the tissues uptown of it also benefit.

Reflect

1. Do your feet feel wider? Flatter? More arched?
2. Does your posture feel different?
3. Finish this statement: I feel _____.

Sequence 3: Ankle & Lower-Leg Treat

Setup

Roll Model Balls:
Original YTU, PLUS,
or ALPHA Twins in tote

Mat

Stretch strap or belt

Block or stool

EmbodyMap

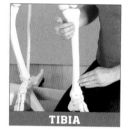
TIBIA

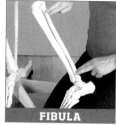
FIBULA

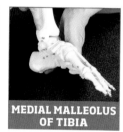
MEDIAL MALLEOLUS OF TIBIA

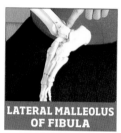
LATERAL MALLEOLUS OF FIBULA

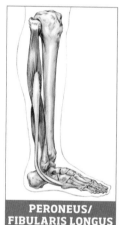
PERONEUS/ FIBULARIS LONGUS

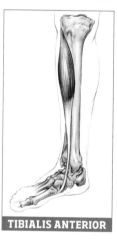
TIBIALIS ANTERIOR

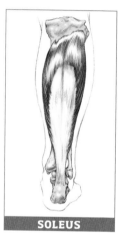
SOLEUS

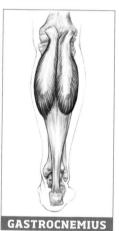
GASTROCNEMIUS

Basic Ball Stops

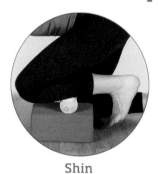
Shin

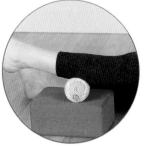
Calf

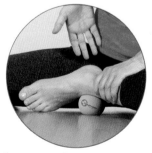
Inner and outer ankle

Check In:
Sitting Seza with Strap

- **(1)** Wrap a stretch strap or belt around your ankles and **(2)** pull it taut like an Ace bandage (don't fasten or buckle it). **(3-4)** Position your feet in dorsiflexion so that the bottoms of your feet are stretched long, and sit on your heels while pulling the strap as snug as possible. (If you are unable to manage the pressure on your feet and ankles, lean forward and place your hands on the floor to relieve some of the pressure. If you have bunions that are painfully squashed, place a soft towel between your feet. If your knees dislike this position, place a rolled towel or blanket behind your knees before sitting.)

- **(5)** Take 5 to 10 Abdominal-Thoracic Breaths.

- **(6-7)** Point (plantar flex) your feet so that the tops of your feet and ankles are stretched. Pull the strap snug again if your inner ankle bones (medial malleoli) have drifted apart.

- Take 5 to 10 Abdominal-Thoracic Breaths.

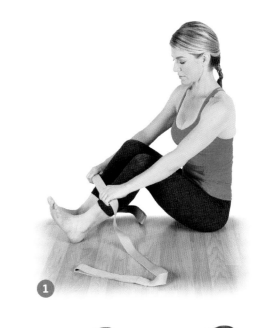

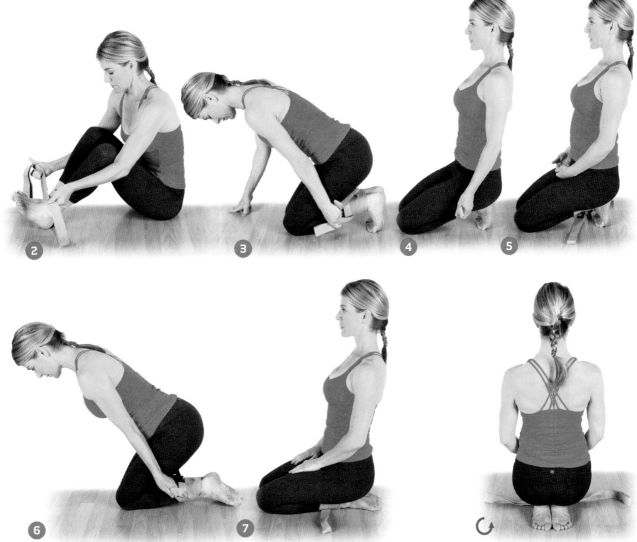

Roll Sequence

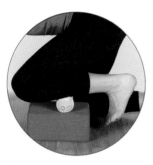

SHIN-ROLL

Action 1:

(1) Place a pair of toted balls on a block on top of a mat or other nonslip surface. (2) Settle your left shin in between the balls. (3–4) Roll your shin up and down the balls, from the bottom of your knee to the top of your ankle, in order to strip your anterior tibialis and peroneus/fibularis longus.

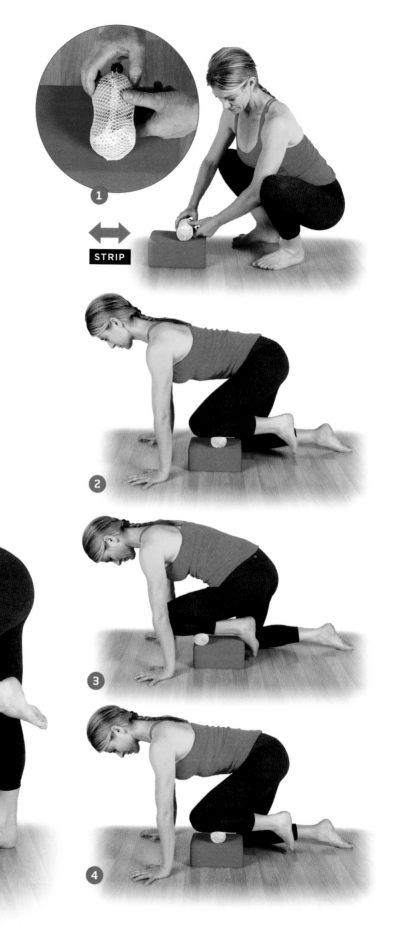

STRIP

modify

Actions 2-3:

- (1) Lock the upper half of your shin into the balls. (2-3) Pin & stretch by pointing and flexing (plantar flexing and dorsiflexing) your foot. (4-6) Then make circles with your ankle.

- Roll the balls into the lower half of your shin and repeat these actions.

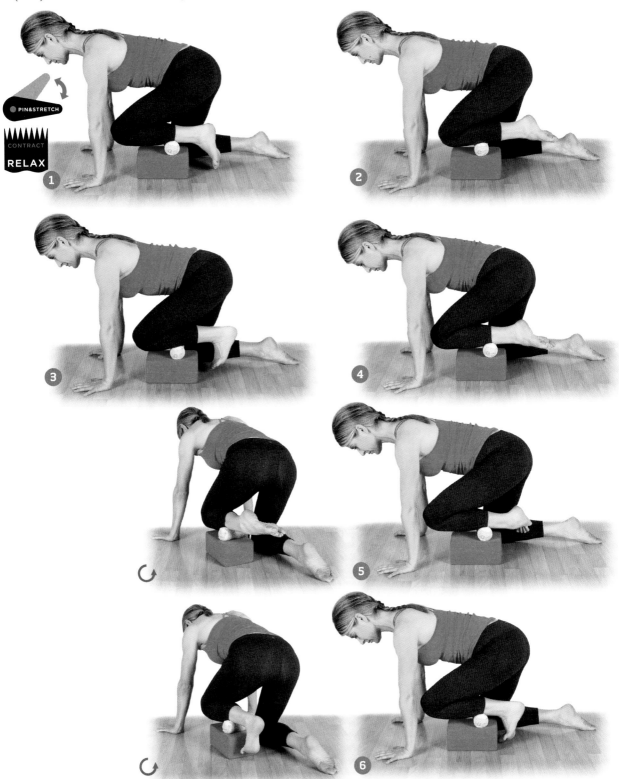

Action 4: "Screwball"

(1) Select any point along your shin for some extra shear. (2) Shift your body weight and load your right shin on top of your left calf. (3-6) Then twist your lower body from side to side to spiral the toted balls deep into the soft tissues they are contacting. Pause from time to time and mobilize your left ankle. Select another point along your shin and repeat.

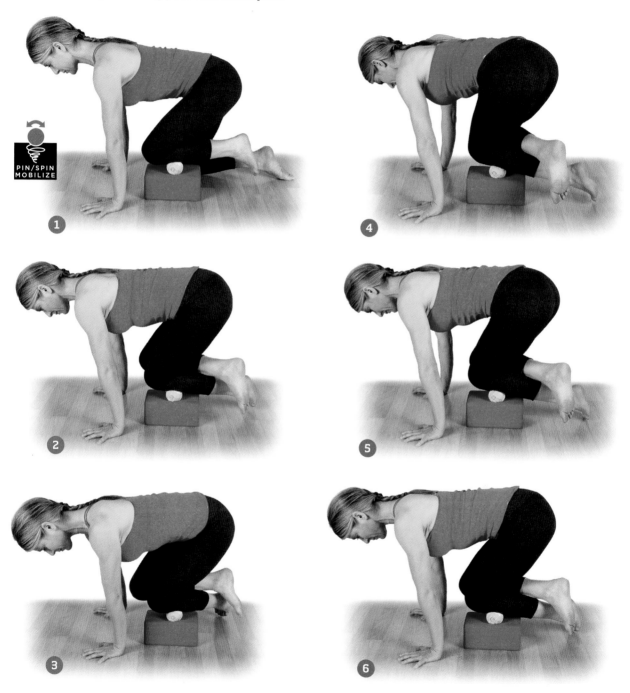

Action 5: Ball Plow

(1) Keep the balls in the tote, but position one ball where your lower leg meets your foot (the talocrural joint). (2) Nuzzle the ball into this junction and lean your body weight to the left. The ball will plow your tissues toward the lateral malleolus. (3) Keep tension on the soft and hard tissues here, and point and flex your foot.

SWITCH LEGS AND REPEAT ACTIONS 1-5.

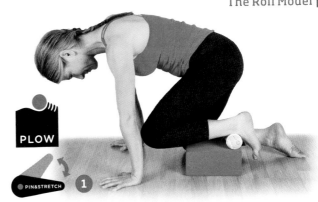

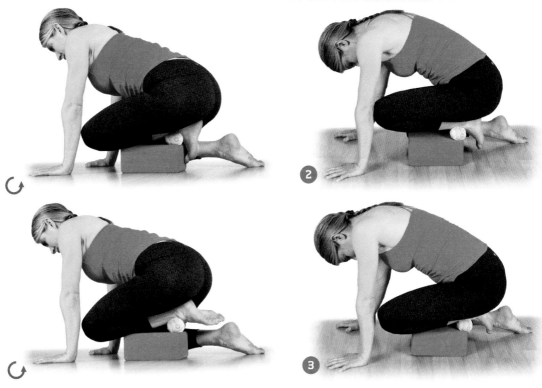

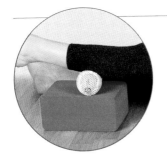

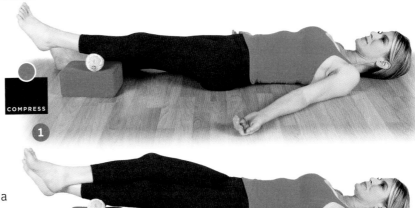

CALF MASH

Action 1:

(1) Place your toted balls on top of a block and lie on the ground. Mount the bulk of your left calf between the balls, then (2) cross your right calf on top of your left shin. Take 5 to 10 Abdominal-Thoracic Breaths.

Action 2:

Rock your calves from side to side to CrossFiber the thick planes of tissue. Then add a bit more pressure (if manageable) by driving more weight into the balls while lifting your pelvis 1 or 2 inches off the floor. Continue to rock your calves.

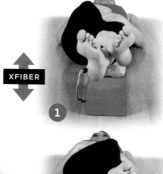

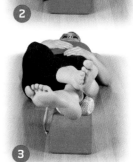

XFIBER

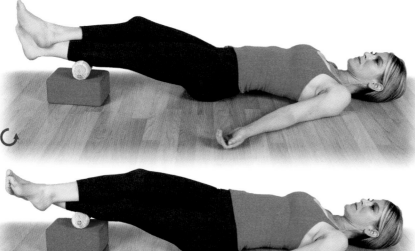

STRIP

Action 3:

Strip your calves by bending and straightening your knees. The balls will roll up and down the length of your lower leg, from the bottom of your calf to just below your knee.

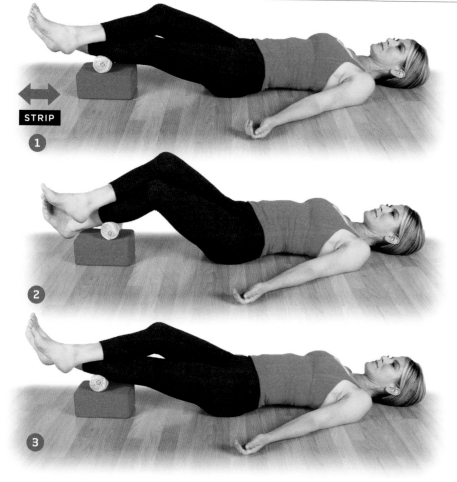

Action 4:

(1-2) Lock the balls in place at any point along the back of your calf, then flex and point your foot.

(3-5) Also try pivoting your ankle at different angles while flexing and pointing, or rolling it in circles.

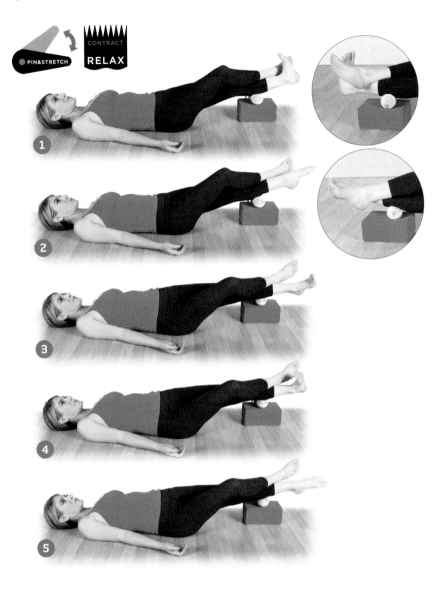

Bonus Technique: Calf Stack

Stack any size balls on either side of your calf to bring slide & glide to this dense myofascial zone. Point, flex, and circle your foot, then re-stack the balls higher or lower along your calf.

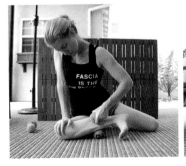
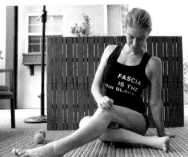
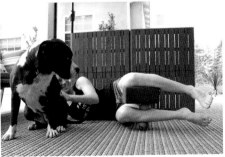

RETINACULUM RESET

Action 1:

(1) On your left foot, hook one ball in front of your lateral malleolus (the bony bump on the side of your ankle, the end of the fibula bone) and (2) angle your foot so that the ball can grab your fibula and plow it toward your Achilles tendon. (3) Sustain this pressure using one or both hands.

COMPRESS PLOW

Action 2:

(1) Maintain the compressed/plowed pressure from Action 1, and (2) point and flex your foot. (3) Then use your right hand to pry your heel bone (calcaneus) downward toward the floor, which will mobilize the subtalar joint (one of the three joints of the ankle).

PIN&STRETCH

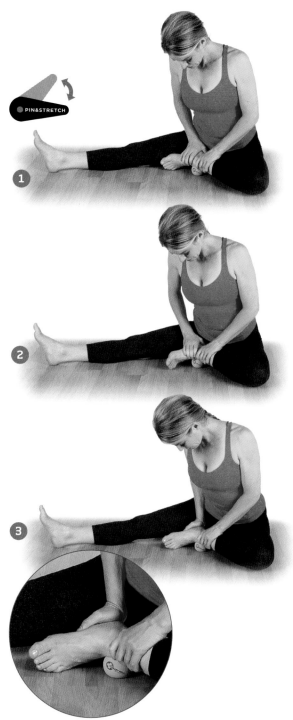

Action 3:

(1-3) Maintaining your new position, use your right hand to spin the ball firmly into the tissue. Continue to lean pressure into the ankle and ball from above with your left hand and arm. (4-5) Attempt to maneuver and mobilize your heel bone with your right hand by twisting and pivoting it in all directions. Then try spinning the ball in the opposite direction.

PIN/SPIN
MOBILIZE

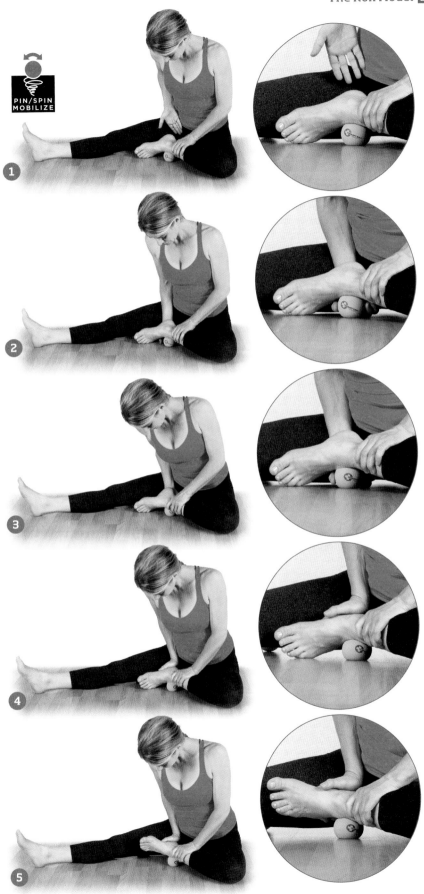

Action 4:

Create a ball stack by pinning the tissues on either side of the lateral and medial malleoli. Try to sandwich the ankle joint with pressure from the balls. Find as many movements as possible.

SWITCH LEGS AND REPEAT ACTIONS 1-4.

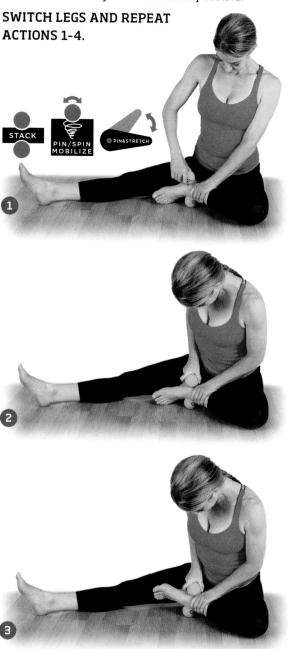

ReCheck: Sitting Seza with Strap

Reset the stretch strap around your ankles and spend 2 Abdominal-Thoracic Breaths in dorsiflexion (soles facing behind you) followed by 2 Abdominal-Thoracic Breaths in plantar flexion (soles facing up). Notice any changes in your ankle range of motion and your level of comfort.

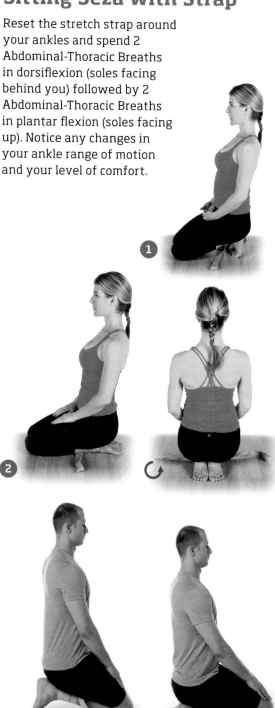

Reflect

1. How does it feel to walk?

2. Try walking on your tiptoes and notice how that feels.

3. Finish this statement: I feel _____.

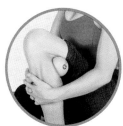

Sequence 4: Kneed to Knead

Setup
Roll Model Balls: Original YTU, PLUS, or ALPHA

Mat

2 blocks or stool

EmbodyMap

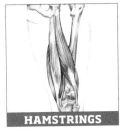

PATELLA

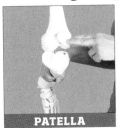

HAMSTRINGS

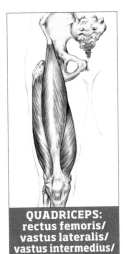

IT BAND

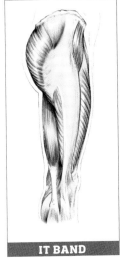

QUADRICEPS:
rectus femoris/
vastus lateralis/
vastus intermedius/
vastus medialis

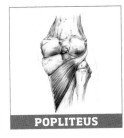

GASTROCNEMIUS

POPLITEUS

Basic Ball Stops

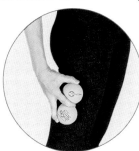

IT band and
vastus lateralis

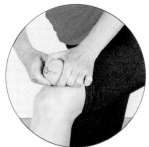

Suprapatellar
pouch

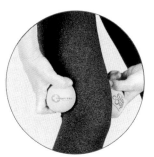

Vastus medialis
and lateralis

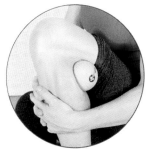

Hamstring
tendons

Check In: Child's Pose

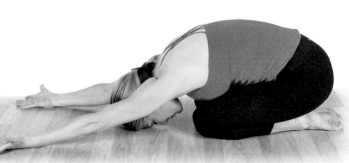

- Place yourself facedown on the floor and fold your body at your knees and hips. Reach your arms overhead with your palms facing up. Notice how close your buttocks descend toward your heels. If your buttocks cannot touch your heels, that's fine; this stretch is simply a way to check the range of motion of your knees.

- Take 5 to 10 Abdominal-Thoracic Breaths.

Roll Sequence

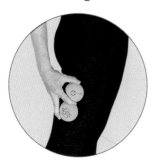

IT BAND MELTDOWN

Action 1:

- (1) Lie on your right side with your head propped on a block or pillow. Place 2 untoted balls underneath your right thigh, and scissor your left leg behind you slightly to minimize pressure on the balls at first. Breathe deeply and let your thigh conform to the balls. (You can also do this sequence standing up, leaning against a wall with toted balls.)

- (2-4) Slowly begin to slide your right thigh forward and backward to help the balls cross the grain of the IT band and vastus lateralis.

- (5-6) Add more pressure, if tolerable, by placing your left thigh on top of your right and continue to CrossFiber.

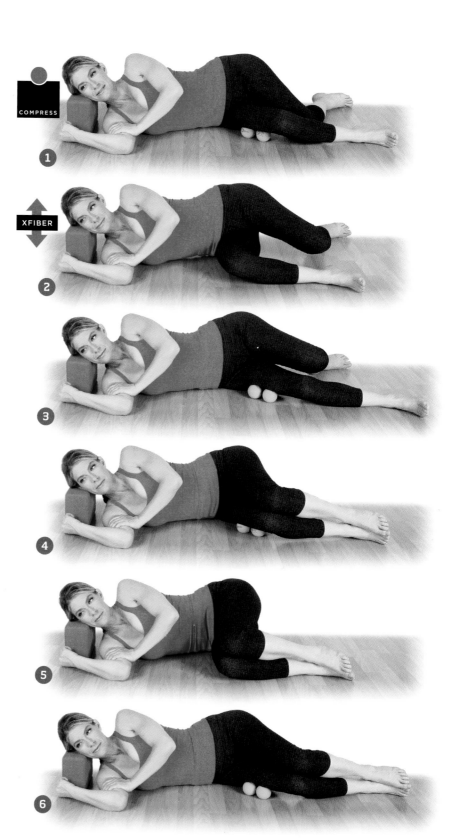

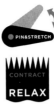

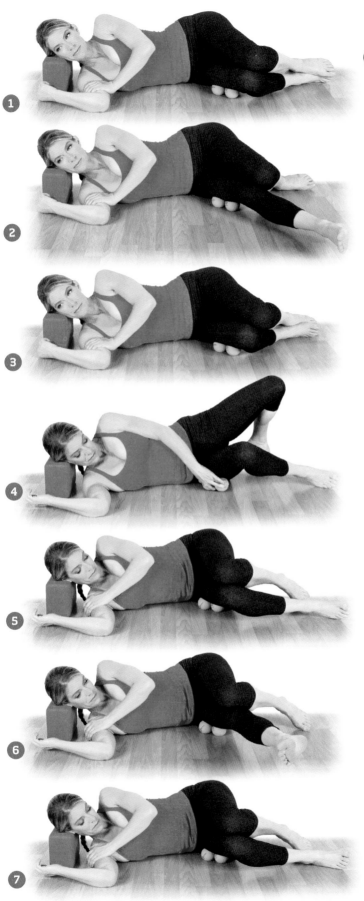

Action 2:

(1-3) Remain in the same position and bend and straighten your knee several times. (4-7) Move the balls higher or lower on your thigh and continue to pin & stretch.

(1-2, below) Modify by removing one ball, or sit up to drive more body weight into the ball(s). Pin & stretch 2 or 3 different points along your outer thigh.

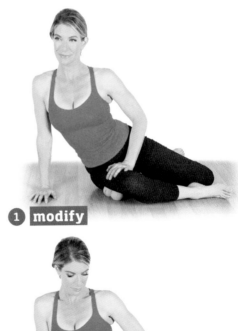

① **modify**

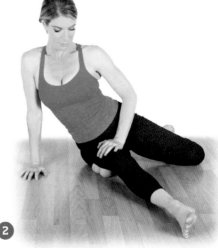

Action 3:

Sit up to load the balls with your body weight. Lock the balls against the side of your thigh and, with a broad, flat left hand, guide your quadriceps group as a whole in a plow-like action as the balls slowly shift toward your hamstrings. It's as if you were moving the bulk of the myofascial sleeve of all the muscles around your thigh bone (femur) and prying it off the bone.

SWITCH LEGS AND REPEAT ACTIONS 1–3.

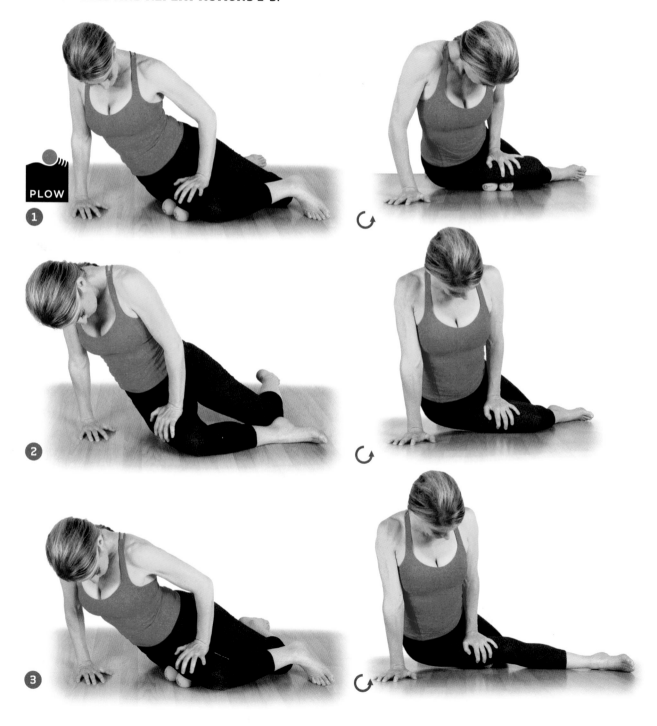

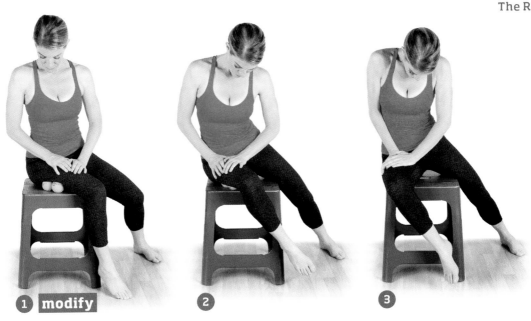

1 modify 2 3

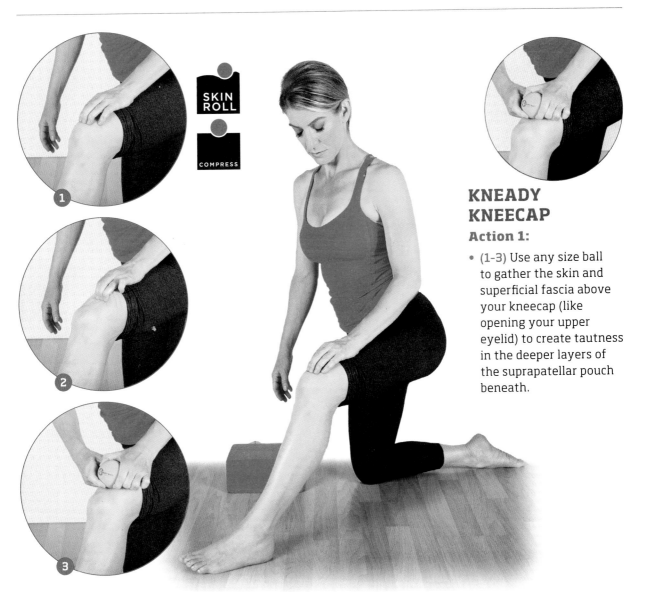

SKIN ROLL

COMPRESS

KNEADY KNEECAP

Action 1:

- (1-3) Use any size ball to gather the skin and superficial fascia above your kneecap (like opening your upper eyelid) to create tautness in the deeper layers of the suprapatellar pouch beneath.

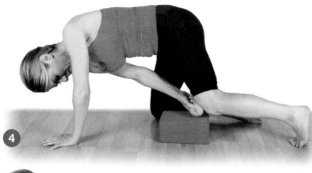

- **(4-5)** Plunk your knee on top of the ball on a block or stool.
- **(6-8)** Wave your lower leg slowly from side to side to CrossFiber the tendons converging above your kneecap.

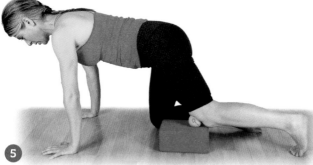

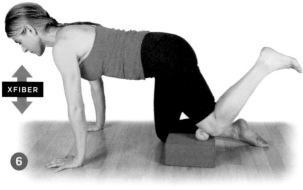

XFIBER

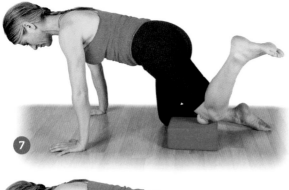

Action 2:

Keeping the ball in place, **(1)** slowly contract your quadriceps by opening your knee, and then **(2)** stretch the same area by bending your knee.

SWITCH LEGS AND REPEAT ACTIONS 1 AND 2.

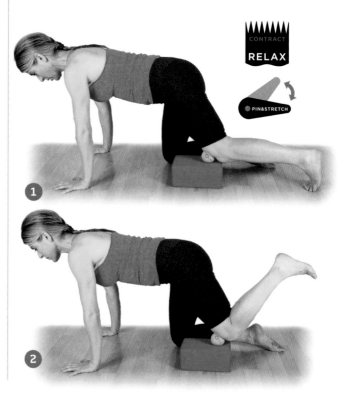

CONTRACT
RELAX

PIN&STRETCH

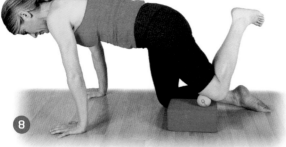

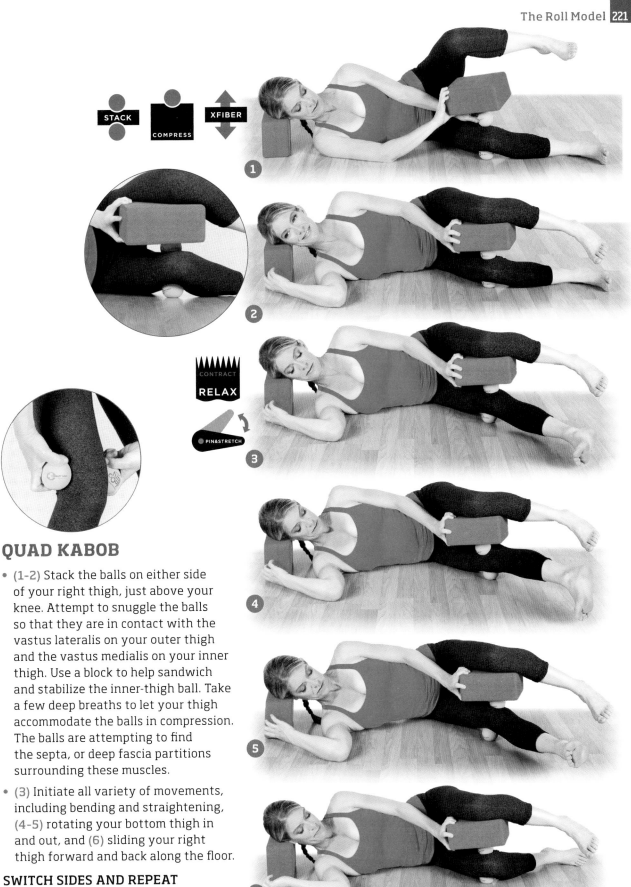

STACK • COMPRESS • XFIBER

CONTRACT • RELAX • PIN&STRETCH

QUAD KABOB

- (1-2) Stack the balls on either side of your right thigh, just above your knee. Attempt to snuggle the balls so that they are in contact with the vastus lateralis on your outer thigh and the vastus medialis on your inner thigh. Use a block to help sandwich and stabilize the inner-thigh ball. Take a few deep breaths to let your thigh accommodate the balls in compression. The balls are attempting to find the septa, or deep fascia partitions surrounding these muscles.

- (3) Initiate all variety of movements, including bending and straightening, (4-5) rotating your bottom thigh in and out, and (6) sliding your right thigh forward and back along the floor.

SWITCH SIDES AND REPEAT ACTIONS 1 AND 2.

KNEE CHEW

Action 1:

(1-2) Place a ball behind your bent knee, toward the outside of the knee. Use your hands to add compression as your tolerance permits. It will make your calf bulge. Pause for a few breaths, then initiate the following movements:

- (3-6) Slide your foot and ankle from side to side.

- (7) Point and flex your foot.

- (8) Contract and release your calf and hamstring muscles by trying to squeeze the ball and then releasing the pressure.

COMPRESS

CONTRACT

RELAX

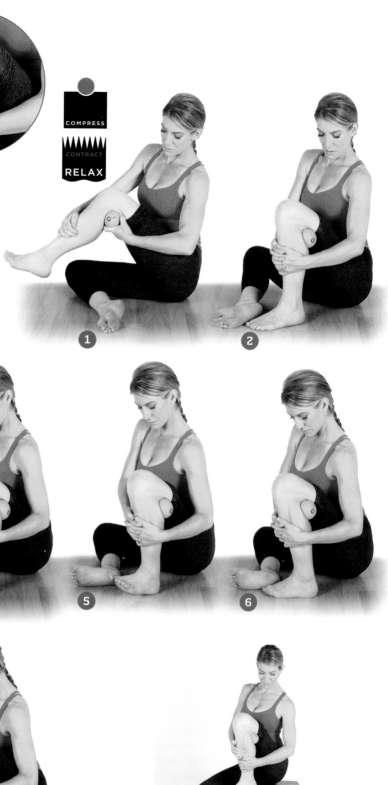

1

2

3

4

5

6

7

8

9 modify

Action 2:

- (1-2) Grip the ball and spin it into your tissues, grabbing as much excess skin and connective tissue as possible, then mobilize your ankle and foot in every possible way.

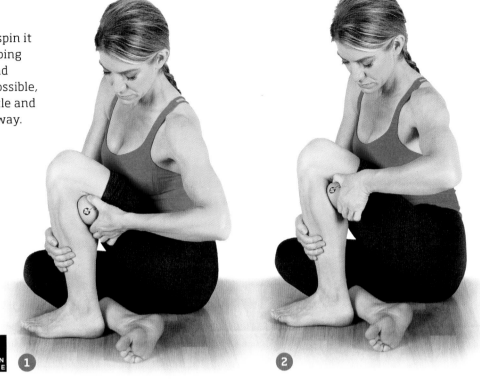

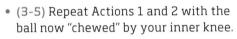

- (3-5) Repeat Actions 1 and 2 with the ball now "chewed" by your inner knee.

SWITCH LEGS AND REPEAT ACTIONS 1 AND 2.

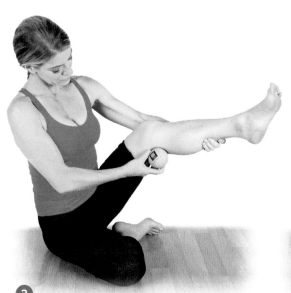

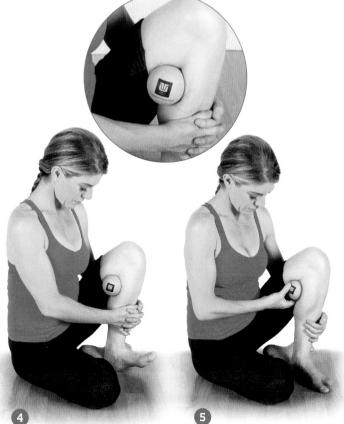

CHILD'S POSE ON BALLS

(1) If your knees permit, place a ball behind each knee, then roll the balls about 1 inch toward your calves. (2) Bring your buttocks toward your heels while the balls dig into your calves. The balls will be sandwiched between your calves and hamstrings. (3-4) Breathe deeply, then CrossFiber by shifting your weight from side to side.

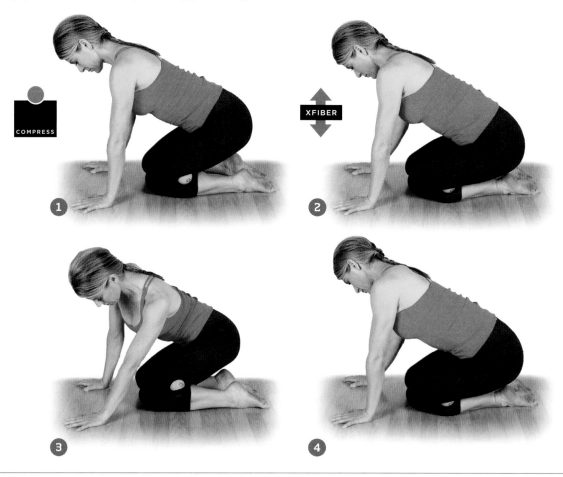

ReCheck: Child's Pose

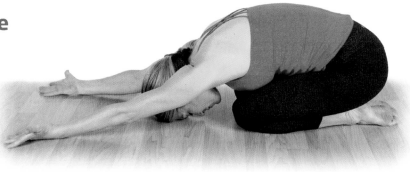

- Lie facedown on the floor and fold your body at your knees and hips to check the range of motion of your knees. Notice how close your buttocks descend toward your heels. Are your hips closer to your heels now? Do you feel less strain in your knees?

- Take 5 to 10 Abdominal-Thoracic Breaths.

Reflect

1. Contract your quadriceps. Do they have more power?

2. Try squatting and notice how that feels.

3. Finish this statement: I feel _____.

The ACL Tear That Wouldn't Heal: When Surgery and Recovery Don't Resolve the Issue

Tiffany Cresswell-Yeager, 37
Director of Student and Enrollment Services, Penn State Lehigh Valley
Orwigsburg, Pennsylvania

Tiff Cresswell-Yeager was always an athlete. In high school, she played basketball and golf and ran track. She currently oversees every aspect of extracurricular life for the students at Penn State Lehigh Valley, including activities, counseling, conduct, health, diversity—you name it. However, as her career brought on greater responsibilities and stresses, she found that she wasn't playing sports anymore, and she missed the identity that being an athlete gave her. She earned a PhD in sociology in 2012, completing a grueling seven-year dissertation research project on first-generation college students. About a month before it was time to defend her dissertation, she took up CrossFit for stress relief.

Tiff fell in love with CrossFit from the very first WOD (workout of the day). Previously she had tried "every new workout craze," like Zumba, step aerobics, and kickboxing, but she always got bored and was never really challenged. CrossFit "felt like it was meant for me," and she even got her brother and 60-year-old mom to join in her workouts. At 36, she had thought her athletic days were behind her, but now she loved feeling strong and young again and pushed herself to reach new goals. In

January 2013, in a goal-setting exercise (popular in CrossFit), she wrote on a white board, "I want to do a pull-up, I want to run a mile"—and, most important—"I want mental toughness" to be able to do more intimidating movements, like thrusters (squats with an overhead barbell press), which still scared her. Little did she know that her mental toughness was about to be challenged in a totally different and far more painful way.

One day, about a month after setting her goals, Tiff was driving to the CrossFit "box" (what CrossFit gyms are called), excitedly anticipating her workout. She had had a particularly stressful day—her job involves a lot of putting out fires in various departments at the university—and as she headed to the box she thought to herself, "I'm going to crush this workout." That day's WOD was called Fight Gone Bad after a professional boxer described the experience of doing it "like a fight gone bad." True to its name, it became a fight gone bad for Tiff.

Tiff had been a long jumper and triple-jumper in high school and had coached track and field, so when it came time for the timed box jumps (jumping up onto metal stages), she wasn't worried. Jumps were fun for her, and she likes to push herself, so when her coach told her with eight seconds left to "Get one more!" she yelled back, "I'm getting two!" On the second jump, Tiffany landed on a totally hyperextended knee. She heard a pop, but it didn't hurt too badly, so she thought that she might have sprained a muscle or that it was an "over-35 injury." Over the next week or two, she saw her chiropractor a few times, but he didn't think anything was torn. With her strong thigh muscles, Tiff was able to keep working out, but her knee wasn't feeling any better. Finally the athletic director at school convinced her to go to an orthopedic surgeon, who took one look at her knee and said, "You have a torn ACL."

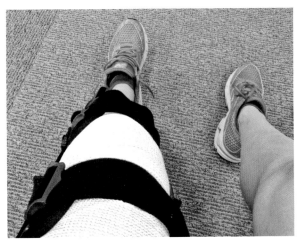
Tiffany's left knee on her first day of rehab.

Tiff's response? "No, I don't!" She couldn't believe it, because she'd done a little online research into knee injuries, and the people she saw with ACL tears couldn't even walk. An MRI confirmed not only the ACL tear, but also a 20 percent tear of her medial meniscus (the cartilage on the inside of her knee). Tiff was so upset by the damage she saw on the MRI that she had to lie down for the rest of her appointment. She knew what an ACL tear meant in terms of recovery, and while she had prepared herself for a few days away from her workouts, she couldn't fathom the months off that this injury would require.

She agreed to have ACL repair surgery just one week later, as she wanted to be able to run and work out again. The first week post-surgery she felt pretty mentally strong about her path of recovery, but after the medication wore off and she realized how weak and painful her knee felt, the reality of her situation hit her. She went to excruciating physical therapy sessions that attempted to force her unbending knee into extension and left her in tears, but the therapy wasn't making her knee better. She couldn't control her leg at all, and her formerly strong quads felt weak and useless. She couldn't straighten her leg all the way, which made going up and down stairs and even taking a shower awkward and difficult. At meals she had to sit with her leg propped up on a chair. She couldn't drive comfortably or sit in church for very long, and she wore a knee immobilizer over her pants "at first because I needed it, but then out of fear that someone might bump or trip me."

For a physically active person like Tiff, having to be almost totally sedentary was an immense psychological burden. After a few weeks with little change, it was all beginning to weigh her down, but her dad told her, "Listen. My birthday is April 25. You'll be fine by then." Tiff resolved to stay strong until that date, convinced that she would magically be healed by then, but when the birthday came and went and she wasn't any better, she became deeply depressed. "I was starting to lose my identity–I had put so much into my athletic ability and the stress relief that I got from CrossFit–and even my identity at work. I was really struggling," she says. To top it off, Tiff got whacked with a $2,000 out-of-pocket bill from her physical therapist. It turned out that her early chiropractic visits had been counted as part of her rehabilitation, and after the twenty-four insurance-approved visits, the PT office had begun charging her full price for her sessions.

Tiff was devastated, frustrated at her lack of improvement and angry with herself for choosing to have the surgery at all. She started to believe that her knee would never be functional again. She was in constant pain inside her knee, and it felt like she was being stabbed by knives in the back of her knee and tight calf. She cried every day.

As a CrossFitter, Tiff followed Kelly Starrett's MobilityWOD on Twitter, and sometime in mid-May of 2013, she recalls him mentioning me and Yoga Tune Up. Tiff tweeted me, "I tore my ACL. Where do I start?" I replied with a few suggestions, including my KneeHab DVD from the Yoga Tune Up website. Tiff had used lacrosse balls for massage before (a popular technique in the CrossFit world), so she understood what myofascial release might do for her. But this was something of a last-ditch effort: by now she had lost so much faith she was skeptical that anything could help at all.

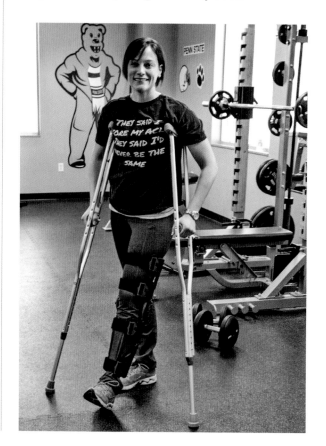

At first she was scared to roll, afraid of damaging the graft and of the lingering inflammation in her calf, but I allayed her fears, explaining that I had constructed the KneeHab DVD in stages. The DVD would guide her through different phases of her pain and recovery cycle. I encouraged Tiffany to go at her own pace and not to rush through any of the sections.

Tiff trusted my expertise and dove in. She appreciated the clear explanations, and the very first time she did the exercises, including the Prehab section that includes the Roll Model techniques, she felt "instant relief, better than any of the physical therapy I had done." Her pain was so much improved that she stopped taking Aleve, and she gained the best range of motion she'd had since her injury in just one session. That first experience brought her so much respite from the constant pain that a glimmer of hope resurfaced for Tiff. After that, she began to diligently use the Therapy Balls every day to roll out her shin, tight IT band, and hip, teasing out the difference between "good pain" and "bad pain" and pushing each day for a little less bad pain and a little more mobility and knee extension.

That whole summer, Tiff rolled and practiced her KneeHab exercises daily, regaining strength and mobility in her quadriceps. Most important, she regained her usual optimism and was able to return to her beloved CrossFit in the fall. Since her return to CrossFit, she has blasted through her old PRs (personal records), shaved 20 seconds off her mile run, and lost the 15 pounds she gained after surgery (helped by a clean, anti-inflammatory Paleo diet). Tiff carries the Therapy Balls with her everywhere ("I have six pairs of the Original YTU Balls stashed all over the house") and has convinced her whole family, as well as her colleagues at work, to start rolling with her. She also uses the Roll Model Balls to soothe her aching shoulders, neck, and upper back from her twice-daily hour-long commute. Recently, she and her husband bought road bikes and went on a 10-mile ride.

Tiff's a proponent of the Roll Model Method, even attending one of our Roll Model Therapy Ball trainings in New York so that she could better understand the science behind her fascia. "I feel like this injury recovery is actually injury prevention—the Therapy Balls are helping me stay supple and soft so that I never have to go through anything like this again, because I don't think I could do it. I really feel like the Therapy Balls gave me hope again, and it's so important when you're dealing with pain and recovery. Your experience and expertise saved me from a dark place. I feel like I'm me again."

Tiff's brother and sister-in-law recently welcomed a new baby boy into the family, and she can't wait to run and jump and play with him. She feels rejuvenated and young again—"I don't feel a day over 25," she says—and she now has the tools to stay healthy at any age.

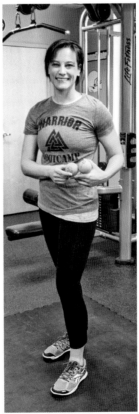
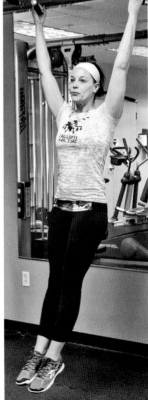

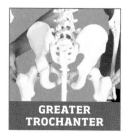

Sequence 5: Pliable Thighs

EmbodyMap

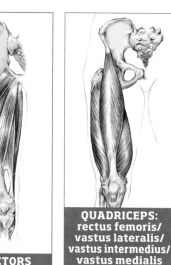

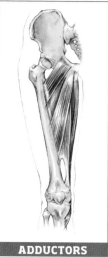

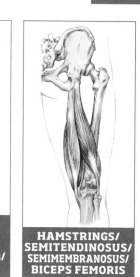

GREATER TROCHANTER

ISCHIAL TUBEROSITY

ADDUCTORS

QUADRICEPS: rectus femoris/ vastus lateralis/ vastus intermedius/ vastus medialis

HAMSTRINGS/ SEMITENDINOSUS/ SEMIMEMBRANOSUS/ BICEPS FEMORIS

Basic Ball Stops

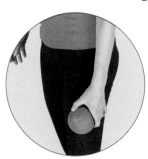

Quadriceps group

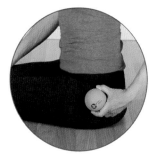

Greater trochanter

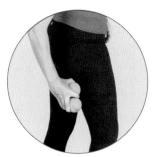

Hamstrings

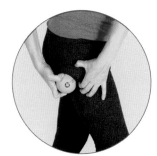

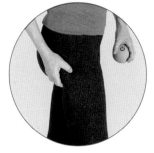

Gluteus maximus meets IT band

Check In: Twister with Block (or Stool)

- (1-2) Step your feet 2 to 3 feet apart and bend forward with your braced spine remaining neutral (no rounding other than the natural spinal curves). Depending on your flexibility, you may need to place your hands on a block or stool.

- (3) Slide the block or stool to the right in order to spin your head and feet around to face the opposite direction. (4) Stop when your thighs and hips won't permit any more motion. Your right leg will be in front of your left.

- Hold for 5 to 10 Abdominal-Thoracic Breaths.

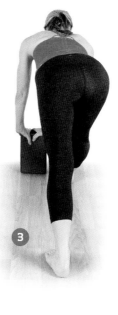

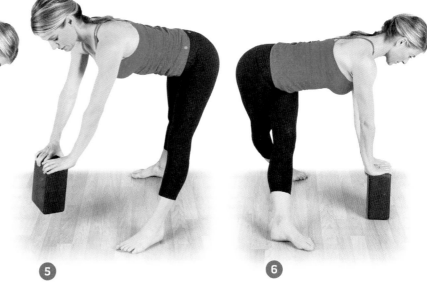

- (5-6) Unscroll and wind in the opposite direction. You will now be trapped in a twist with your left leg in front of your right.

Roll Sequence

HAMSTRING FLUFF

Action 1:

(1-2) Sit on a chair or stool, place one ball just below your left sit bone (ischial tuberosity), and nestle it into your hamstrings. Take several deep breaths to get used to the pressure. (3-4) Then CrossFiber your hamstrings by sliding your left knee from side to side.

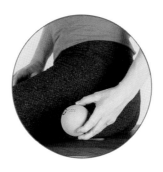

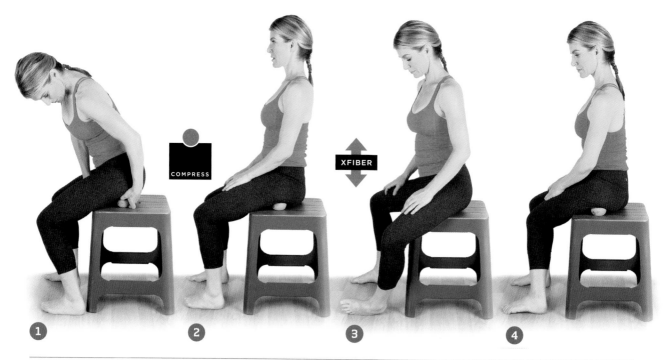

Action 2:

Add contract/relax to the mix by actively pivoting your left knee in and out, awakening your inner thigh and outer buttock muscles. This will change how your left foot is positioned on the floor. Keep your thigh in these new positions and increase the intensity of your contractions and relaxations while the ball pushes up against your inner or outer hamstrings.

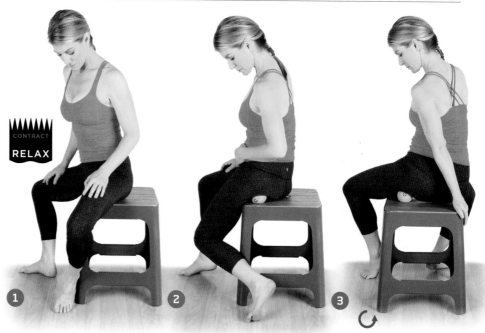

Action 3:

(1–2) Cross your left ankle on top of your right thigh and then (3–6) attempt to track the ball into the seams between the gluteus maximus, IT band, and hamstrings.

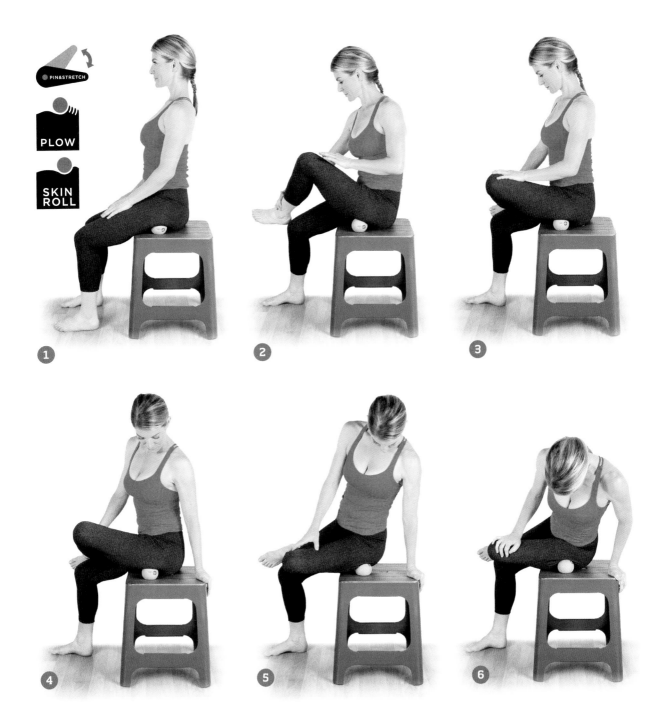

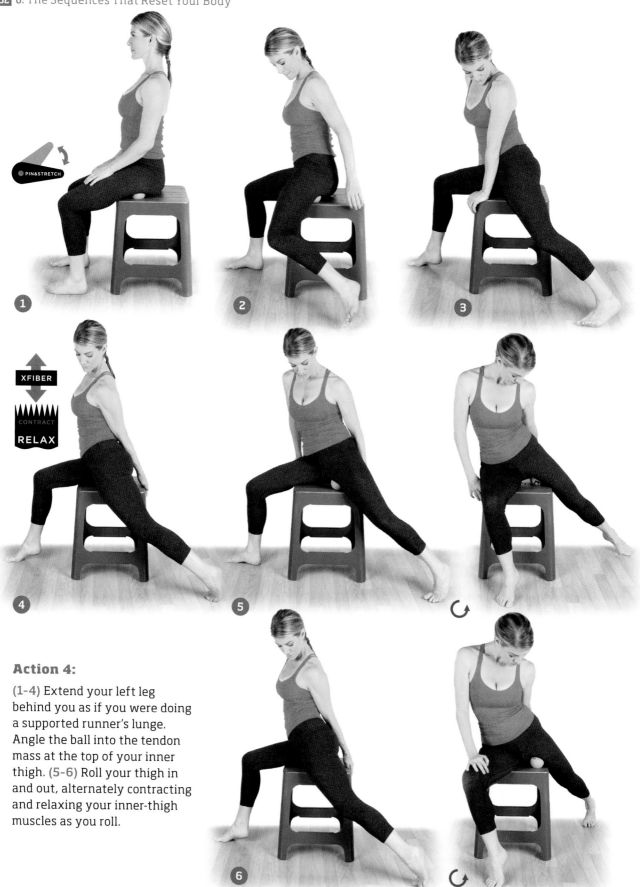

● PIN&STRETCH

XFIBER

CONTRACT

RELAX

Action 4:

(1-4) Extend your left leg behind you as if you were doing a supported runner's lunge. Angle the ball into the tendon mass at the top of your inner thigh. (5-6) Roll your thigh in and out, alternately contracting and relaxing your inner-thigh muscles as you roll.

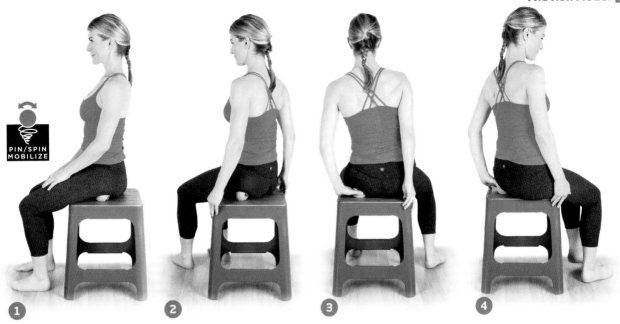

Action 5:

(1-2) Reset the ball in any area of your left hamstrings. (3) Lock the ball in place with your left hand, then twist your body and buttocks around the ball so that your tissues are wrung to the maximum. Once you can no longer find twisting motion, (4) mobilize your left thigh in as many ways as possible, then wind up the tissues a bit more, mobilize again, and unwind in the other direction.

SWITCH SIDES AND REPEAT ACTIONS 1-5.

ADDUCTOR KABOB

(1) Lie on your right side with a block or pillow underneath your head for support. (2) Place an ALPHA Ball underneath your right thigh and a PLUS pair between your thighs to create a ball stack. (3-4) Pause and rest with deep Abdominal-Thoracic Breathing for 1 to 2 minutes.

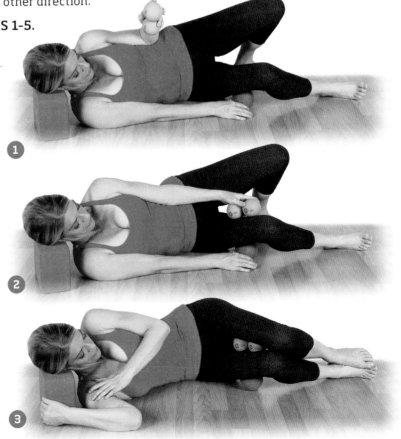

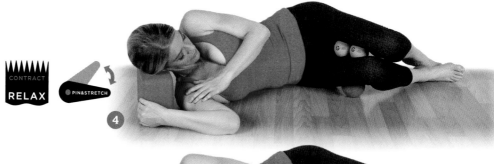

Once your tissues are more compliant:

- **(5)** Explore bending and straightening your bottom knee.

- **(6)** Contract and relax all the tissues that are in contact with the balls.

- **(7-8)** Slide and scissor your thighs past one another.

- **(9)** Lift and lower your right foot off the ground.

- Repeat all of the above actions with the balls a few inches lower or higher on your thighs.

SWITCH SIDES AND REPEAT.

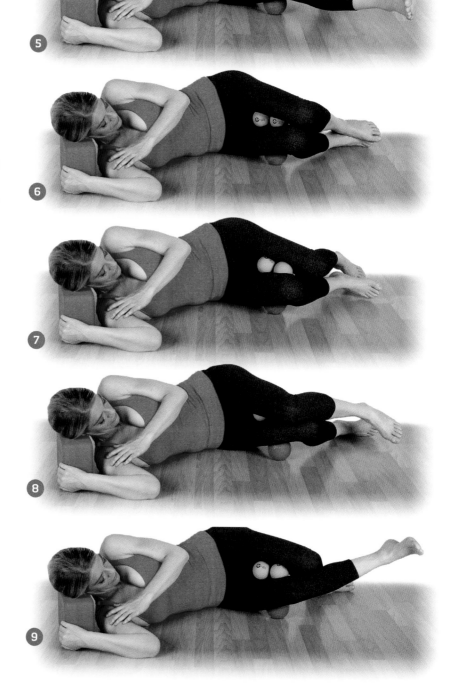

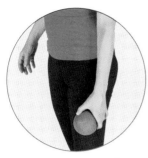

QUADRICEPS KERFUFFLE

Action 1:

- (1-2) Using any size ball, lie facedown with the ball tucked between the floor and your left quadriceps group. Spend 1 minute with Abdominal Breathing.

- (3) Alternately contract and relax your quadriceps. Try 2 or 3 different locations to contract/relax. Once the tissue feels more supple, (4-6) begin a super-slow CrossFiber action with your left thigh, breathing deeply as you move.

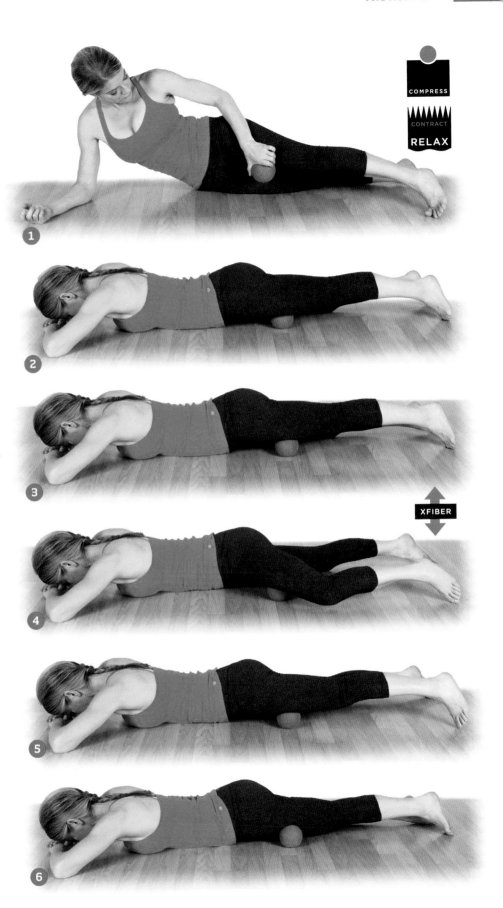

Action 2:

Slowly pull your body forward while the ball CrossFibers your thigh. This creates a serpentine pattern on the front of your thigh as you combine stripping and CrossFiber and tousles the interface of the rectus femoris and vastus intermedius. Once you are close to your knee, reverse your direction and move the ball up your thigh.

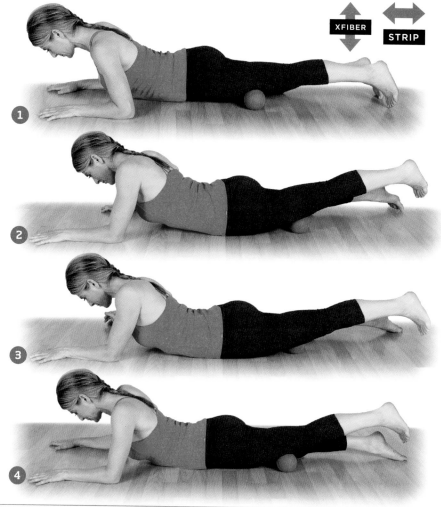

Action 3:

(1-2) Continue to CrossFiber, and (3) add pin & stretch by bending and straightening your knee. Actively roll your thigh from side to side, wagging your lower leg like a windshield wiper.

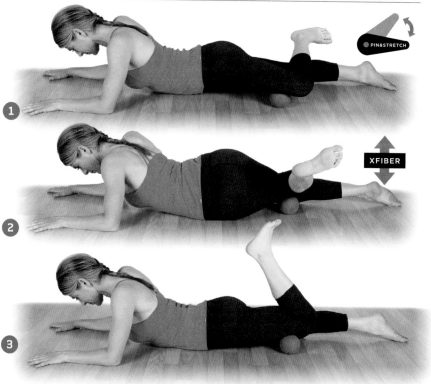

Action 4:

(1) Use your hand to wind the ball deep into your thigh (try this on bare skin), then (2-3) attempt to mobilize your hip or knee to encourage slide & glide among the quadriceps tissues. Try 2 or 3 different locations on your thigh.

SWITCH SIDES AND REPEAT ACTIONS 1-4 (OR, TO SAVE TIME, TRY DOING BOTH THIGHS AT ONCE).

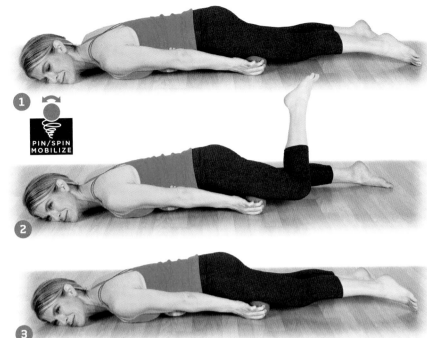

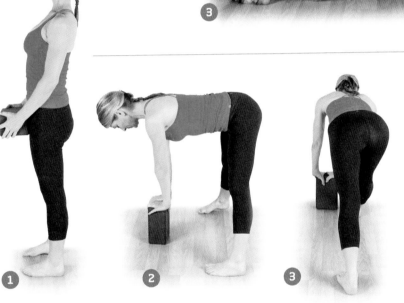

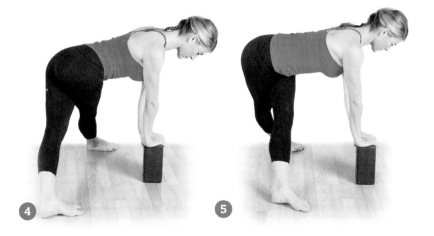

ReCheck: Twister with Block (or Stool)

- (1-3) Reset the same stretch and sense whether your twisted legs permit a bit more range of motion with less restriction.
- (4-5) ReCheck each side for 5 to 10 breaths.

Reflect

1. Consider the ReCheck stretch. Did you feel a difference as you twisted in one direction or the other?

2. Does your posture feel altered?

3. Finish this statement: I feel _____.

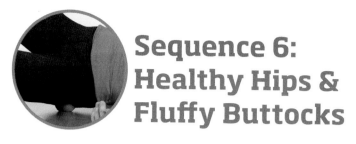

Sequence 6: Healthy Hips & Fluffy Buttocks

Setup

Roll Model Balls: Original YTU, PLUS, or ALPHA

Mat

Block or pillow

EmbodyMap

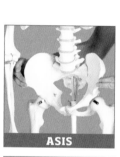

ASIS

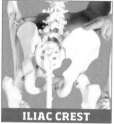

GREATER TROCHANTER

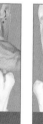

PSIS

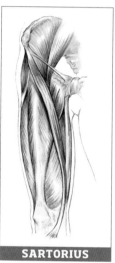

SARTORIUS

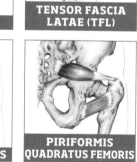

TENSOR FASCIA LATAE (TFL)

SACRUM

ILIAC CREST

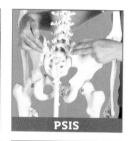

GLUTEUS MAXIMUS, MEDIUS

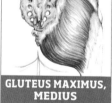

GLUTEUS MINIMUS

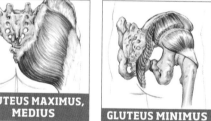

PIRIFORMIS QUADRATUS FEMORIS

Basic Ball Stops

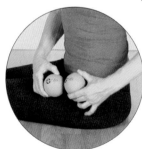

Tensor fascia latae (TFL)

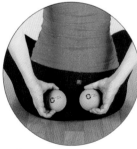

Buttock muscles

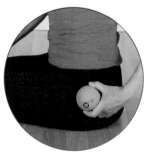

Greater trochanter

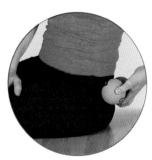

Gluteus medius

Check In: Double Pigeon

- Sit on the floor and stack your lower legs on top of one another, attempting to place your right ankle on top of your left knee and your right knee on top of your left ankle. Keep your feet locked in dorsiflexion (in other words, don't let your ankles sickle or bend).

- If this position forces your spine to lose its neutral position, prop yourself up on a block or stool. You can also check one hip at a time rather than stacking both at once.

- Sit for 5 to 10 Abdominal-Thoracic Breaths, then switch sides.

NOTE: *I have a large range of motion in my hips, which is why this shape fits my body so well.* **Please do not force yourself to look like me in this picture (or any picture),** *but feel for your own range of motion as it exists each time, before and after rolling.*

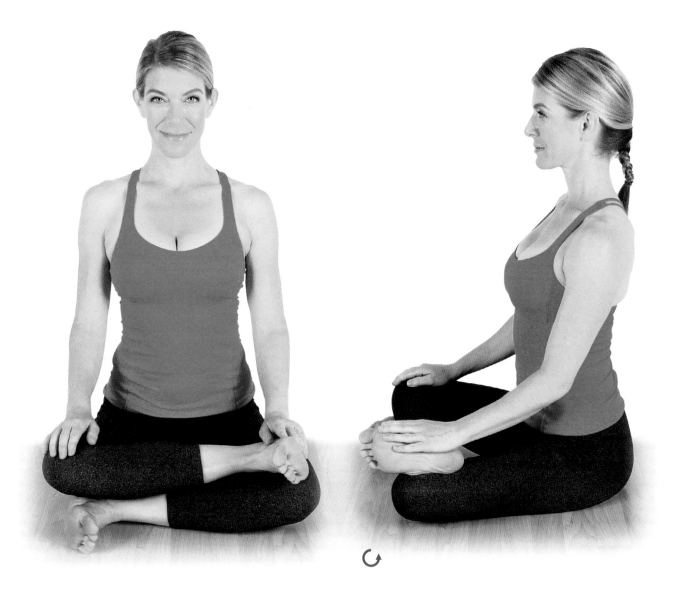

Roll Sequence
PIRIFORMIS PLAY

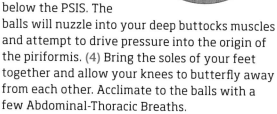

Action 1:

- **(1-3)** Lie on your back and place one ball on each buttock, just below the PSIS. The balls will nuzzle into your deep buttocks muscles and attempt to drive pressure into the origin of the piriformis. **(4)** Bring the soles of your feet together and allow your knees to butterfly away from each other. Acclimate to the balls with a few Abdominal-Thoracic Breaths.

- **(5-6)** Contract/relax by tightening your buttocks for a few seconds and then releasing, 5 to 8 times.

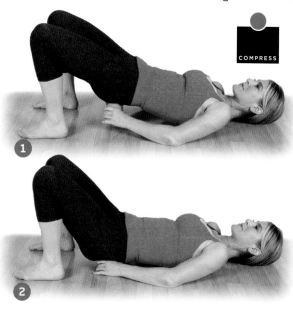

COMPRESS

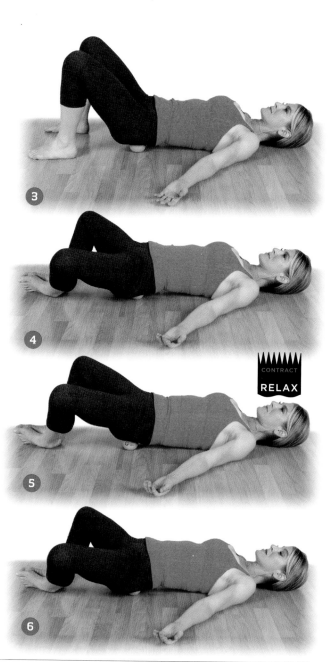

CONTRACT
RELAX

Action 2:

Remove the right ball, place the sole of your right foot on the floor, lean into the left buttock and ball, and begin to strip your piriformis. To do so, consider its line of pull, running from the sacrum to the greater trochanter– basically a "line" across your buttock. This move simultaneously CrossFibers all the muscles that lie on top of your piriformis.

STRIP   XFIBER

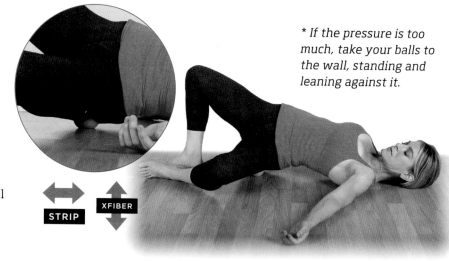

* If the pressure is too much, take your balls to the wall, standing and leaning against it.

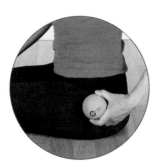

Action 3:

(1-2) Use a ball to locate your left greater trochanter (the bony protrusion on the side of your upper thigh). (3-6) Maneuver your pelvis and hips so that the ball draws a circle around that bony landmark and travels across its tendons and the other soft tissues that connect here. Circle in one direction, then reverse.

SWITCH SIDES AND REPEAT ACTIONS 1-3.

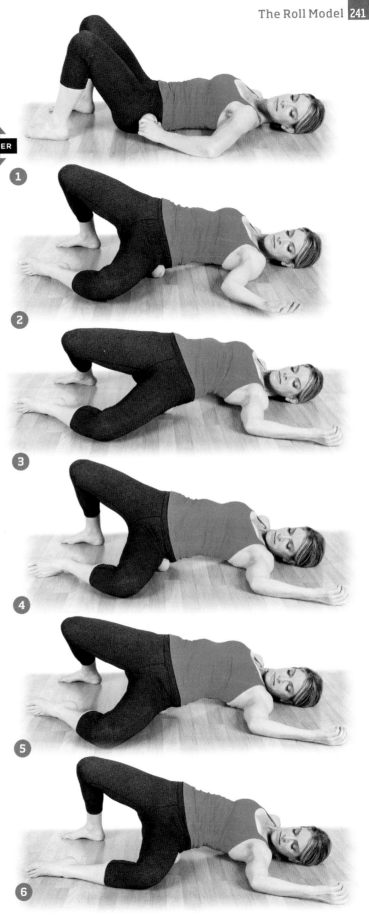

MOM JEAN POCKET

Action 1:

- (1-3) Place 2 balls side by side at the upper margin of your gluteus medius. Lie on your left side, rest your head on a block or pillow, and let the balls sink in for several breaths.

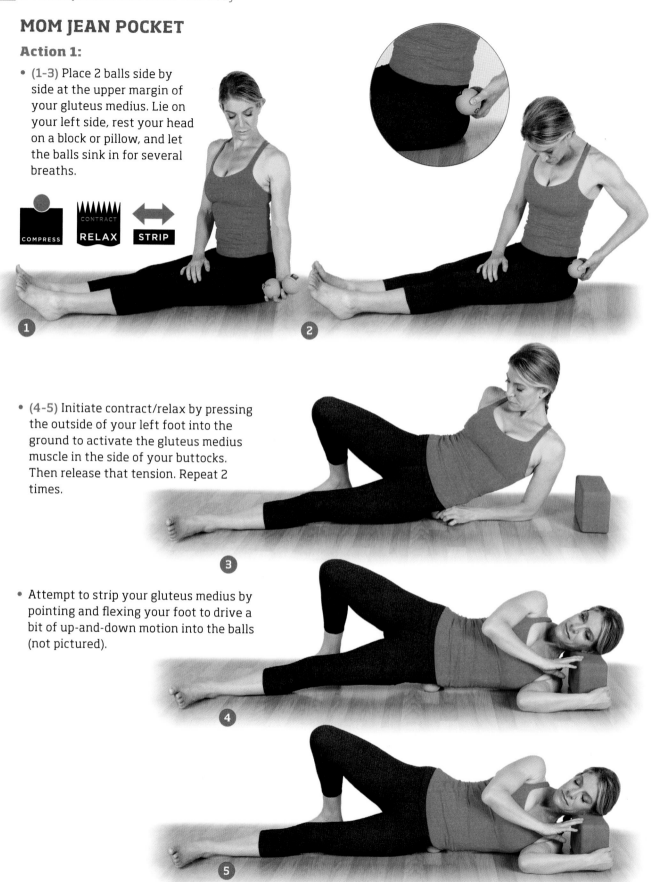

- (4-5) Initiate contract/relax by pressing the outside of your left foot into the ground to activate the gluteus medius muscle in the side of your buttocks. Then release that tension. Repeat 2 times.

- Attempt to strip your gluteus medius by pointing and flexing your foot to drive a bit of up-and-down motion into the balls (not pictured).

Action 2:

- Initiate a CrossFiber action by tucking and untucking your pelvis (anterior and posterior tilt).

- Intensify this action by spinning one or both balls deeper into your upper buttocks before initiating the tucks (not pictured).

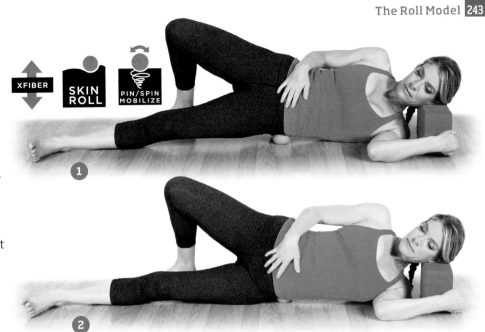

Action 3:

- (1-3) Pin & stretch and create a taffy-pull action of these tissues by lifting and lowering your left thigh toward the ceiling and back to the floor several times.

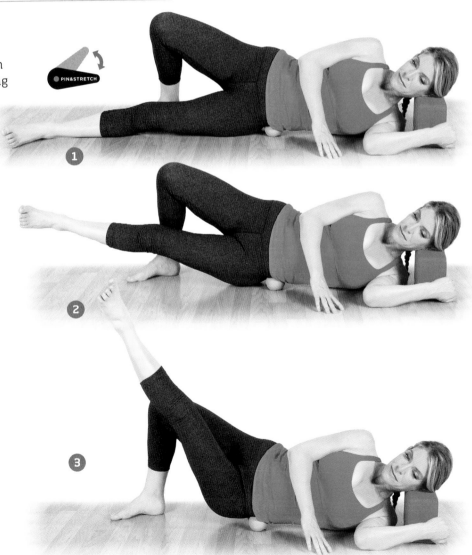

- **(4-8)** Follow that with a bicycle pedal action, hovering your left leg a few inches above the floor. Cycle a few times in one direction, then switch directions.

SWITCH SIDES AND REPEAT ACTIONS 1-3.

SKIN ROLL

CONTRACT RELAX

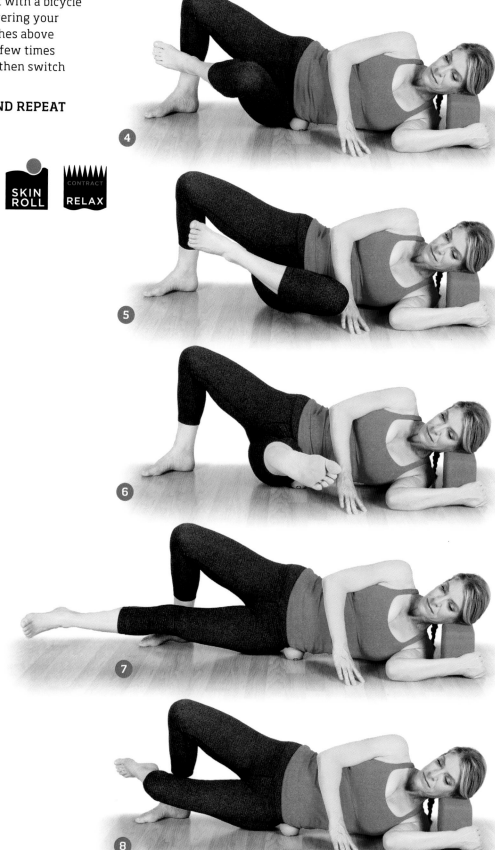

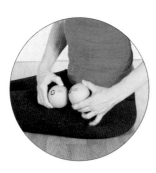

TENSOR FASCIA FILET

Action 1:

- (1) Place 2 balls vertically along your left tensor fascia latae (TFL), which is located where your front trouser pocket rests on your outer thigh. Find it just below and to the side of your ASIS.

- (2-3) Cross your right foot in front of your left thigh to pin the balls in position. Take several deep breaths and let the balls impress themselves into your tissues.

- (4-5) Initiate stripping by pointing and flexing your left foot into the floor to propel the balls up and down your TFL. This is a very small motion.

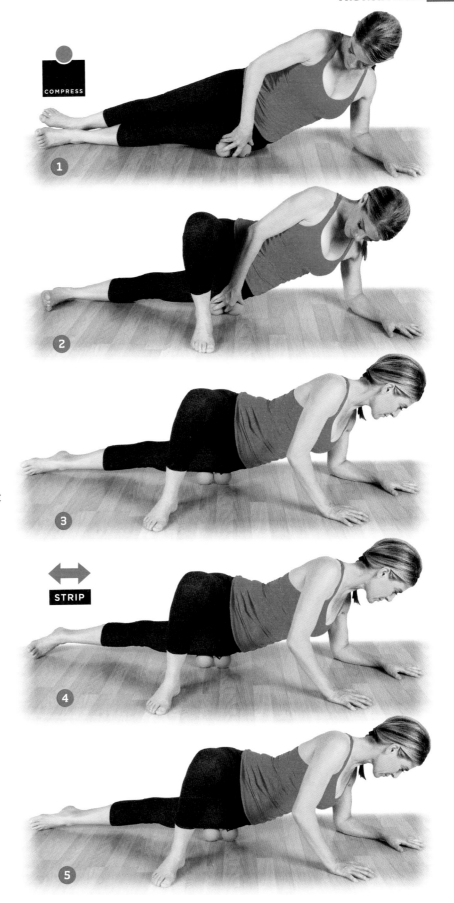

Action 2:

Pivot your body and thigh over the balls to create CrossFiber friction across this small myofascial tissue. Repeat 5 to 8 times.

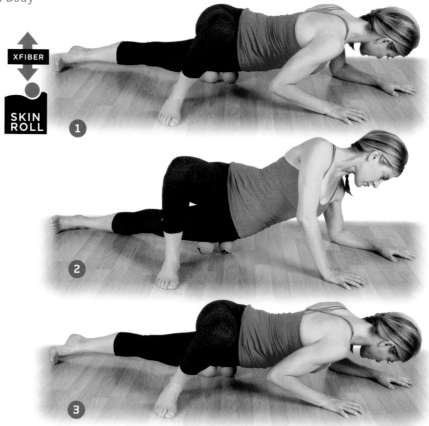

Action 3:

Pin & stretch your TFL by flexing and extending your knee.

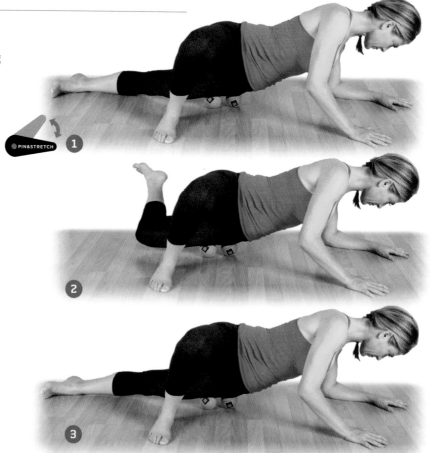

Action 4:

(1-3) Track the ball(s) down to the center of the side of your left thigh on your IT band. Keep your knees bent, and, if you can tolerate the pressure, stack your right thigh on top of your left. (If not, keep your right leg scissored behind the left.) (4-5) Slide your left thigh forward and backward to encourage the balls to cross the IT band and vastus lateralis. (For detailed IT band rolling, work your way through Sequence 4, Kneed to Knead, starting on page 215.)

SWITCH SIDES AND REPEAT ACTIONS 1-4.

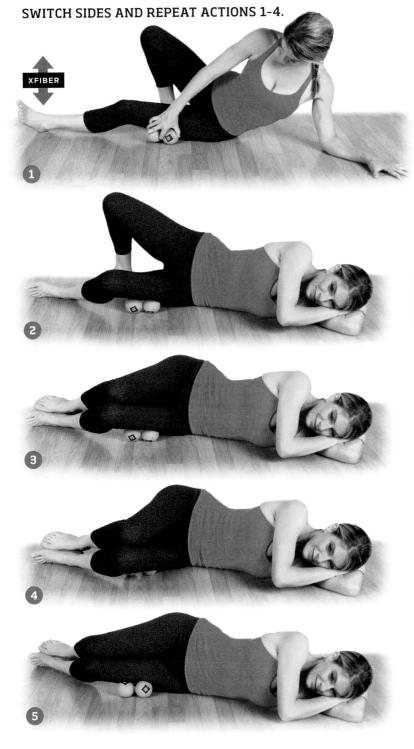

ReCheck: Double Pigeon

Reset your stretch position and notice if you have more range of motion available in your hips, and if it is easier to keep your spine neutral.

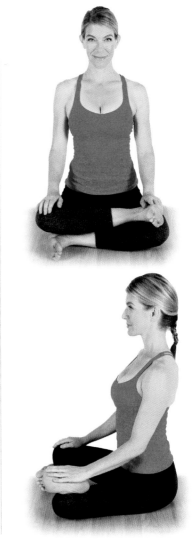

Reflect

1. Was there more or less tension on one side of your buttocks?

2. Take a walk and notice if you feel your buttocks firing as you step.

3. Finish this statement: I feel

_____.

Sequence 7: Pelvic Funnel

Setup

Roll Model Balls:
ALPHA or Coregeous

Mat

EmbodyMap

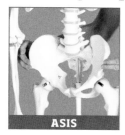

ASIS

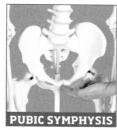

PUBIC SYMPHYSIS

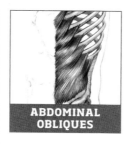

ABDOMINAL OBLIQUES

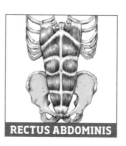

RECTUS ABDOMINIS

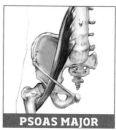

PSOAS MAJOR

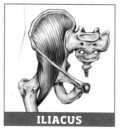

ILIACUS

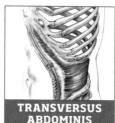

TRANSVERSUS ABDOMINIS

Basic Ball Stops

Iliacus (front of pelvic funnel)

Check In: Half Frog/Half Cobra

- Lie facedown and actively tighten your abdomen and buttock muscles.
- Swing your bent left knee out to the side as if you were initiating a crawl. Flip your right foot into dorsiflexion, as pictured.
- Maintain the tension in your buttocks and core and slowly attempt to pull your spine forward and upward in order to stretch and lengthen through the front of your right hip.
- Take 5 to 10 Abdominal-Thoracic Breaths, concentrating on sensing the iliacus and psoas on the front of the right pelvis.

SWITCH SIDES AND REPEAT.

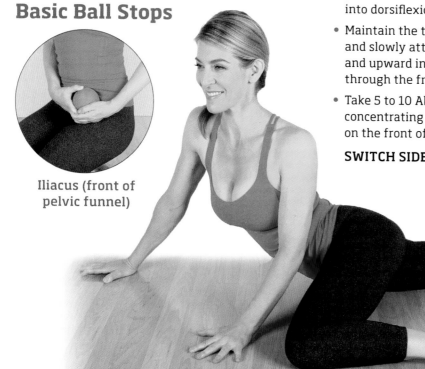

Roll Sequence

Action 1:

- (1-3) Place an ALPHA or Coregeous Ball on the front left side of your pelvis and slowly proceed to lower your body until you are resting facedown on the ground. (See the warning at right.) If the pressure is too intense, lean more of your body weight into your right side. Rest for 2 to 3 minutes with deep Abdominal Breathing, letting the ball gently burrow into this often ignored area.

- (4) Initiate a subtle contract/relax action by trying to pull your left knee directly into your chest, but do not allow that grand action to happen. To an observer, there is no joint motion, just a stiffening of the tissues, followed by relaxing and sinking. Repeat 5 to 8 times.

WARNING: If you have an inguinal hernia or are pregnant, please avoid this sequence. If you have recently had any kind of abdominal surgery, seek permission from your physician. Warm up your entire abdomen with global shear before doing this sequence. Do not apply your full body pressure initially, and do not rush. Gradually apply more pressure as your comfort level permits.

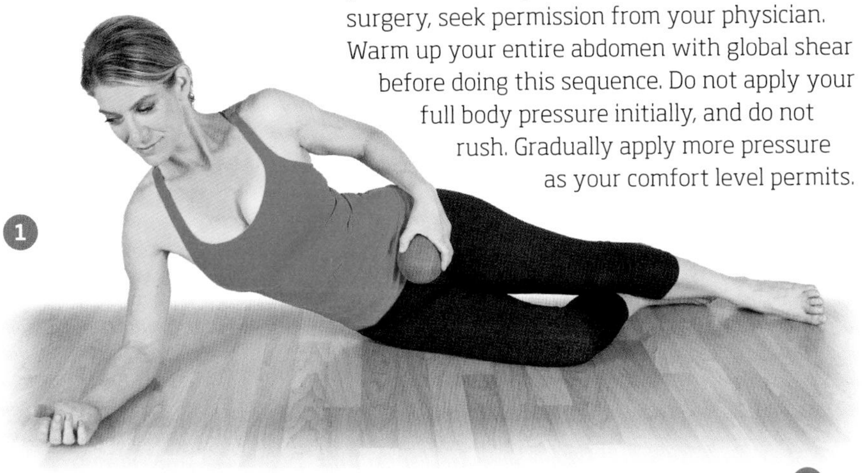

COMPRESS

CONTRACT

RELAX

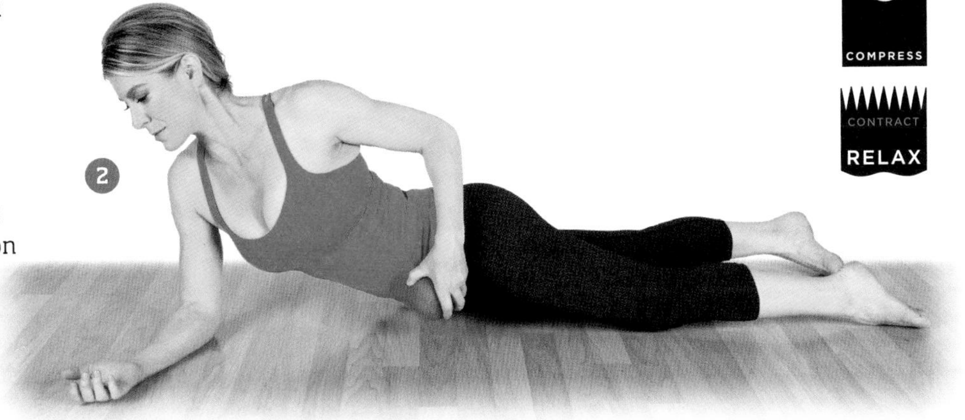

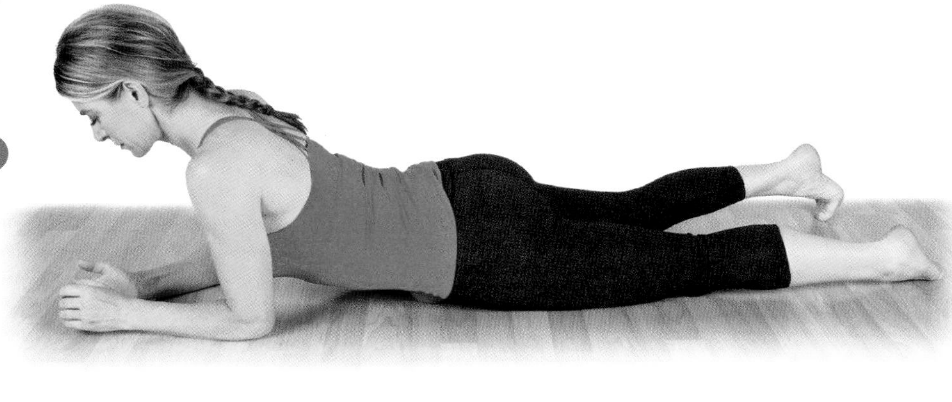

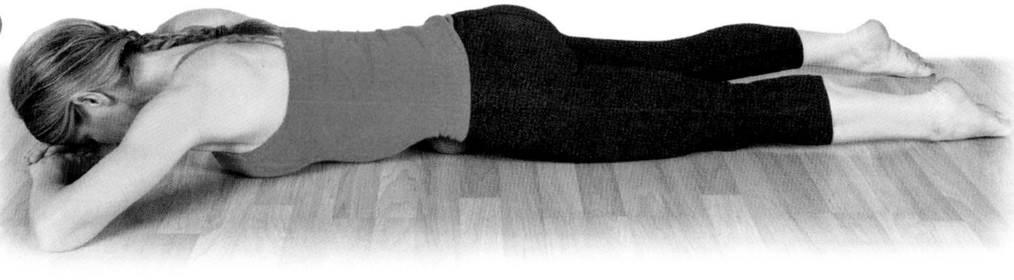

Action 2:

- (1-3) Initiate pin & stretch by bending and straightening your knee.

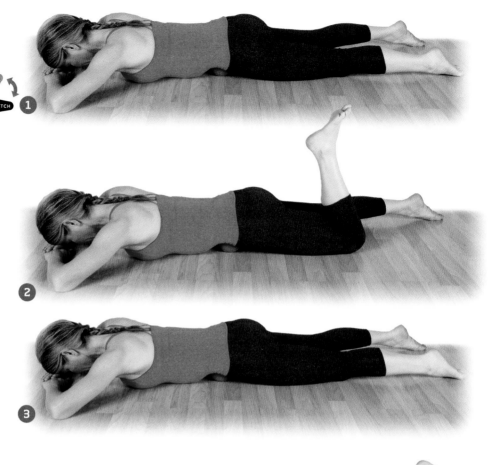

- (4-6) Keeping your whole leg stiff and straight, raise your left thigh off the floor several times.

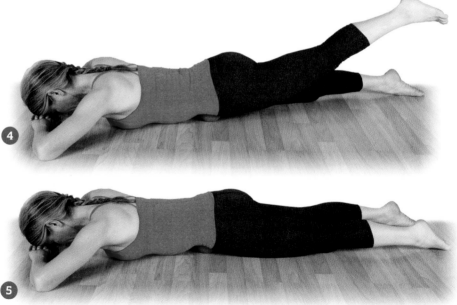

- **(7-9)** Bend your knee and wave your left foot from side to side to roll your hip socket and CrossFiber your iliacus.

XFIBER

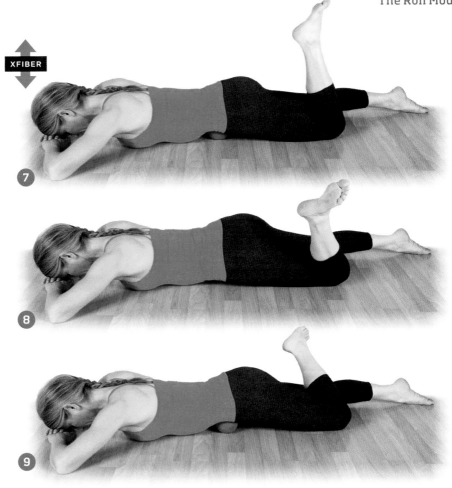

Action 3:

CONTRACT RELAX

- **(1-2)** Bend your left knee and slide it along the floor toward your left armpit in a "frog crawl" move. **(3)** Then slide it back. Try this move a few times.

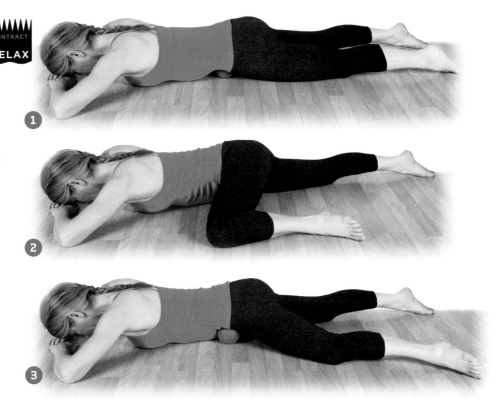

- **(4-5)** If you are able to tolerate more pressure, prop yourself up on your elbows, which pushes more body weight into the ball and iliacus, and **(6-8)** frog crawl a few more times.

SWITCH SIDES AND REPEAT ACTIONS 1-3.

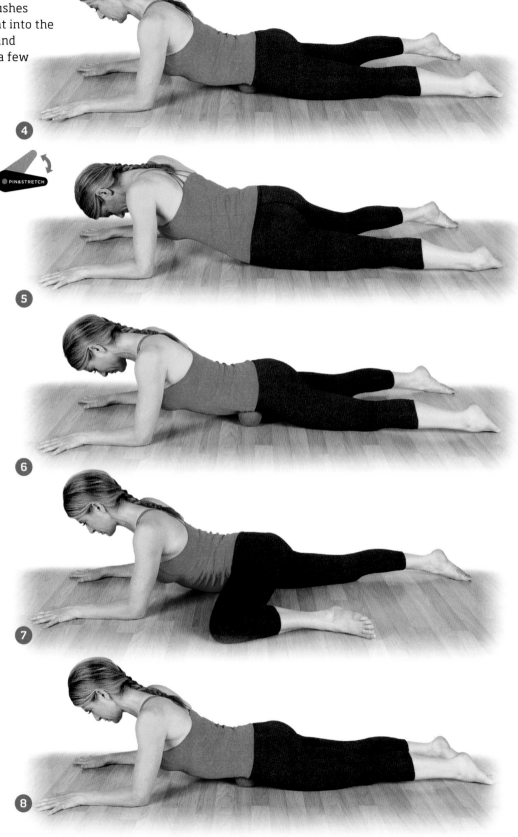

ReCheck:
Half Frog/Half Cobra

- Reset your stretch position and see if there is any change in the amount of soft-tissue resistance in the front of your pelvis.

- Notice any changes in your access to your breathing.

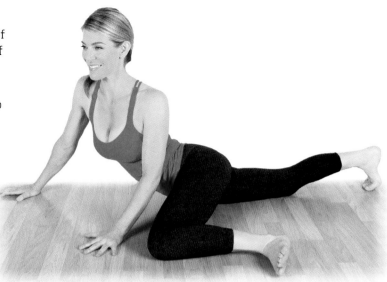

Reflect

1. What was your initial reaction to placing the ball on the front of your pelvis?

2. Did you notice your breath changing throughout the sequence?

3. Finish this statement: I feel _____.

EXTRA-SPECIAL SUBJECT: PELVIC FLOOR MASSAGE

Just about every part of the body can be rolled with the Roll Model Balls. Some parts may appreciate (and be more appropriate for) a smaller, larger, softer, or harder ball, but in most places at least one of the Roll Model Balls can be put to work. In the privacy of my home, I have been able to tackle areas that would seem taboo to "rub" in a public setting. While pregnant last year, I finally shared a "secret rolling place" with the world: the pelvic floor. I was inspired by the work of my friend and pelvic biomechanical goddess, Katy Bowman. I began using the ball on my perineum, the myofascial tissue that lies between the anus and the genitals (performed through clothing), and found that it improved my ability to contract by buttocks, connect to my hips, and align my upright posture. I debuted these techniques in a two-day pregnancy webinar on CreativeLive. com.* The webinar still lives on the website, and I happily refer folks (not just pregnant women) with back pain, pelvic floor issues, sacroiliac dysfunction, and more to this video.

I encourage all my Yoga Tune Up teachers to innovate and explore, and several of them were diving into the pelvic floor at the same time. Todd Lavictoire, a lead YTU trainer in Ottawa, had been experimenting with pelvic floor techniques after suffering multiple low-back grievances that a physiotherapist traced to issues in his sacroiliac (SI) joints. His SI joints had also altered his pelvic floor so that it was riddled with trigger points. Todd rolled the balls into his own pelvic floor dysfunction and found great relief. Then he began fearlessly sharing his Roll Model techniques in his group classes at gyms, yoga studios, and CrossFit boxes. It was a few weeks after instructing these rare moves for the first time that one of his students reached out to me with her remarkable journey of healing from a slew of pelvic surgeries, digestive dysfunction, and chronic bowel disease. She was 22 when she wrote the following letter.

* "Healthy Pregnancy, Healthy Baby: Dispelling Myths of Prenatal Exercise, Diet and Self-Care with Jill Miller," www.creativelive.com/courses/healthy-pregnancy-healthy-baby-jill-miller

Rolling Away Stigma, Shame, and Pain "Down There": Pelvic Floor Self-Massage

Rebecca Moss, 23

Personal Trainer, Yoga Instructor, Zumba Instructor, Registered Holistic Nutritionist

Ottawa, Ontario, Canada

Dear Jill,

As young as age 12, I remember lying on the floor after eating because of digestion pains—cramping colic-type pain, bloating, and constipation. At age 18 I was diagnosed with Crohn's disease (a chronic inflammatory condition of the gastrointestinal tract). In addition, further testing showed celiac disease, osteoporosis, anemia, and cervical cancer. As time progressed I became plagued with excessively frequent bowel movements, upwards of twenty a day, for four years. Then I started to lose control of my bladder. Laughing, sneezing, coughing, or bearing down was enough to make me lose control.

As I approached college and post-college, I was unable to work. I slept 18 hours a day and was looking for a bathroom everywhere I went. It was definitely embarrassing when I lost control of my bowels and bladder and needed a change of clothes. I couldn't live a normal life the way others my age were. This includes things like eating out, staying out late, and having energy for just about anything.

For a while, I blamed myself for my issues: what I had eaten in the past, not managing stress correctly, and so on. It was exhausting trying to balance a perfect diet as well as graduate from school. Thankfully my teachers were understanding as I missed many weeks for hospitalizations. My biggest hurdle was my passion for track and field. I was a cross-country athlete in high school, but my body was deteriorating. I was 125 pounds at 15, and when I was 22, I weighed 88 pounds at my lowest. While the incontinence was already a problem, I have had three LEEP* procedures for cervical cancer as well. This didn't improve things for me either; it made them worse with both urine and bowel movements. This continued right up until and post-operatively.

> NOTE: Rebecca studied a bit of anatomy and tried to understand her condition from every possible dimension. Not content that diet or her disease were the only contributing factors, she wanted to understand how and why she would lose control over the muscles and sphincters (round muscular outlets) of her pelvic floor. She recognized that all those tissues had been severely compromised by multiple surgeries and procedures.

Since I was constantly contracting my sphincter with the bowel movements, I assume I had imbalances in my pelvic floor and things weren't quite working how they should. At 22 years old, this was very

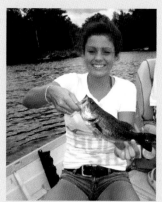

Rebecca, pre-diagnosis at a healthy 120 pounds.

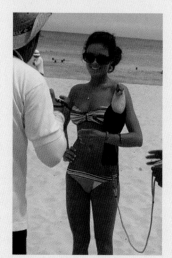

Her smile covers up an unstoppable 30-pound weight loss during her worst times with Crohn's disease. She weighed close to 90 pounds here.

frightening to me. I had been working with a physiotherapist for two months before Todd introduced self-pelvic floor massage in a Yoga Tune Up class. But the physiotherapist's treatment plan was basic, including kegels and relaxation techniques. She said this might be an ongoing problem since I had Crohn's disease.

In Todd's class, we had worked with pelvic floor exercises in the past, and I get totally excited for innovative and different work. In the first class when we sat on the smallest Roll Model Ball—man, it was excruciating at the beginning, but it felt great afterwards. I stopped the kegels upon Todd's reasoning that adding more kegels only makes a tight pelvic floor tighter. This made sense to me.

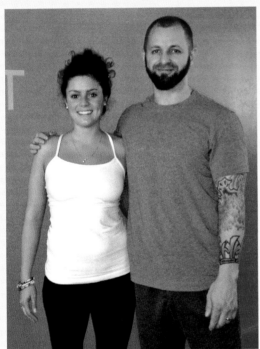

Rebecca with her innovative teacher, Todd Lavictoire.

I purchased some of the Roll Model Therapy Balls, stopped seeing the therapist, and continued to come to class.

At home, every other morning, I made sure that when eating my breakfast I would sit on one Therapy Ball. It was very painful at the beginning. I wanted to scream the majority of the time, and I couldn't last more than a minute. But as I relaxed, I was able to sit for longer periods of time. I can currently sit on the ball for 10 to 15 minutes. I move my body in circles from left to right. I contract my pelvic muscles against the ball and then relax them, all while doing deep breaths for further relaxation. The more I sat, the more relaxed things felt. I didn't notice any benefits immediately, however the past week I have made shocking improvements. Laughing, coughing, and sneezing no longer results in me wetting my pants. The bowel movements haven't been a problem since my Crohn's disease is now in remission after partial bowel removal surgery, but I have never been so impressed.

NOTE: Rebecca's initial letter to me was seven weeks after she started using the balls on her pelvic floor. In less than two months, while sitting on her ball at breakfast, she changed five years of incontinence. Rebecca has also used the other Roll Model Balls for some of her other issues and has reaped tons of benefits.

I own the ALPHA and the two smallest balls. I also have the Coregeous Ball that I use on my stomach for the scars, as well as deep abdominal scar tissue where the bowel was removed and gets general inflammation. I use the small balls and the ALPHA for ankles, knees, IT band, adductors, piriformis, glutes, and hip flexors. I use Coregeous for my stomach and chest and the smaller balls for shoulders, forearms, and my entire spine. The benefits are amazing and impossible to ignore; they have made a huge difference in my posture.

I feel relieved and happy knowing this won't be a forever thing I am stuck with. Before, it was a hard pill to swallow, thinking this was going to be my life moving forward. Honestly, knowing my body

---

*The loop electrosurgical excision procedure (LEEP) uses a thin, low-voltage electrified wire loop to cut out abnormal tissue in the cervix.

and wanting it to be optimal is likely why I was so receptive to Todd's work and taking it to my own level at home. I think if your health is that far gone, you're willing to do whatever you can to improve your life, and I wouldn't take no for an answer.

I know there is a need for more literature on such specific problems that a number of people experience, especially in my case, which can be a sensitive topic for many. [The Roll Model Method] is the kind of work that actually works, but not many have heard of using self-manual therapy for these types of issues. I would love to take your course and spread the knowledge to those who suffer as I did.

This work has greatly influenced my life. Something I was so embarrassed, frustrated, and angry about was fixed with what seemed like something so small yet amazing! I can't thank you and Todd enough for pursuing this avenue! I hope many other women and men with pelvic floor imbalances will try this work, because it really, truly works.

Incontinence doesn't have to control your life. There is a lot to be said for self-manual therapy and the ability to work toward your optimal health on a budget, time restraint, and without a specialist. You can become the specialist of your own ailments and trust the possibility to returning to optimal health—for those with incontinence, this means being in control of your own bladder and bowels. Trust your body and your mind!

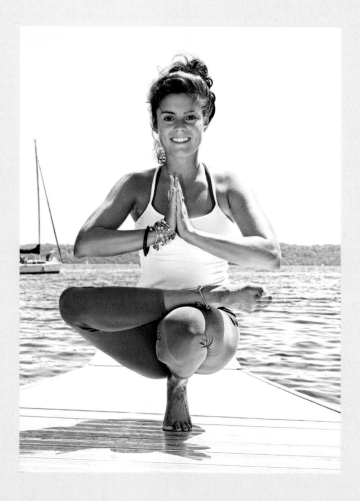

A Postscript from
Teacher to Teacher

Todd Lavictoire, 40

Movement Educator,
Yoga Tune Up Teacher Trainer,
Yoga Teacher Trainer

Orleans, Ontario, Canada

Dear Jill,

People don't often associate their low-back or hip pain with SI and pelvic floor dysfunction.

In my case, I believe that my back issues were exacerbated by some of the fears my wife and I have around my 12-year-old son's health; he was found to have nonspecific brain lesions at age 8.

I am always aware and mindful when presenting the Coregeous Ball and pelvic floor work in class. Coregeous work often is much too challenging and emotional for many people, let alone someone with a clinical digestive disorder like Rebecca. But from her studies she understood how the work can help reduce inflammation in the gut, how it would temper tensions in the musculature of the midsection, free up the diaphragm for better movement, and help her whole central nervous system to better down-regulate and encourage a healing parasympathetic response.

The original pelvic floor Therapy Ball sequence that I taught was developed between my physiotherapist, Shane Maley, and me in order to address some of my own pelvic floor dysfunction, but it was easy to scale it to classroom work once I had worked with it enough on myself. I was aware that introducing self-massage for such a personal and "private" body part in a group setting could be considered "odd." But over my years of teaching with the Roll Model Balls, I've found that people come to expect out-of-the-box thinking and amazing results.

Working through pelvic floor tension can help free up a lot of hip tension. One client of mine was a CrossFitter whose squat was locked at a certain height. He kept blaming his ankles. After we did some pelvic floor work, he retested his squat. The look on his face as his new squat fell through his old standard position was like someone had opened a trapdoor beneath him. He was completely surprised by how quickly this change had occurred.

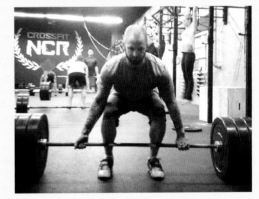

I've found when rolling on the pelvic floor, less is more. In other words, if there is any pain, less pressure is better. Deep breathing is a must to help the pelvic floor relax. If the pelvic floor is chronically contracted or adhered and tight, the breath will be restricted. Contract/relax techniques, including kegel exercises, while using the ball can often speed up the process of reducing tension in the pelvic floor. My pelvic floor is so much freer and more responsive to my breath since I started doing this work.

I hope my suggestions, and the results my students have seen, will encourage readers to "get on the ball!"

Sincerely,
Todd

Spotlight on the Pelvic Floor

This topic merits its own book, but I want to give you some basic reasons why you *should* consider rolling "down there." For many, the floor of the pelvis is totally taboo. Its taboo-ness keeps many people from learning about its muscles, bones, and perforations. You may let your doctor or a sexual partner have access to this area, but have you done your own pelvic self-care? There's no reason to let others safeguard the seat of your power. Get to know its tensions, and you might unlock pains that you've unknowingly trapped.

More than one-third of women in the U.S. have pelvic floor disorders. And while pelvic prolapse, pain, and urinary incontinence are not exclusively female problems, their numbers are expected to rise over the next several decades, according to the National Institutes of Health.* Tension in these myofascias affects the organs nestled in the pelvis, bowels, bladder, and sexual organs. These tensions are not isolated, but are interconnected to neighboring tissues and can be a cause or a result of dysfunctions relating to your hip, back, and abdominal myofascias. Decades of sitting or standing with poor pelvic position (see chapter 3) set up the pelvis for its fair share of unhappy accidents.

* www.nichd.nih.gov/health/topics/pelvicfloor/conditioninfo/pages/risk.aspx

HOW TO ROLL YOUR PELVIC FLOOR: A SHORT PRIMER

The muscles of the pelvic floor sling like a tarp between four of the bony landmarks you learned about in chapter 5. They are attached to:

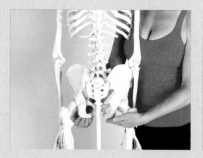

Ischial tuberosities

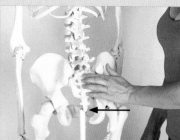

Coccyx

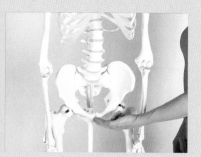

Pubic symphysis

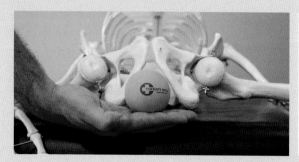

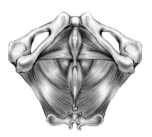

Restore your floor with an extra-pliable Roll Model Ball.

1. For your first few explorations into the pelvic floor, you will get the best benefits by massaging your abdominals and psoas using the Coregeous Ball for global shear for 3 to 5 minutes (see page 144). Then treat your gluteals using Sequence 6, Healthy Hips & Fluffy Buttocks (beginning on page 238) for 3 to 5 minutes. This will help relax the associated myofascias of the entire pelvic floor.

2. Sit on a chair, a stool, or the floor and try circling the entire area with the Coregeous Ball to locate each landmark through your clothing.

3. Then use a soft, broken-in Original Yoga Tune Up Ball to tour the soft tissues around the ischial tuberosities.

4. Place the ball in the center of your pelvis with compression and deep breathing. The ball should rest on the toughest tendon band that crosses the bulk of the muscular pelvic floor, called the perineum, which is between the vaginal opening and the anal sphincter for women and behind the testicles and in front of the anal sphincter for men.

5. Activate your pelvic floor around the ball by using contract/relax techniques. Your pelvic tissues will squeeze and release the ball (this is a similar activation to a kegel).

6. Once you feel a bit more receptive to the ball's pressure, move from side to side and trace the small tarp of tissue at the base of your pelvis. Spend between 3 and 10 minutes, or as your comfort level dictates.

7. When these muscles are palpated (through clothing) with the pliable balls, they become better residents in your interconnected body.

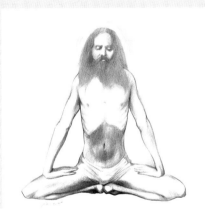
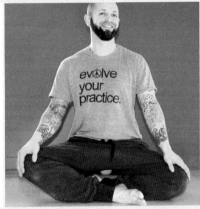

A stone tablet engraving dating to 2500 BCE shows a yogi with his feet rotated backward and his heels pushed into his perineum. While I do not endorse this extreme position for your ankles, a small rubber ball is just the right fit!

CAUTIONS FOR PELVIC FLOOR SELF-CARE

• As with any technique presented in this book, if you are unsure of precisely how and where to place your Roll Model Balls, please seek professional assistance. The structures of the pelvic floor are delicate, and it would be irresponsible of me not to ask you to **proceed gingerly and with caution.**

• Do not place a ball directly on your:

1. Coccyx

2. Testicles

3. Anal, vaginal, or urinary sphincters

Spine Sequences

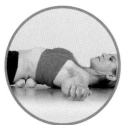

Sequence 8: Lower Back

Setup

Roll Model Balls: Original YTU, PLUS, ALPHA

Mat

Stretch strap

Block or wall (to lessen pressure)

EmbodyMap

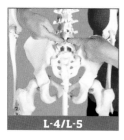

L-4/L-5

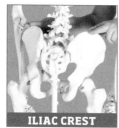

ILIAC CREST

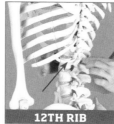
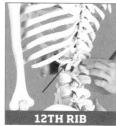
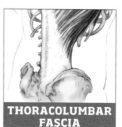

12TH RIB

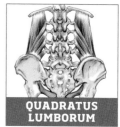

THORACOLUMBAR FASCIA

QUADRATUS LUMBORUM

Basic Ball Stops

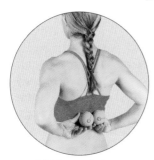

12th vertebra

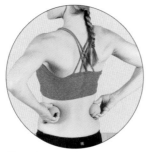

Quadratus lumborum

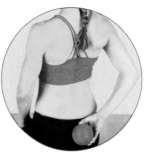

Sacrum

Check In:
Leg Stretch #3 with Strap

- (1) Lie on your back and wrap a strap or belt around the instep of your right foot.

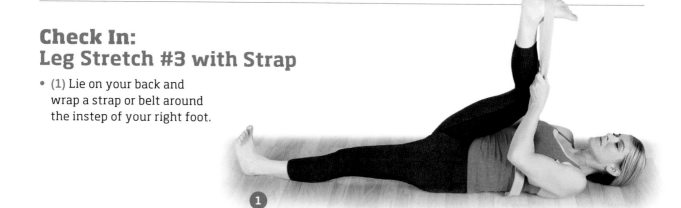

1

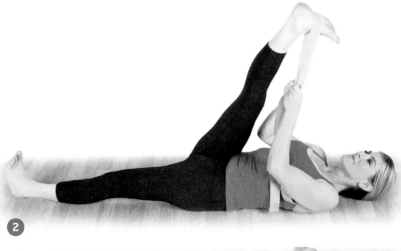

2

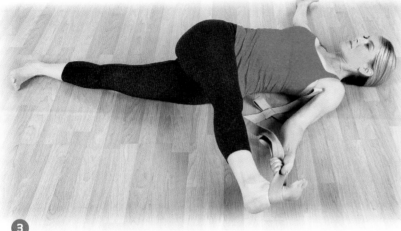

3

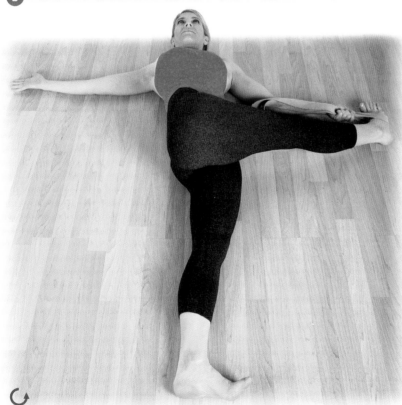

- (2) Attempt to straighten that leg. Maintain a bit of tension throughout your body to stabilize your posture.

- (3) Cross your right leg over your body and rotate your lower back so that your right foot lands at your left side. (If you are very mobile, you will not need a strap; use your left hand to hold your right foot in place.) Your left foot will now be on its side. Make sure that your spine stays in a straight line (good posture) with your left leg–if you are not very mobile, you may have to slacken the strap to avoid curling your spine.

- Once your right foot and thigh have traveled as far over as possible, descend (depress) your right hip and buttock so that they are flush with your left hip and buttock. You may feel a deep stretch in the side of your right hip, hamstrings, and lower back.

- Allow your spine to rotate back toward the floor, and reach your right shoulder toward the floor.

- Hold for 5 to 10 Abdominal-Thoracic Breaths.

SWITCH LEGS AND REPEAT.

Roll Sequence

HOT WATER BOTTLE

Action 1:

- **(1-2)** Lie on your back and place a pair of Roll Model Balls in or out of the tote horizontally across your low back, on either side of your spine. With your knees bent and your feet on the floor, place your forearms on the floor so that your spine curves in a C-shape.

- **(3-5)** Use the balls like a rolling pin to strip up and down your low back, rolling out your thoracolumbar fascia. If the untoted balls start to wander, reset them together. Roll up and down for 2 minutes.

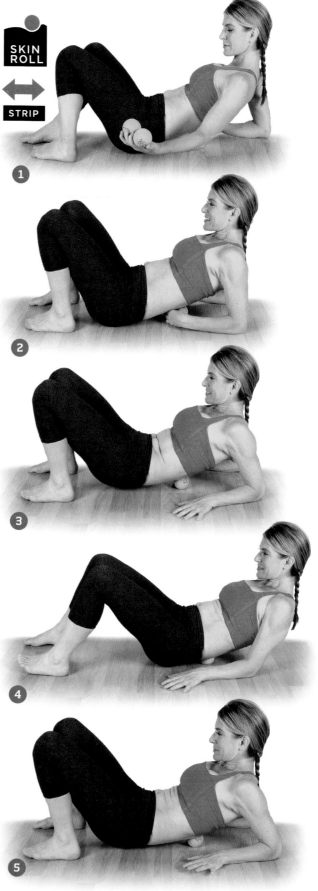

SKIN ROLL ⟷ **STRIP**

toted balls

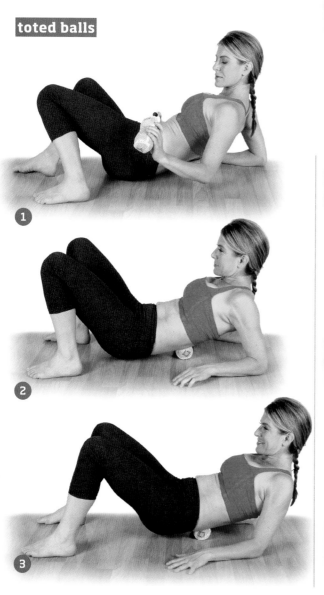

Action 2:

(1) Let the balls settle into any area of your low back, then (2-3) pin & stretch your myofascias by tucking and untucking your pelvis (posterior/anterior tilt) as your low back pivots over the balls.

Action 3:

(1) Remaining on your back, reposition the balls so that they are vertical. (2) Place them on the far left side of your waist, and then (3-5) swipe your low back across the balls to CrossFiber and ball plow the quadratus lumborum.

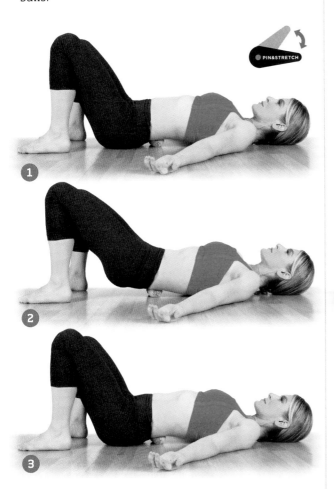

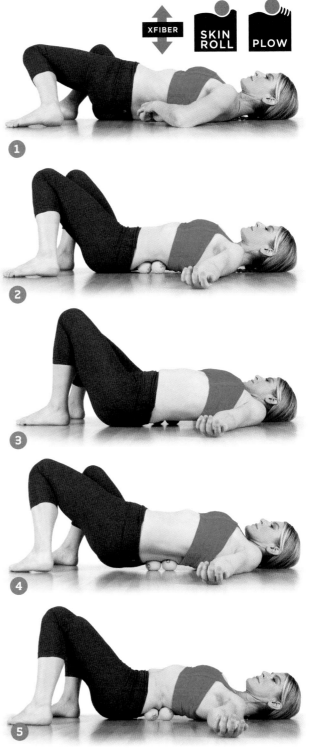

Action 4:

- (1) Place a ball on your sacrum and (2-3) scrape from side to side across the ball to CrossFiber the termination of your thoracolumbar fascia. Do this for 1 to 2 minutes.

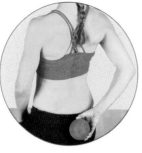

- Remove the ball and rest. Take 5 to 10 Abdominal-Thoracic Breaths. Feel the warmth you've uncorked from your connective tissues.

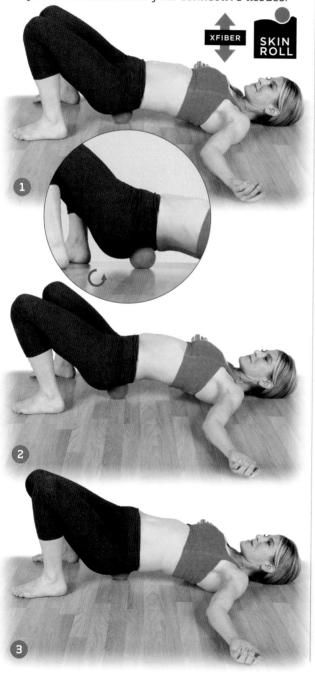

QUADRATUS LUMBORUM MASSAGE

Action 1:

- Choose a Roll Model Ball (please see the modifications on page 268) and either:
  1. Lie flat on the floor.
  2. Lie with your pelvis/low back propped up on a block.
  3. Lean against a wall.

- (1-3) Tuck one ball just above your left iliac crest, then (4) allow your knees to fall to the left. This twists your pelvis toward the ball and presses the ball into the tendon insertion of the quadratus lumborum (QL).

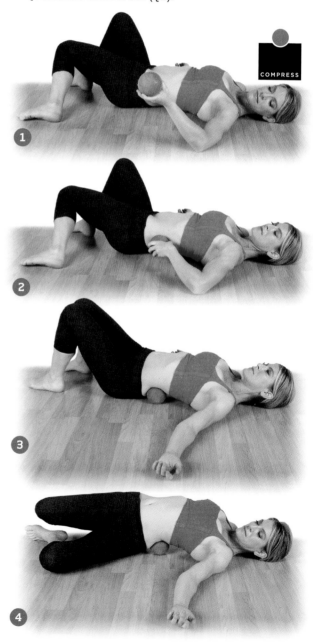

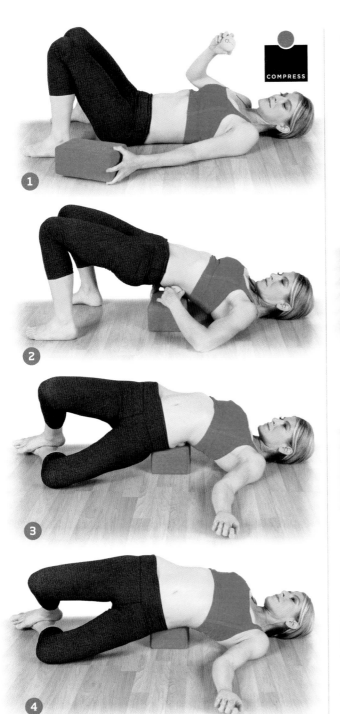

Action 2:

- (1-2) Initiate a CrossFiber motion by gently rocking from side to side across the ball. The ball will pluck at your QL tendon. Breathe deeply into your abdomen as you rock.

- (3-4) Tuck and untuck your pelvis to create a pin & stretch action.

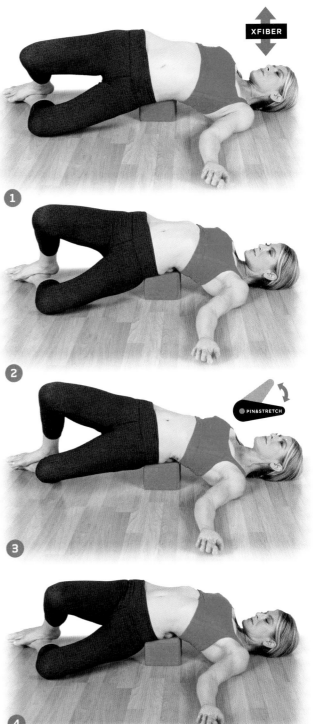

Action 3:

Activate a contract/relax by bending your waist into and away from the ball, as if you were trying to take a bite out of the ball with your waist.

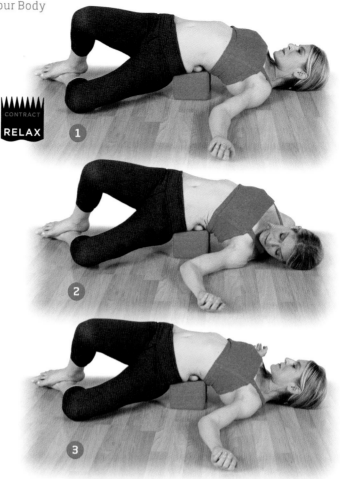

Action 4:

(1-2) Stretch your left leg, shoulder, and arm as far away from your torso as possible, breathe deeply into your whole body, and (3) gently CrossFiber by rocking left and right into and away from the ball.

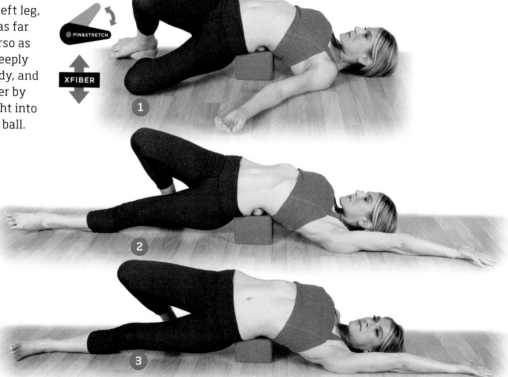

Action 5:

Grab the ball with your left hand and spin it into your low-back tissues. Once it has gathered as much tissue as it can, tuck and untuck your pelvis, rock, bend, and manipulate your low back in any way you can. Then wind up more slack and mobilize your low back again. Then spin the ball in the opposite direction and repeat these actions.

SWITCH SIDES AND REPEAT ACTIONS 1-5.

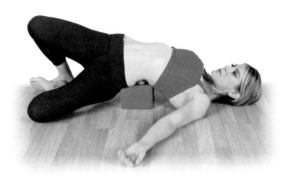

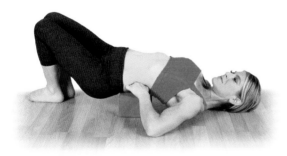

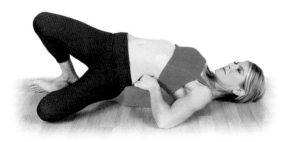

ReCheck: Leg Stretch #3 with Strap

Reset your stretch. Spend 3 to 5 Abdominal-Thoracic Breaths on each side and feel for your ability to sense change in your breath, your low back, and even your hips and hamstrings.

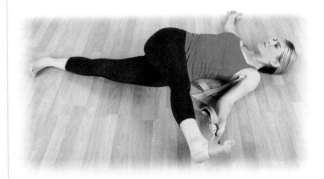

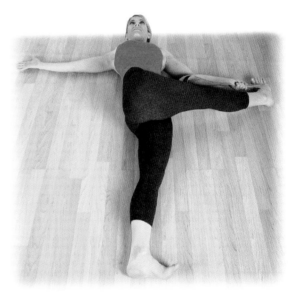

Reflect

1. Stand and feel how your body responds to being upright.

2. Bend to the side and take a breath into the side of your gut. How is your breath mobility there?

3. Finish this statement: I feel _____.

modify lower back

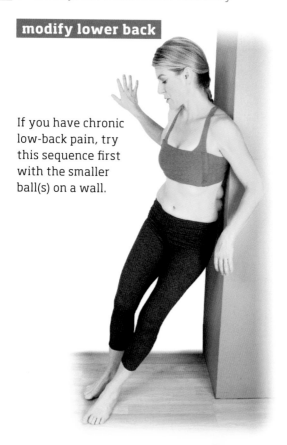

If you have chronic low-back pain, try this sequence first with the smaller ball(s) on a wall.

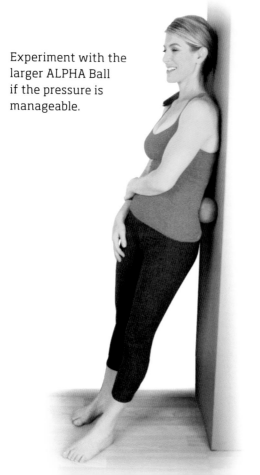

Experiment with the larger ALPHA Ball if the pressure is manageable.

modify lower back

Another option is to use PLUS or ALPHA on the floor without a block.

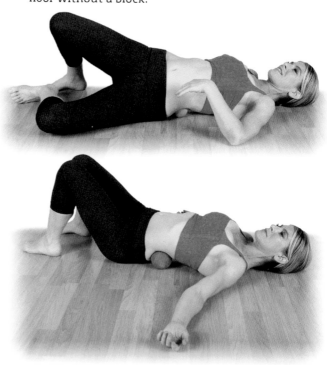

The most intense approach is to use the smallest ball on a block on the floor.

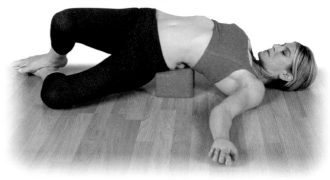

The actions remain the same regardless of which ball you are using or whether you are on a wall, the floor, or a block.

A Soldier's Losing Battle Turns Victorious

Carlton Bennett, 45
U.S. Armed Services Veteran
Hampton, Virginia

As a young man, Carlton Bennett spent five years rising through the ranks of the National Guard. In 1993, shortly after his first son's birth, he joined the Army, retaining his rank of Specialist earned in the National Guard. He reasoned that with the economy not doing so well at the time, it would be a good way to take care of his growing family financially. But he was unprepared for the sheer physical onslaught of active duty. "We wore high-heeled boots and carried 100-pound rucks, sometimes 25 miles at a stretch. Some guys jumped out of airplanes, others carried heavy mortar tubes during marches. We weren't sleeping right, we weren't eating right, everyone was dehydrated—you wouldn't believe the number of injuries. It seemed like every day a knee or a back blew. Three other guys in my group ended up getting surgery."

Carlton can't pinpoint one event that started it, and in all likelihood it was a buildup of different unhealthy stresses on his body, but after four years in the Army he began to experience a tingling sensation in his toes that quickly developed into numbness and pain in his legs. The Army physical therapist said that it was caused by nerve impingement in his lower back and treated him with ultrasound and an epidural, but the treatment didn't help, and the numbness and tingling worsened. Carlton finally visited a neurosurgeon at the Wright-Patterson Air Force Base in Dayton, Ohio, who recommended a laminectomy (removal of part of a vertebra) and a discectomy (removal of part of the cartilaginous disc between vertebrae) in his lower back, between L-5 and S-1. The surgeon told him nonchalantly that the forty-five-minute procedure would relieve the pressure on the nerve and that all his symptoms would go away. Carlton couldn't quite believe that spinal surgery could be that casual, but the surgeon seemed confident, so in 1995 he had the two procedures done. "Knowing what I know now," he says ruefully, "I could have taken care of it with a Therapy Ball."

Unfortunately, the surgeries were just the beginning of Carlton's problems. After leaving the Army, he took a job in software development, which meant sitting for hours in hard, uncomfortable chairs. Before he could even complete the company's training program, his lower back went into spasm and became massively inflamed. "I looked disfigured," he recalls. His doctors at the VA told him to take it easy and do some stretches and he'd be fine. Carlton complied, and the spasm eventually subsided. But it didn't take long before his back spasmed again, and then again.

This was the start of a pattern that would annihilate the next twenty years of Carlton's life. Something as simple as getting up from the dinner table would cause his back to spasm. The doctors would give him muscle relaxants or pain relievers and send him on his way, and the spasm would subside somewhat only to seize up again, sometimes just days later. These debilitating episodes could drag on for days or weeks at a time and would leave him immobilized, bent in half, and wracked with pain. Carlton tried to remain positive that this marathon of pain would come to an end

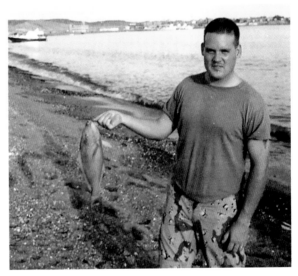

Carlton on duty in Egypt before his spine deteriorated.

at some point, but episode after episode became a psychic assault, leaving him physically depleted and frozen with fear about his future.

"I always felt that there was a dark figure standing behind me with a Taser in his hand, loud and overpowering. Whenever I would get a muscle spasm, it felt like an electric shock, and I imagined this man was hitting me with his Taser," Carlton says. He lived in constant fear that one wrong move–even standing up from a chair or getting out of a car–would send his back into spasm and lay him out for days. "The worst is when it would happen and I couldn't move. I'd be lying on the couch and I'd have time to think about the whole situation. I'd start to beat myself up about it, getting mad at myself for going into the military." Prior to the two spinal surgeries, Carlton had been able to bend over and do simple movements, even though he felt numbness and tingling in his legs. He was positive that the surgeries were to blame for his condition. "The mental health classes I took at the VA suggested getting a hobby to stay upbeat, but all I could think about was how much of a burden I was on my wife and family."

He hated that he couldn't participate in his sons' lives. If he tried to go out for a meal at a restaurant, he could sit with the family for only fifteen or twenty minutes, and then he'd have to spend the rest of the time waiting for them in his van, as most restaurant chairs would give him a back spasm if he sat too long. He couldn't take his family on vacation: cramped airplane seats made flying impossible, and he could no longer manage the eight-hour drive to visit his wife's family.

Carlton tried more physical therapy and pain-blocking injections but was reduced to walking with a cane, unable to stand up straight. Eventually he lost his job, unable to string together more than a few days of work at a time. He was left with no choice but to file for long-term disability. Getting his veteran's benefits took nine frustrating years before they were finally approved in 2005. After so many years of physical and emotional depletion, having to battle the government to prove that he was, in fact, disabled and deserving of benefits took another massive toll on his health that left him deeply depressed. His life barely felt like a life.

While his family remained supportive, a lot of Carlton's friends disappeared when he went on disability, bored with only being able to hang around his house and being unable to get him to "snap out of it." Carlton continued to seek relief with physical therapy and a barrage of medications, from methadone to morphine, as well as antidepressants, but the medical professionals treating him were unable to do anything more than attempt to manage his pain. He continued to grow weaker, a shell of the man he had once been.

In 2007, a neurosurgeon recommended that Carlton repeat the laminectomy and discectomy surgeries on the disc and vertebra directly above the previous site. When Carlton expressed skepticism about the efficacy of the surgeries, the surgeon suggested that he didn't want to get better and that, like a lot of other people on disability, he was too comfortable with the handout and didn't want to contribute to society. Carlton was furious, but this attitude was nothing new.

Then in 2010, after fifteen years of continuous physical trauma, Carlton was rushed to the emergency room with searing stomach pain. The ER staff dismissed it as stomach flu, but Carlton knew that it was far worse than a bug and demanded more tests. A CT scan revealed gallbladder damage and an umbilical hernia, and he needed emergency abdominal surgery. This compromise to his already weak abdominal muscles did nothing to help Carlton manage his pain and movement, and his fear of back spasms brought him to the point of almost total immobility.

Through the years, as Carlton battled frustration, anger, and hopelessness, he continued to seek out therapies that might help him. In 2012 his desperation reached a peak, and he had a facet rhizotomy on six nerves of his lower-back facet joints. This procedure uses heated electrodes to burn the nerve endings and deaden all sensation in the area. The doctor who performed the procedure told Carlton that his back was weak and that he needed physical therapy to get strong again. Though he had repeatedly tried PT with little effect, Carlton was still willing to try. He returned to PT in September 2012, and on the first day, incredibly weak from almost two years of immobility, he sprained both of his thumbs trying to do weight-bearing exercises. That Thanksgiving, as he was getting up from the dinner table, his back spasmed again.

"That was the absolute lowest point. Not only could I not walk, but I couldn't use my hands. I was beyond miserable. Everything was in slow motion. Getting out of bed took fifteen minutes. Getting dressed, showering, everything took forever."

Finally, Carlton's best friend from his military days, Paul Alkoby, suggested that he look up Kelly Starrett, a well-known physical therapist based in San Francisco. Carlton Skyped with Kelly and lifted his shirt to show him how his stomach muscles had started to bulge. Kelly told him that the muscles were weak and had separated, and that he should watch the "Gut Smash" video that Kelly and I collaborated on. Carlton dutifully practiced rolling on a prototype of the Coregeous Ball, and within a week the bulge in his stomach went away.

Encouraged, Carlton reached out to me, and I suggested that he follow more of the ball-rolling videos and use the Roll Model Balls for his back.

"I finally broke down and bought a set of the Yoga Tune Up Balls after a few months of seeing them. At first touch I thought, 'There is no way this squishy ball will help my twisted and knotted muscles!' I lay down on the ball near a major knot in my lower back and was very nervous because I was afraid it would cause my back to spasm. After about thirty seconds I relaxed and felt the ball start to melt into that muscle. My first reaction was to tense a little because this new sensation scared me. But the muscle continued to release, and it was one of the best feelings I'd had in nineteen years. I went searching for more knots in my back and spent a good fifteen minutes working on them. Afterwards I stood up and felt taller. The knots were mostly gone, and I knew that this was my key to a better life."

Carlton eagerly "dug in," thrilled not only at the possibility of softening the layers of tight tissue in his back that were filled with tension and pain, but also that he was finally able to take his health into his own hands. Carlton fell in love with the soft rubber Roll Model Therapy Balls and quickly became an avid roller. "I started using them on my lower back to release the muscles. There were so many knots–and the more I used them, the more my back started to relax." Even better: after rolling his lower back, Carlton was able to stand up straight for the first time in twenty years.

Kelly also told Carlton to find someone to teach him how to brace his core. Carlton found that person in Dr. Stuart McGill, who diagnosed him as flexion intolerant–whenever Carlton bent over, his vertebral disc would push against his spinal nerves, setting off the spasms in his back. It finally made sense why sitting and standing movements were the source of his problems. Dr. McGill taught Carlton how to organize his movement to avoid setting off spasms and encouraged him to continue rolling on the Therapy Balls.

The combination of exercise, correct movement, and ball therapy has literally given Carlton his life back. "I knew that a lot of my problems were movement based. Between Kelly, Dr. McGill, and Jill, my eyes were opened to a whole new world. I would lie in bed after a severe back spasm and wonder if my life would ever get better. Now I feel stronger with knowledge and tools to fix myself

Carlton took complete control of his healing after working with Dr. Stuart McGill (near right), Dr. Kelly Starrett (far right), and the Roll Model Therapy Balls.

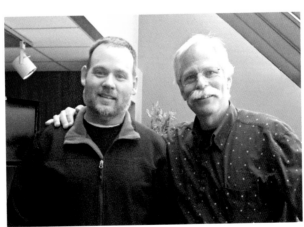
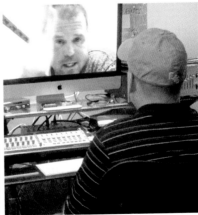

that I can use so I don't have to reach for the med bottle."

Carlton can now go out with his family, go shopping with his sons, even sit in a restaurant for a full meal without being afraid that he'll suffer the embarrassment of being incapacitated in public. He loves being able to stand up straight and proud again, once more the head of the family. If he wakes up with some stiffness, he rolls against the wall in the living room, often concentrating on his neck, lower back, and hips, and then gets on with his day, enjoying the simple pleasure of running errands that most of us take for granted. "I carry them everywhere with me. One time I had one in my pants pocket and forgot. I walked into a store, and the looks I got were priceless."

Now he takes the Therapy Balls everywhere he goes. If he's on a long road trip and feels his back begin to tighten, he pulls over and uses the back of the van as a wall to roll on–there's even a groove in the panel that fits the ball perfectly. "One time I was picking my son up from school, and there's always a half-hour wait in the car line, so I got out and started rolling my back on the van. Someone asked me if I was singing, because I was swaying back and forth!" When he went back to the physical therapist at the VA, he brought the balls with him, and the PT was so impressed with Carlton's recovery that he bought his own supply of balls to give out to his other clients.

Carlton has been able to stop all pain and depression medications completely. He still takes a medication to help with digestion after his gallbladder removal, but he's free of the other meds and their debilitating side effects. And, after almost ten years, he no longer uses a cane.

It's been a long and arduous journey for Carlton, and he describes it as a miracle to have gone from feeling scared to death all day to being able to participate in life again. He's not yet at a point where he has begun to incorporate more vigorous exercise, and he's not sure if the long-term damage done will ever permit it, but he's grateful for the team of people who brought on his recovery–"Jill, Kelly, and Dr. McGill–they're the best people in the world right now with this stuff." Carlton lived for twenty years with pain, disability, psychological demons, and a bleak future. In eight short months,

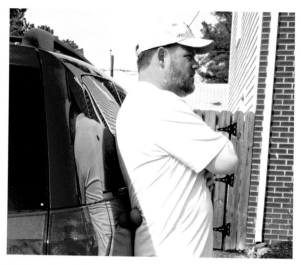

Carlton has pioneered his own "Van Roll" techniques.

he won a victory that no bandage, pill, or surgery could deliver.

Carlton knows that he still has to be careful with his movement–"That guy with the Taser never totally goes away," he says–but those dark thoughts aren't nearly as bad as they used to be, and he's able to ward off any incoming micro-spasms with the Therapy Balls. With the help of his new toolkit, Carlton feels like himself again, empowered with knowledge of how to take care of himself after decades of being at the mercy of passive, reactionary, and ineffective therapies.

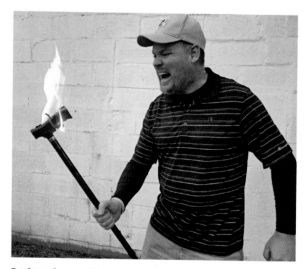

Carlton burns his cane on January 8, 2014, less than ten months after beginning daily use of the Roll Model Balls.

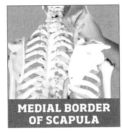

Sequence 9: Upper-Back Unwind

Setup

Roll Model Balls: Original YTU, PLUS

Mat

EmbodyMap

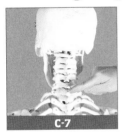

C-7

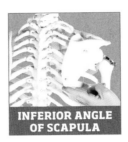

MEDIAL BORDER OF SCAPULA

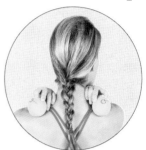

INFERIOR ANGLE OF SCAPULA

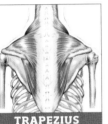

TRAPEZIUS

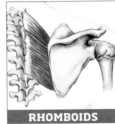

RHOMBOIDS

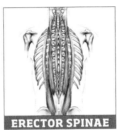

ERECTOR SPINAE

Basic Ball Stops

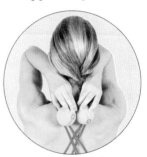

Upper trapezius

Rhomboids

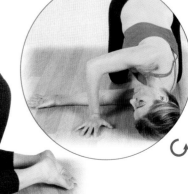

Check In: Thread the Needle

- (1) Get on the floor on your hands and knees. (2) Slide your left arm between your right hand and right knee and reach as far to the right as your back will allow you to twist.

- (3) If they reach, rest your head and left arm on the floor and take 5 Thoracic Breaths into the back of your ribcage.

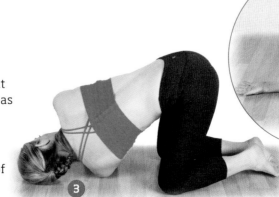

SWITCH SIDES AND REPEAT.

Roll Sequence

LOOSEN THE NOOSE

Action 1:

- **(1-2)** Lie on the floor and place the balls on either side of your upper trapezius–on the upper inner corners of the scapulae, at the top of the medial border. **(3)** Bridge your pelvis off the floor (with support from a block if needed) and sustain compression for 5 to 10 Abdominal-Thoracic Breaths.

- **(4-5)** CrossFiber your trapezius by using your feet to create a push-and-pull action that travels through your whole body. Your upper shoulders will chug over the balls, and your head will "nod" as a result.

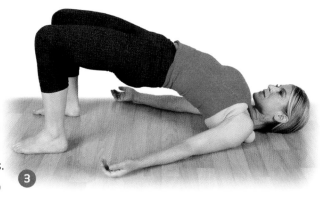

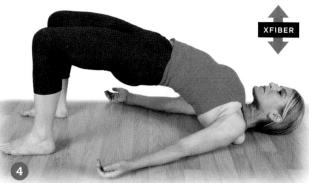

XFIBER

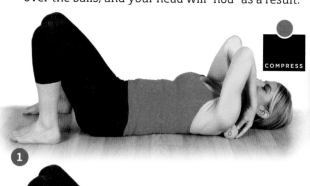

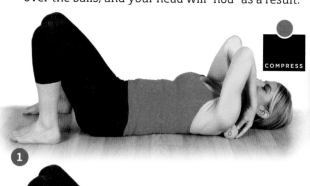

COMPRESS

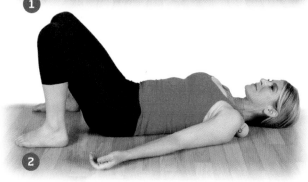

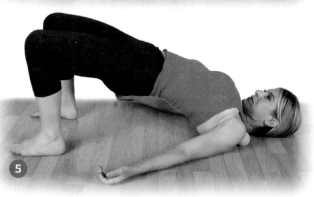

Action 2:

Let your upper-body mass continue to collect into the balls and reach your hands toward the ceiling, allowing them to float as if you were underwater. Contract your upper trapezius and shrug your shoulders into the balls, then relax. Repeat 3 times.

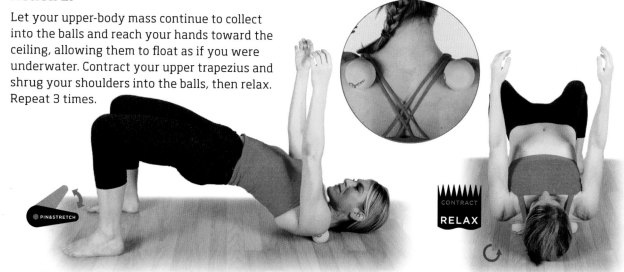

PIN&STRETCH

CONTRACT

RELAX

Action 3:

- Initiate pin & stretch combined with stripping by waving your arms from side to side and scrolling the balls into the "shelf" of your shoulder tissues. Your arms should move lightly as if they were underwater, like swishing seaweed. Use your ribcage to help maneuver the balls over as much upper-shoulder territory as possible.

- If the pressure is too intense, take your balls to the wall.

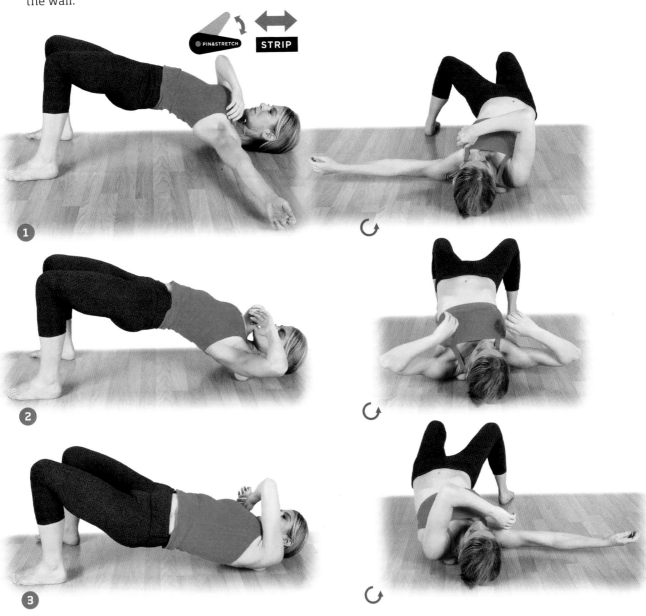

UNZIP THE BONY CORSET

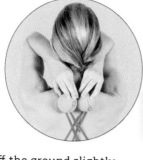

- **(1)** Lower your body and reset the Original YTU or PLUS Balls on either side of your spine, just below C-7. **(2)** Cradle your head in your hands, and lift your head and pelvis off the ground slightly so that only your feet are in contact with the ground. **(3)** Use the pressure of your feet to create a small push-and-pull motion that drags the balls and strips up and down your back in an approximately 2- to 3-inch range.

- **(4-5)** Lean your body more deeply into the left ball while stripping a few strokes, then deeper into the right ball for a few strokes. (Feel the difference between the two sides of your rhomboids and erectors.)

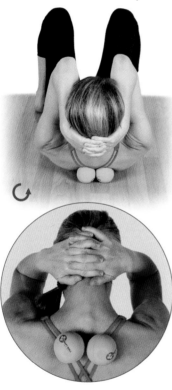

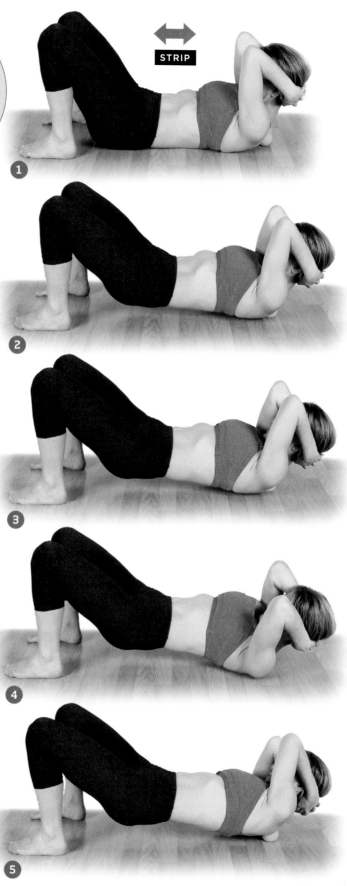

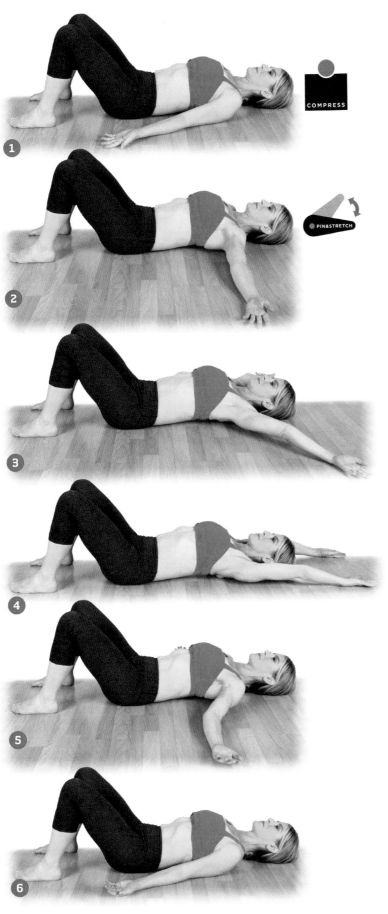

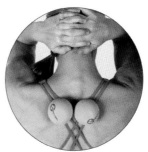

SNOW ANGEL ARMS

- **(1)** Shift your side-by-side balls a bit lower on your spine so that they are between the scapulae at the very top of the medial border (in the T-3/T-4 area). Place your head and pelvis on the ground. (If you lack a lot of extension in your upper back, you may need to place a pillow or folded towel underneath your head to reduce the pressure on your neck.) Rest with 5 deep Thoracic Breaths.

- **(2-6)** Initiate a grand pin & stretch by swiping your arms out to the sides along the floor and all the way up over your head, as if you were making snow angels.

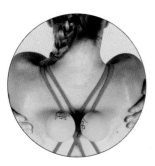

PUPPET ARMS + HUG ROLL

Action 1:

Slide the balls down your spine 1 more inch. They will land on either side of your spine at T-5/T-6. Continue to let your body weight compress the balls while breathing thoracically. **(1)** Reach your hands up toward the ceiling and separate your shoulder blades on a huge inhale. **(2)** On the exhale, contract your shoulder blades against the balls as if you were trying to crack them like walnuts. **(3)** Inhale and reach to the ceiling again, then **(4)** exhale and contract. Do this 8 more times, as if your hands were connected to puppet strings pulling you up toward the ceiling again and again.

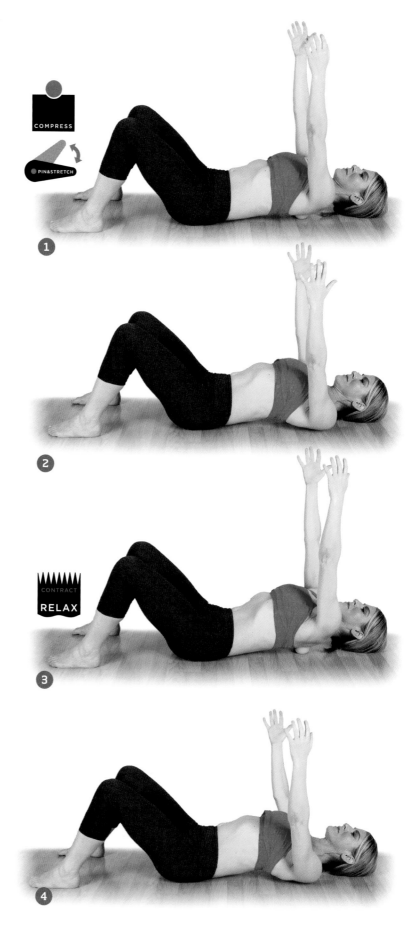

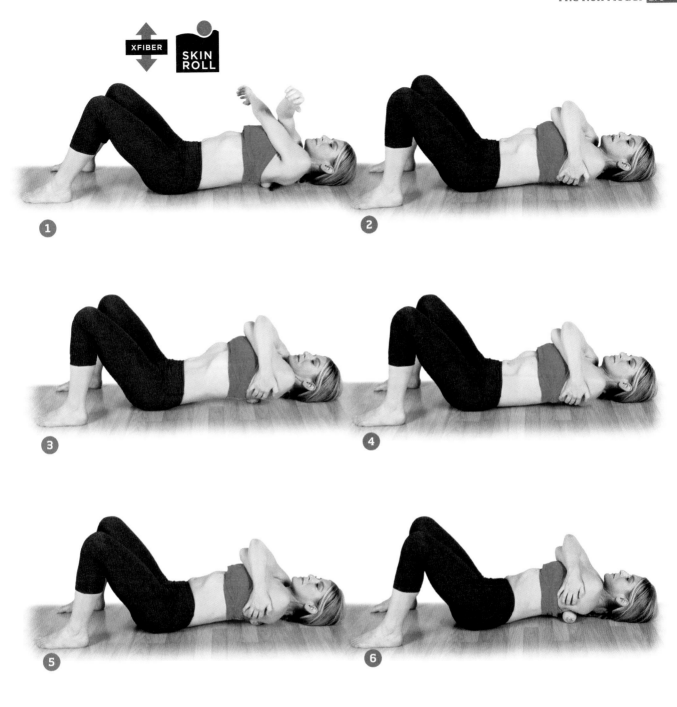

Action 2:

(1) Wrap your arms around your ribs and give yourself a hug. (2) If you have the reach, hold onto the inner edges of your shoulder blades. (3) Begin to increase the size of your Thoracic Breaths as if you were crushing the balls with the exaggerated breaths. (4-7) Maintain this as you wiggle from side to side, hugging, skin-rolling, and CrossFibering all the tissues of your upper back. In the Hug Roll, you roll the balls from shoulder blade to shoulder blade in a "fake makeout session."

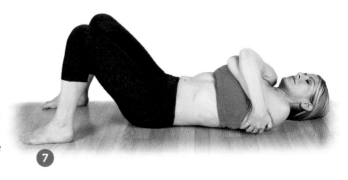

RESUSCITATE BREATH

(1) Strip the balls down your back until they land on either side of your spine around T-8/T-9, below the scapulae. They will rest on your bra strap or, as Katy Bowman says, the "bro strap" for men. This position happens with no rolling, just an intense internal breath sequence:

(2) Inhale a massive ribcage breath.

(3) Exhale and eliminate all the breath from your body by squeezing your ribs together, compressing all layers of abdominal tissue, flattening the balls underneath you, and zipping your pubic bone toward your ribs.

Relax and allow your next inhale to rush in naturally, "resuscitating" you.

Allow your next exhale to exit passively.

Perform all breath steps again. Do 5 complete rounds of this breath strategy. Each round involves 2 distinct breath cycles. The first has an active inhale and an extremely active exhale, and the second has a passive inhale and a passive exhale.

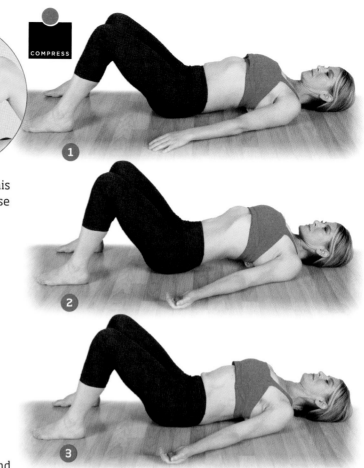

KNEE TO CHEST

- (1) Straighten both legs and help the balls roll down 1 more inch so that they land on either side of your spine at T-10/T-11. (2) Draw your right knee in toward your chest and create a slow bouncing action with your thigh. This is a subtle, not aggressive, pull and release that ricochets an up-and-down movement into the balls. Bounce your knee for about a minute with Abdominal-Thoracic Breathing before (3) switching sides.

- Remove the balls and rest for a few Abdominal-Thoracic Breaths before you perform your ReCheck.

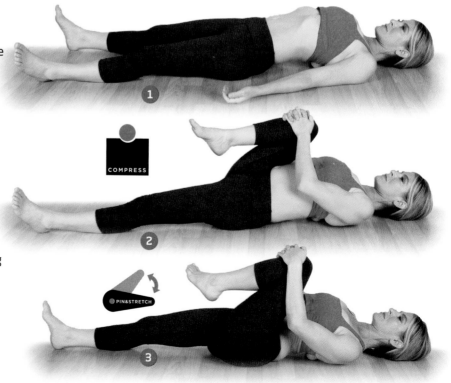

ReCheck:
Thread the Needle

Reset your stretch and notice any changes in your breath access and upper-back rotation. Also assess your level of relaxation.

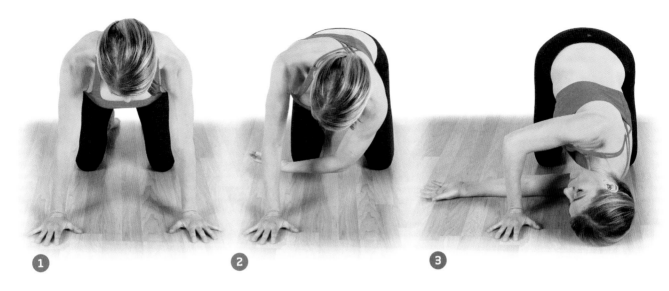

Reflect

1. Notice the contact of your upper back to the floor–has it changed?

2. How does it feel stand up? Is holding great posture easier or more awkward?

3. Finish this statement: I feel _____.

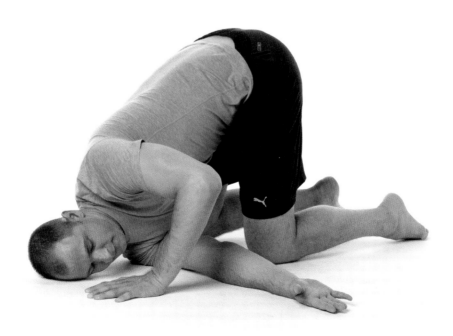

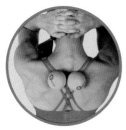

Sequence 10:
Ribcage Rinse & Respire

Setup

Roll Model Balls:
Original YTU,
PLUS

Wall corner

EmbodyMap

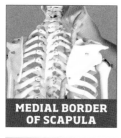

MEDIAL BORDER OF SCAPULA

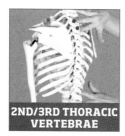

2ND/3RD THORACIC VERTEBRAE

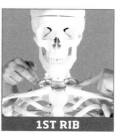

CLAVICLE

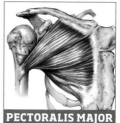

1ST RIB

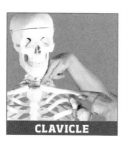

PECTORALIS MAJOR

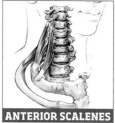

ANTERIOR SCALENES

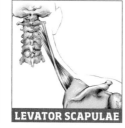

LEVATOR SCAPULAE

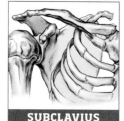

SUBCLAVIUS

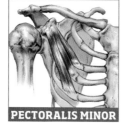

PECTORALIS MINOR

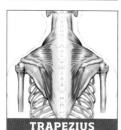

TRAPEZIUS

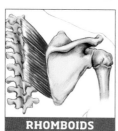

RHOMBOIDS

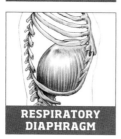

ERECTOR SPINAE

RESPIRATORY DIAPHRAGM

Basic Ball Stops

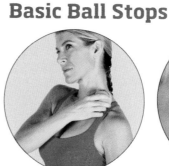

Supraclavicular area

Coracoid process/ pectoralis minor

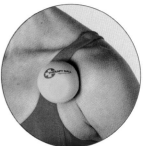

Levator scapula attachment

Trapezius/ rhomboid seam

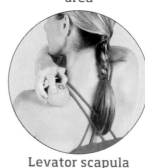

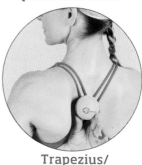

Subclavius

Bra/"bro" strap area

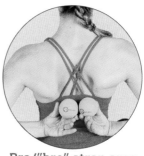

Check In: Abdominal-Thoracic Breath

- (1) Practice Abdominal-Thoracic Breathing by placing one hand on your abdomen and the other on your chest. (Once you have mastered sensing that these areas move as you breathe into them, you will no longer need to place your hands on your body; you can leave your arms resting comfortably at your sides.)

- (2) Feel your belly expand first, then your ribcage like a giant soft-tissue balloon, followed by both areas emptying. Your hands will rise and fall with each inflation and deflation.

- Take 5 to 10 complete breaths.

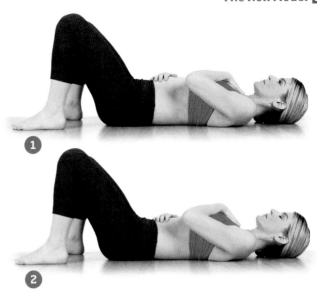

Roll Sequence

SUBCLAVICLE DETANGLE
Action 1:

- (1) Place any size ball on a wall corner or doorway and pin your left subclavius to the ball. (2) Move your torso from side to side to strip all along the underside of your clavicle to target your subclavius and pec minor.

- (3-4) Place your hand on the wall above your head and bend and straighten your knees to scrub the ball across the fibers of your pec minor, directly next to your armpit.

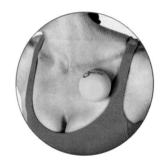

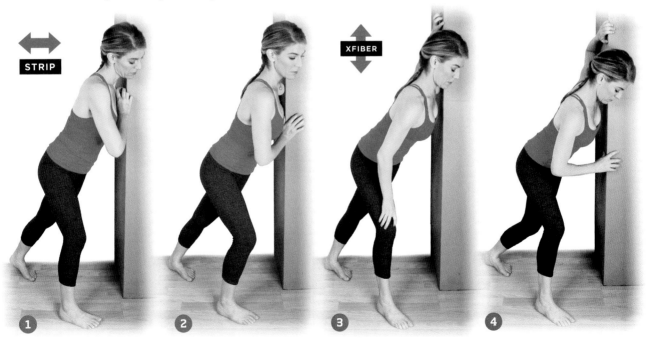

Action 2:

(1–3) Use your right hand to spin the ball into any of the tissues you've been rolling. (4–5) Once you've tightly wound up those tissues, mobilize your neck by turning your head to the right and moving it in as many directions as possible. Wind the ball again and grab even more slack.

SWITCH SIDES AND REPEAT ACTIONS 1 AND 2.

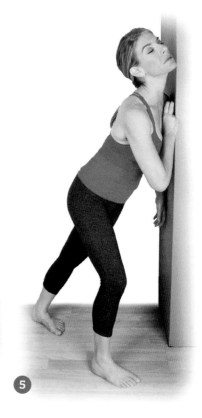
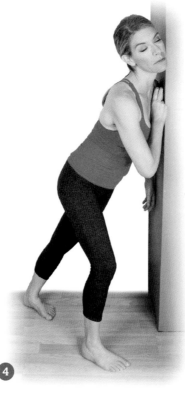
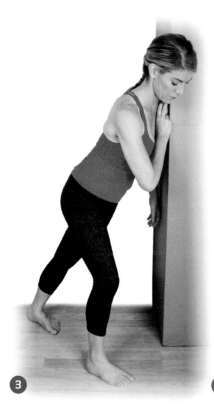
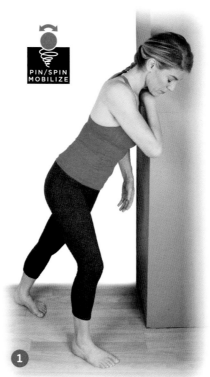
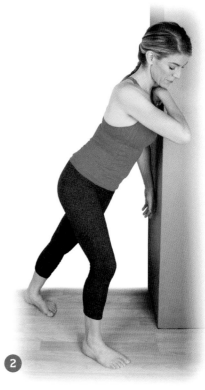

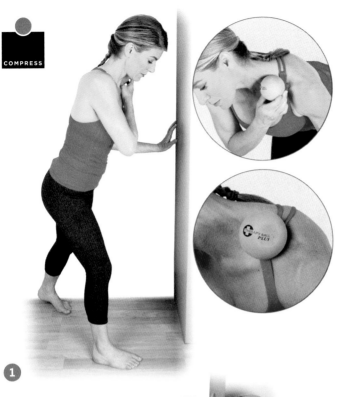

SUPRACLAVICLE SOFTENER
Action 1:

(1-2) Travel the ball above your clavicle and rest it directly on the soft-tissue triangle above your collarbone. (2) Hinge at your hips in order to pin the ball to the wall, making sure that your head is clear of the wall.

(3-7) Take several Thoracic Breaths, then begin a variety of pin & stretch moves that travel your left arm and shoulder behind your back, around the doorjamb/corner.

(8) Then keep the ball pinned in place and stretch your neck by turning it to the right and looking up or down.

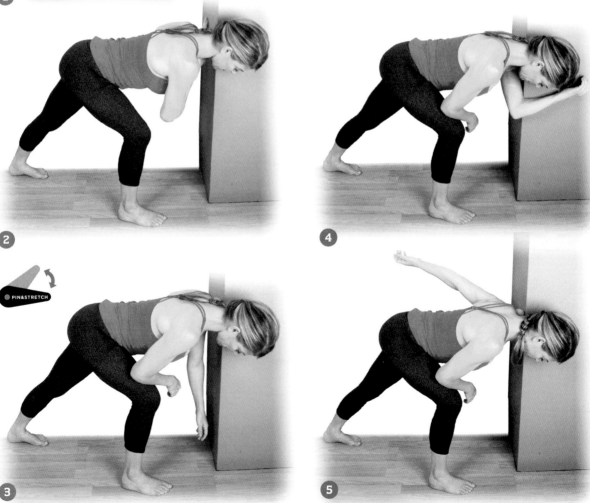

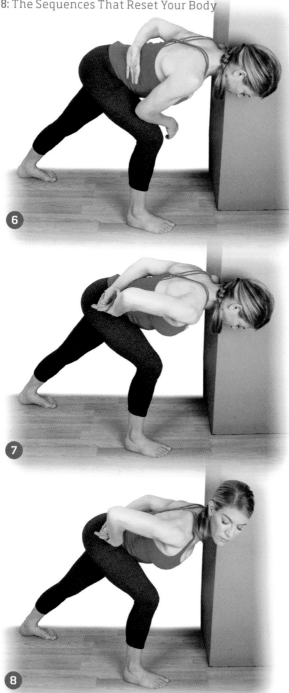

6

7

8

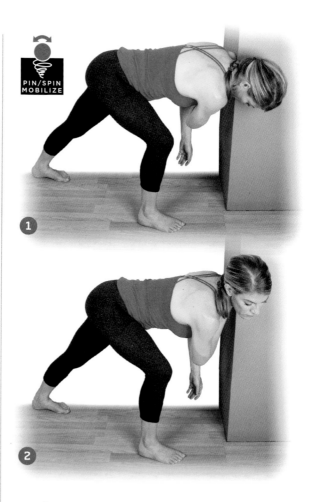

PIN/SPIN MOBILIZE

1

2

Action 2:

Use your right hand to pin & spin the ball while you remobilize your left shoulder, neck, and first rib. Continue to scroll the ball into the supraclavicle area, foraging for areas of tension. Then wind it in the opposite direction.

SWITCH SIDES AND REPEAT ACTIONS 1 AND 2.

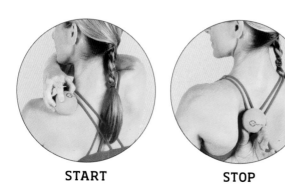

START   **STOP**

TRAPEZIUS TAMER

This movement travels the ball across the fibers of your trapezius and rhomboids. The ball always moves between the upper inner corner of your shoulder blade, at the levator scapula tendon (the medial superior border of the scapula), and travels at an angle down to the third/fourth thoracic vertebrae without crossing over your spine. (The ball literally traces the angle of the straps on my tank top.)

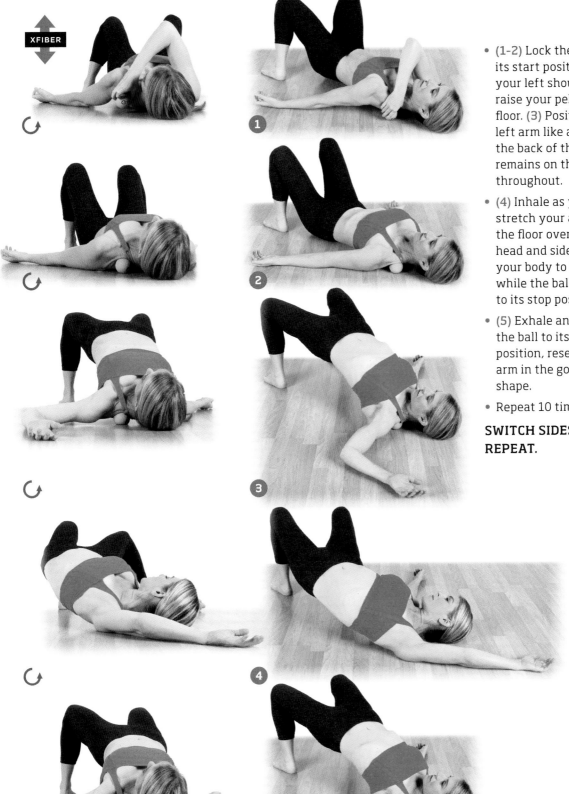

- **(1-2)** Lock the ball into its start position at your left shoulder, and raise your pelvis off the floor. **(3)** Position your left arm like a goalpost; the back of that arm remains on the floor throughout.

- **(4)** Inhale as you stretch your arm along the floor over your head and side-bend your body to the right while the ball travels to its stop position.

- **(5)** Exhale and return the ball to its start position, resetting your arm in the goalpost shape.

- Repeat 10 times.

SWITCH SIDES AND REPEAT.

SKIN ROLL ⟷ **STRIP**

CARESS WAVE

- **(1–3)** Lie on your back and cradle your head with your hands. Lift your pelvis and head off the floor so that your upper back can balance on the balls. Place any size balls on either side of your spine beginning at about T-2, and **(4–5)** slowly roll them down your spine, stripping the erectors until you land at the T-8 (bra/"bro" strap) area. This is a super-slow-motion action—a long, luxurious, deep caress wave. **(6)** Then reverse the motion and return to T-2. Do this slow wave 3 or 4 times.

- If you have a difficult time getting the balls to roll, use a serpentine action by leaning your ribcage from side to side. Another way to promote the motion is to walk your feet toward your body to help push the balls down your back, then walk your feet away from your body to help the balls track back up your spine. Alternatively, you can do this against a wall or with toted balls.

TOTE OPTION

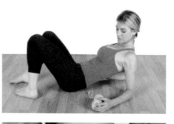

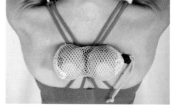

RHOMBOID RINGER

- **(1)** Lodge the 2 balls anywhere between your shoulder blades, keeping your head and pelvis off the floor. **(2-3)** Initiate active skin-rolling combined with a pin/spin & mobilize motion by bending your ribcage and spine from side to side.

- Increase the shear by pinning the balls underneath your back and attempt to walk your feet as far to one side as you can while the balls retain their grip on your tissues. Breathe deeply into your ribs to mobilize, then reverse your spin. This will deeply shear all upper-back myofascial layers (not pictured).

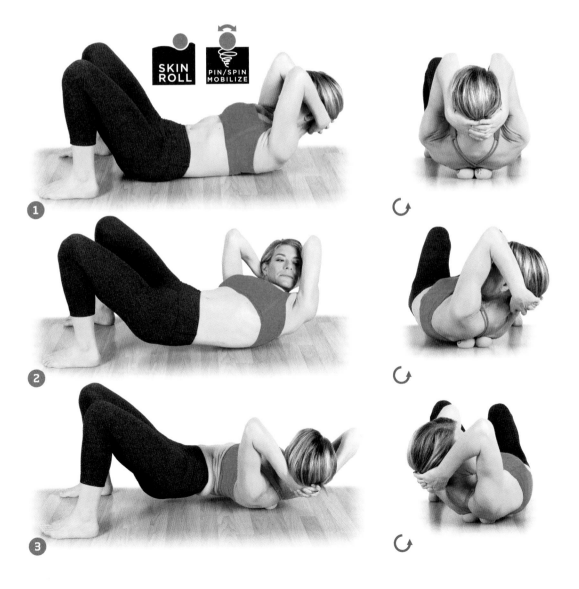

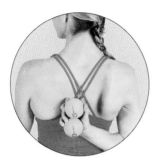

RIB ROCK

(1-2) Place 2 balls vertically against the left side of your spine within your upper back. (3-4) Wrap your left arm across your chest, then (5) hug your right arm across. (6) Inhale into your ribs and simultaneously pull your ribcage toward the left, using the balls as a pivot point on which to hinge and wedging the balls more deeply against your vertebrae. Exhale and return to center. Do this 8 to 10 times slowly.

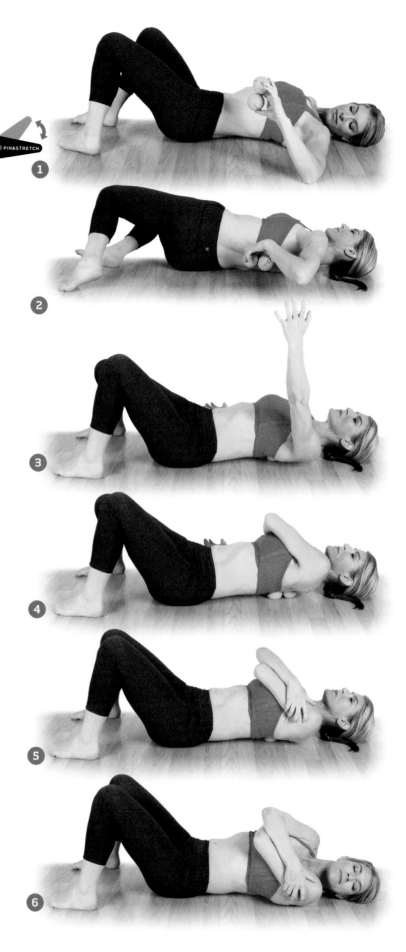

RESUSCITATE BREATH

- **(1)** Strip the balls down your back until they land on either side of your spine at around T-8/T-9 (your bra/"bro" strap area). This exposition happens with no rolling, just an intense internal breath sequence:

  (2) Inhale a massive ribcage breath.

  (3) Exhale and eliminate all the breath from your body by squeezing your ribs together, compressing all layers of abdominal tissue, flattening the balls underneath you, and zipping your pubic bone toward your ribs.

  Relax and allow your next inhale to rush in naturally, "resuscitating" you.

  Allow your next exhale to exit passively.

  Perform all breath steps again. Do 5 complete rounds of this breath strategy.

- Remove the balls and rest, then move on to your ReCheck.

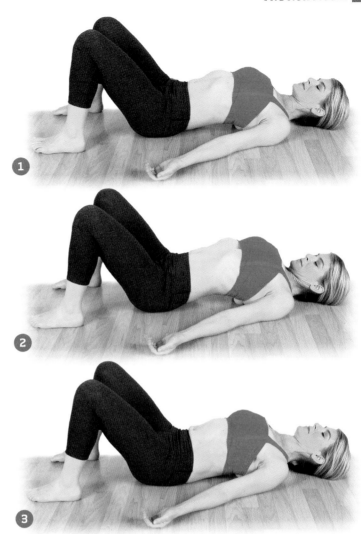

ReCheck: Abdominal-Thoracic Breath

Reset your body to perform Abdominal-Thoracic Breathing. Observe your ability to inflate and deflate your abdomen and chest. Notice your breath's access into the back of your ribs, as well as the rise and fall of your sternum. Notice the quality of relaxation in your body.

Reflect

1. Describe the quality of your breathing.

2. Arch your spine in every possible way and reflect on how it feels to have more upper spinal motion.

3. Finish this statement: I feel

   _____.

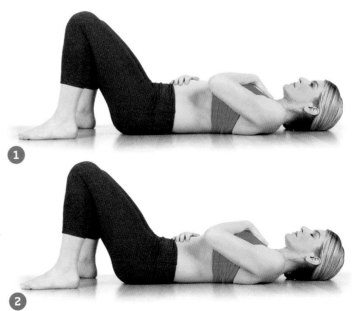

Sequences for Shoulders to Fingers

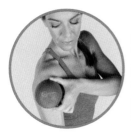

Sequence 11: Shoulder - Rotator Cuff

Setup

Roll Model Balls: Original YTU, PLUS, ALPHA

Mat

Block or wall

Stretch strap or belt

EmbodyMap

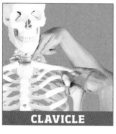
CLAVICLE

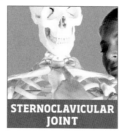
STERNOCLAVICULAR JOINT

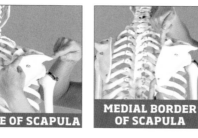
SPINE OF SCAPULA

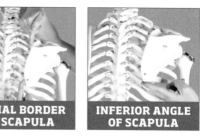
MEDIAL BORDER OF SCAPULA

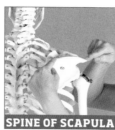
INFERIOR ANGLE OF SCAPULA

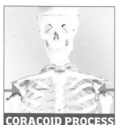
CORACOID PROCESS

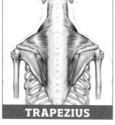
TRAPEZIUS

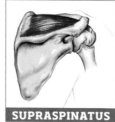
SUPRASPINATUS

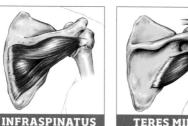
INFRASPINATUS

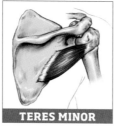
TERES MINOR

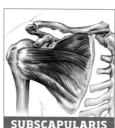
SUBSCAPULARIS

Check In: Shoulder Flossing

- (1) Stand with impeccable posture (see page 84) and hold a strap or belt taut across your hips between your palms, with your palms facing behind you. Your hands will be 2 to 3 feet apart, depending on your shoulder range of motion.

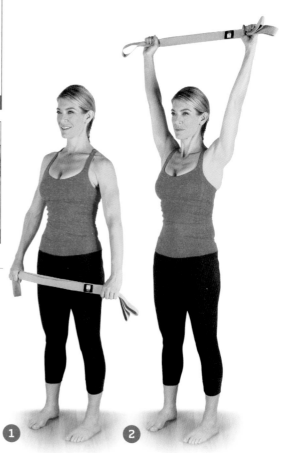

1   2

Basic Ball Stops

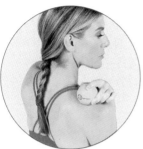

Supraspinatus

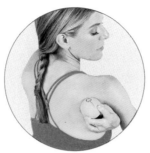

Infraspinatus/
teres minor

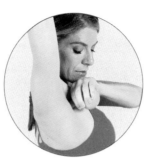

Armpit/
subscapularis

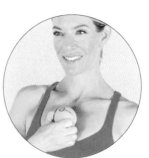

Sternum

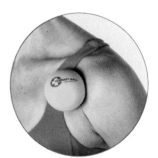

Pec minor/
coracoid process

- (2) Reach the strap overhead and (3-4) roll your left shoulder into internal rotation, which will expose the head of the humerus. Your left hand will drop behind your shoulder, directly behind your upper back.

- (5) Reset your left shoulder by externally rotating it, and then (6-7) roll your right shoulder into internal rotation. Your right hand will drop behind your shoulder, directly behind your upper back.

- Create a dynamic rhythm of rolling through each shoulder and "flossing" around the head of the humerus. Repeat 5 times on each side.

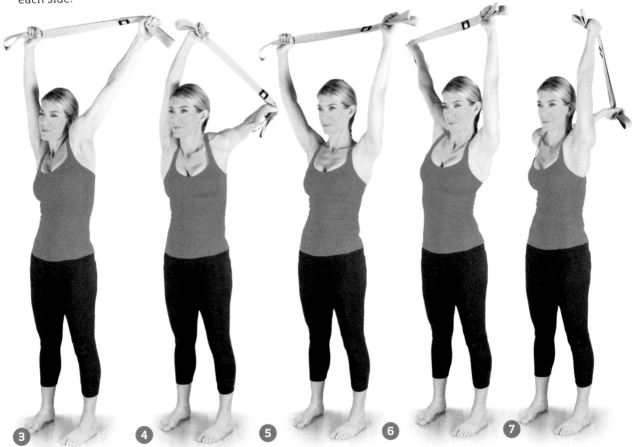

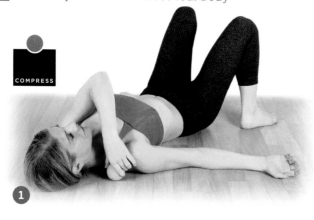

COMPRESS

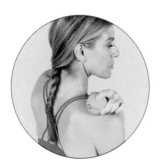

GUTTER-BALL

Action 1:

- (1) Lie on your back and place a ball on your right supraspinatus. (2) Bridge your pelvis off the floor to load the ball with your body weight.

- (3-4) Take several deep breaths, then slowly begin to shift from side to side so that the ball strips the supraspinatus (and the trapezius that lies superficial to it). Do not track the ball into your neck; stay in the region of your upper shoulder blade, above the spine of the scapula.

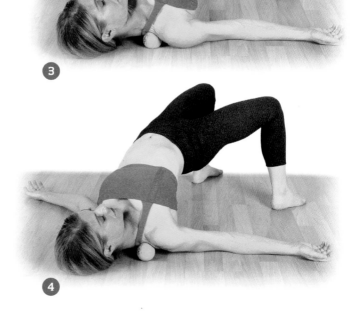

STRIP

Action 2:

Simultaneously pin & stretch and contract/relax by drawing a big half-circle on the floor with your right hand, as if you were making a snow angel. The ball remains pinned, and your shoulder moves through its range of abduction and also rotation if that is available to you. Make 8 snow angels.

SWITCH SIDES AND REPEAT ACTIONS 1 AND 2.

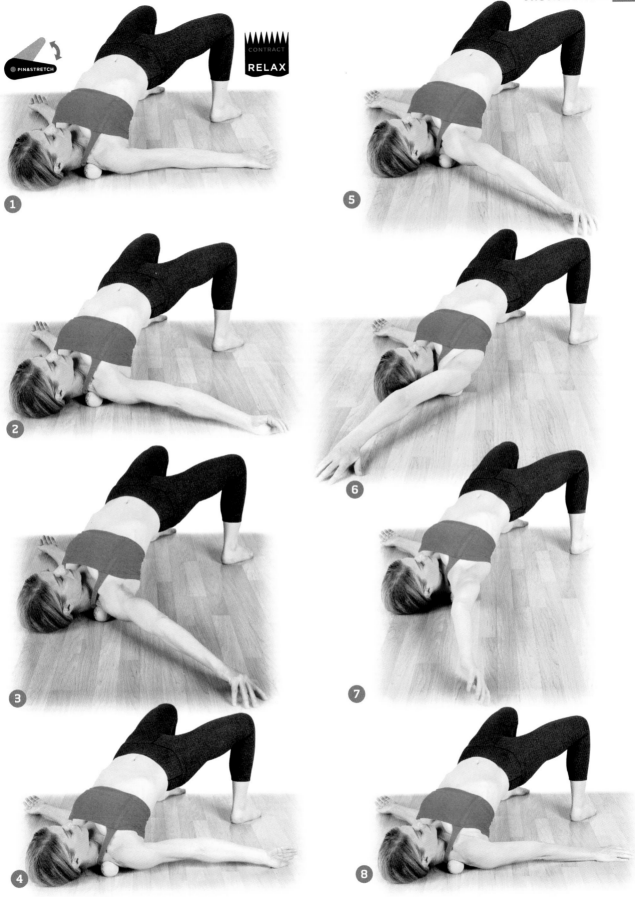

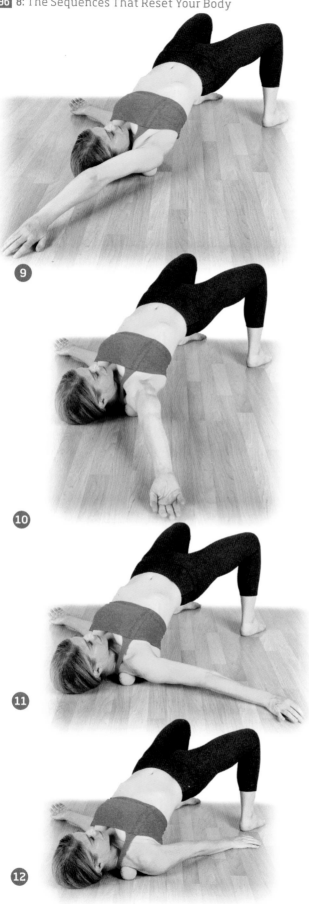

9

10

11

12

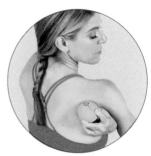

ROTATION REMEDY

Action 1:

- (1) Place a ball on the back of your right shoulder blade below the spine of the scapula and lean your body toward the ball. Breathe deeply.

- (2–5) Strip your infraspinatus and teres minor by moving from side to side, keeping the ball within the boundaries of the triangle-shaped scapula.

- (6–7) CrossFiber those same muscles by using your feet to create a mild thrusting action that rolls the ball up and down your scapula.

COMPRESS

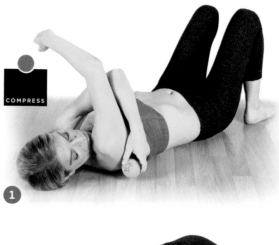

1

2

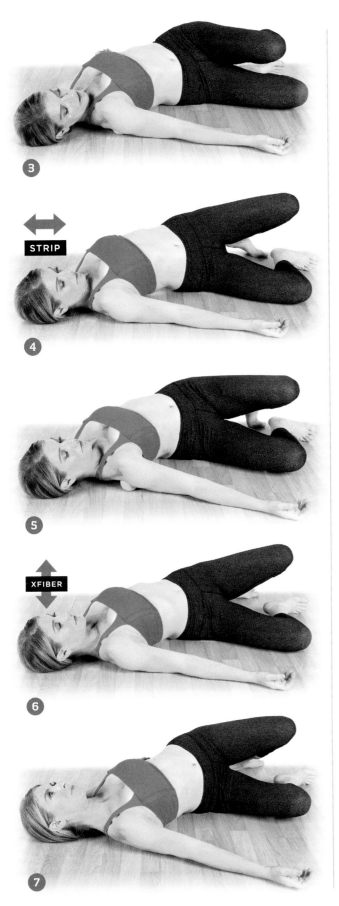

Action 2:

Pin & stretch those same muscles by loosely waving your right arm around like seaweed, traveling through every possible direction.

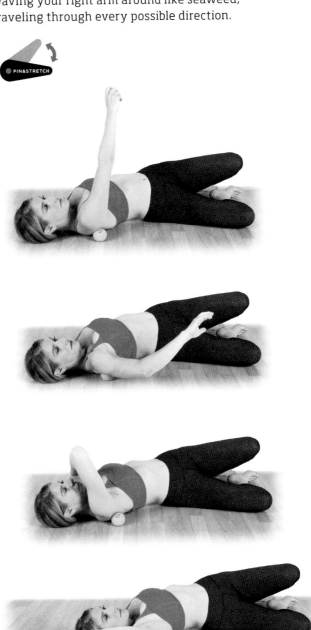

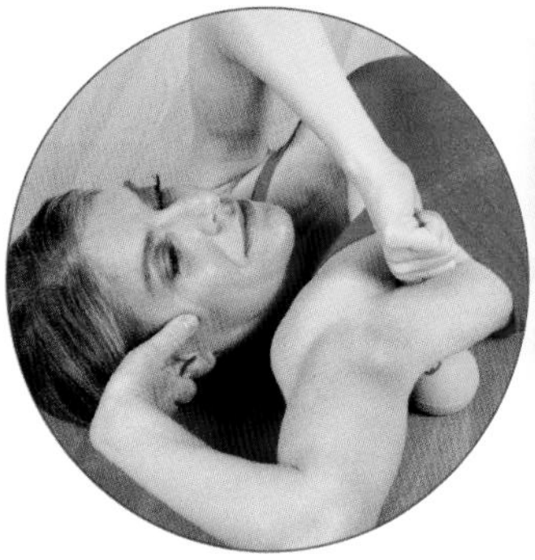

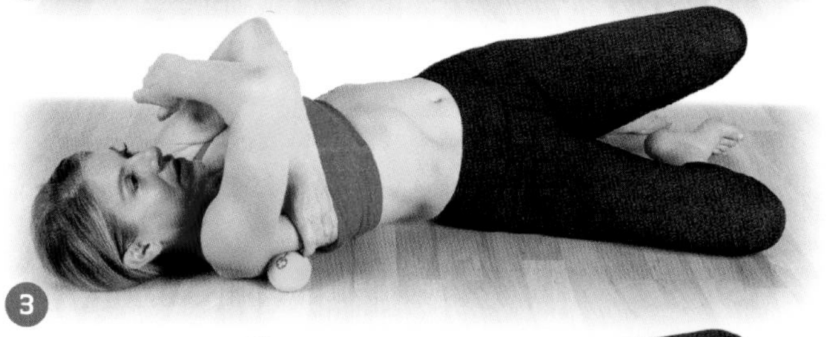

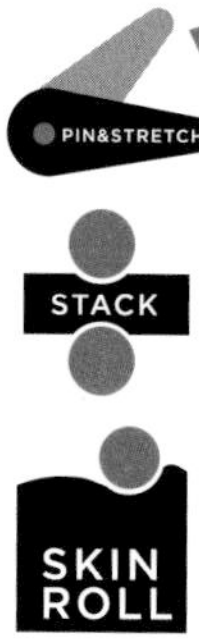

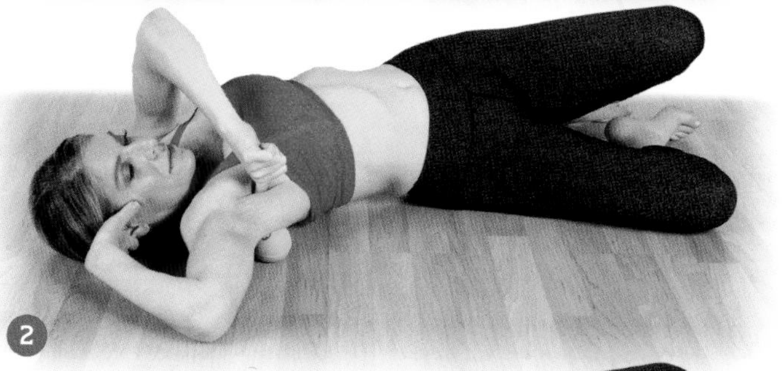

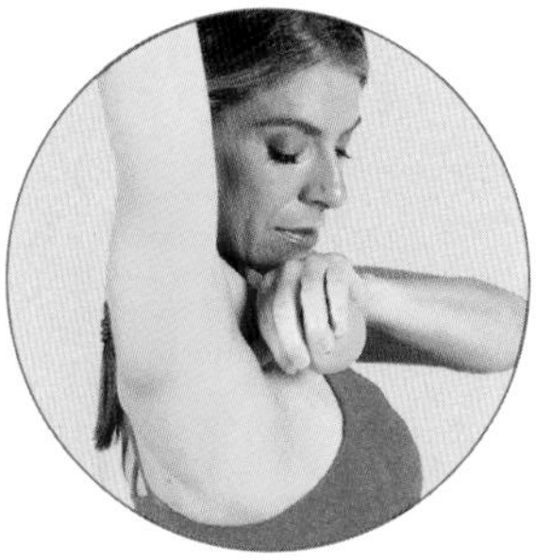

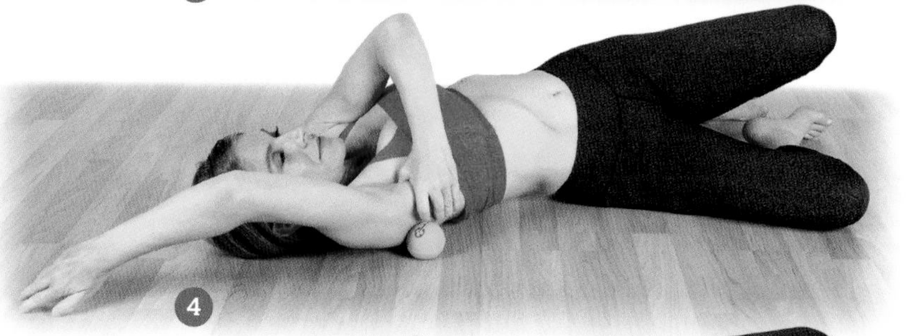

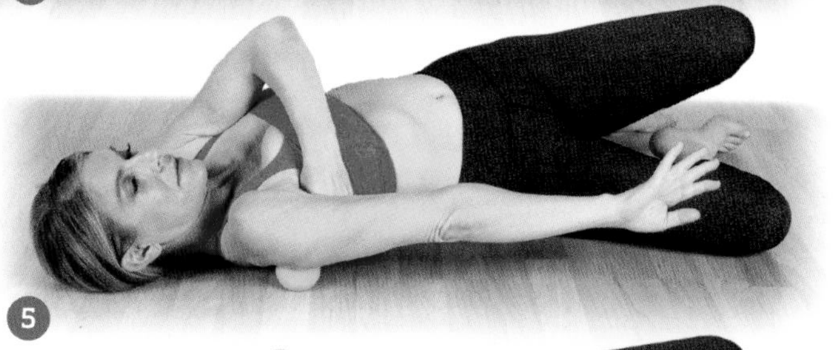

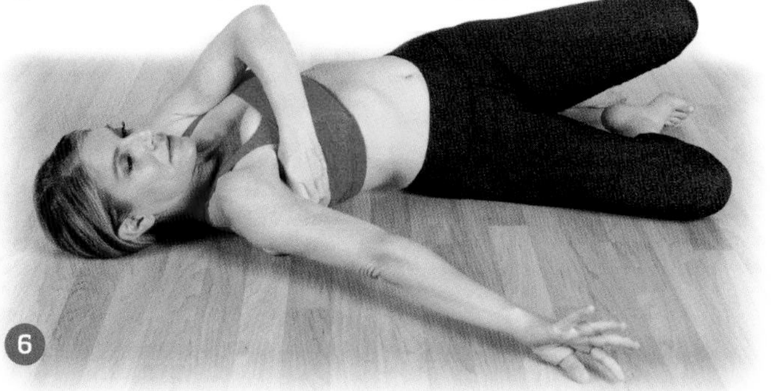

PIN&STRETCH

STACK

SKIN ROLL

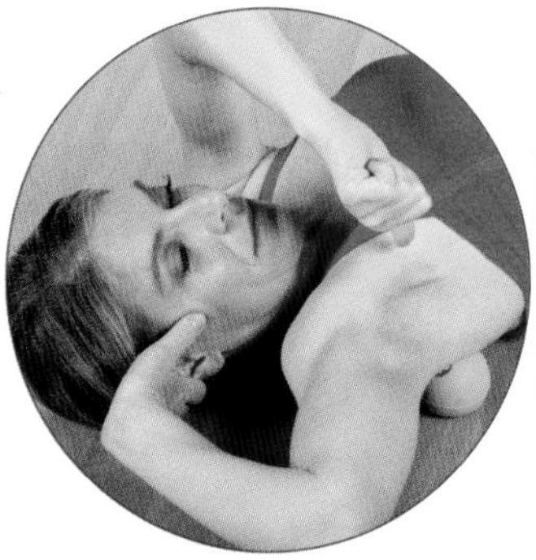

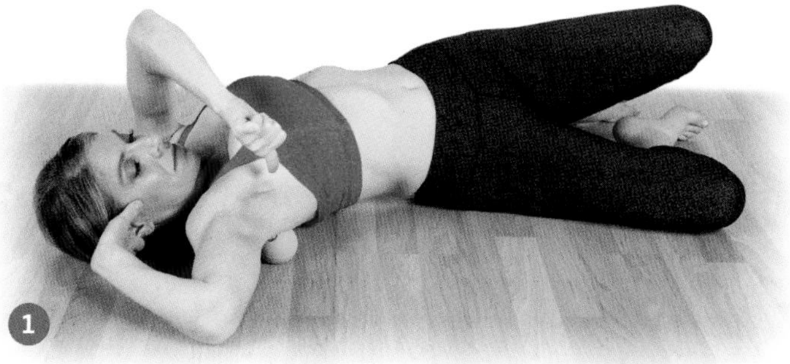

Action 3:

(1) Drive your left thumb deep into your armpit to pin your subscapularis. Push past the latissimus dorsi, and look for the space between your ribcage and the front surface of your scapula for the subscapularis muscle.
(2-9) Continue all actions listed above in Action 2.

SWITCH SIDES AND REPEAT ACTIONS 1-3.

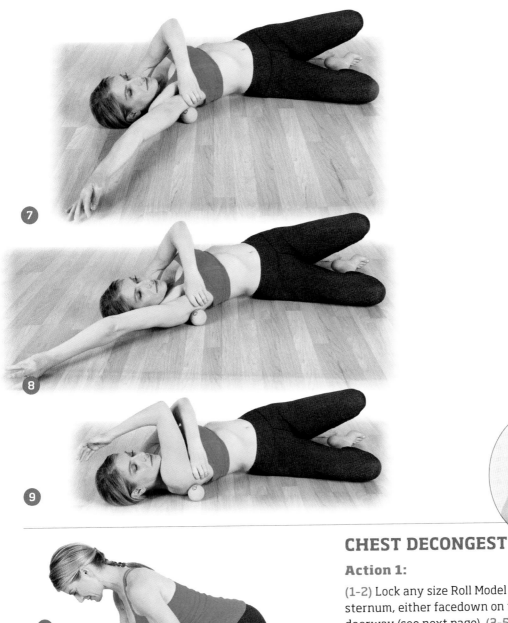

CHEST DECONGEST

Action 1:

(1-2) Lock any size Roll Model Ball against your sternum, either facedown on the floor or against a doorway (see next page). (3-5) Pin & spin the ball against the skin of your sternum and gather as much tissue as possible, then mobilize by moving your neck, shoulders, or ribcage in any direction to effect slide & glide. Gather more slack and mobilize again, then find another spot on your sternum and repeat. This affects all the pectoralis major fascial tissues and the intercostals.

COMPRESS

PIN/SPIN MOBILIZE

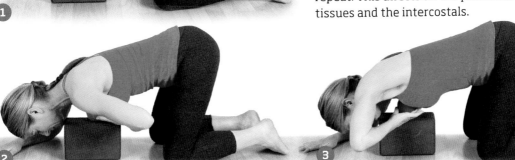

More Options

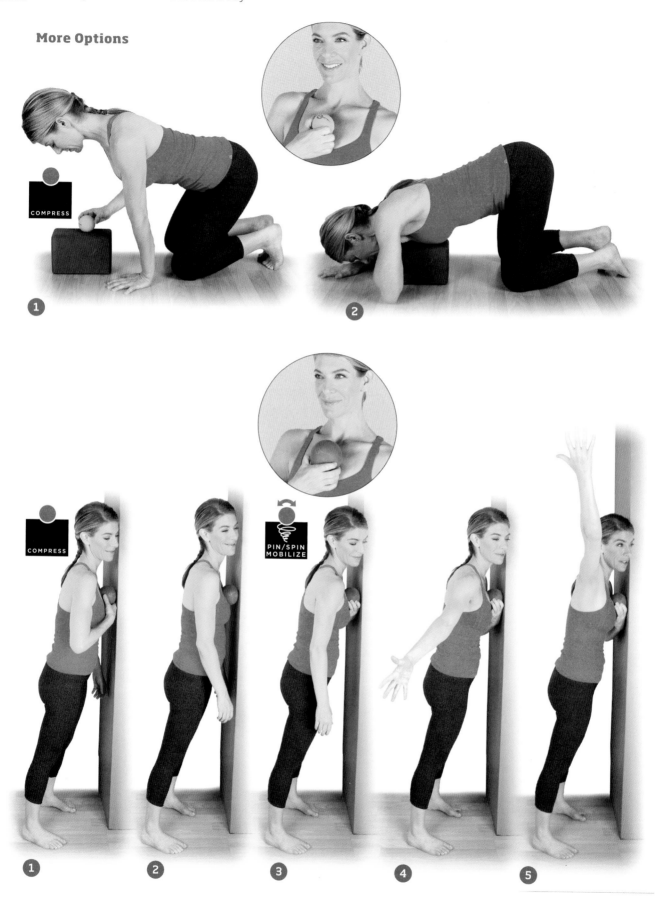

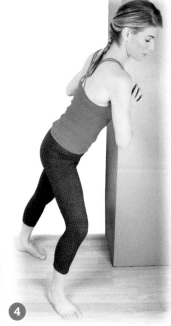

Action 2:

- (1-2) Place the ball underneath your left clavicle and lean into the wall. (3-4) Strip the entire area underneath your collarbone and into the edge of your chest near your shoulder (pec minor). Stroke from side to side, increasing the pressure as needed. (5-7) Then pin & stretch by trapping the ball in place and moving your shoulder, arm, or neck in any available direction.

STRIP

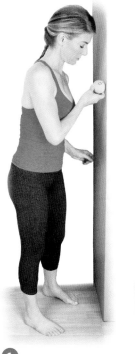

1

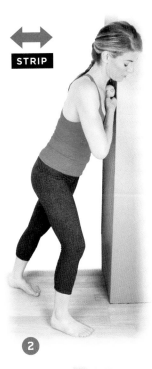

2

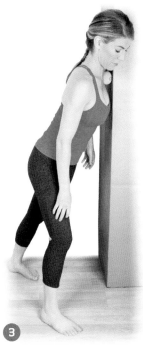

3

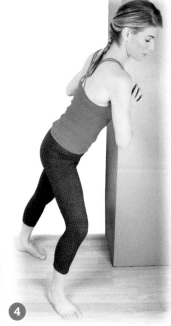

4

PIN&STRETCH

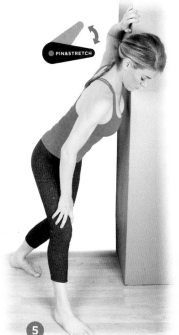

5

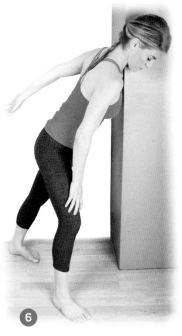

6

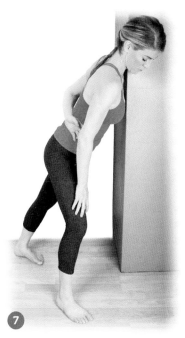

7

• **(8-10)** Accelerate the depth of penetration by pinning & spinning the ball into the same tissues, followed by mobilizing your neck, shoulder, or arm.

SWITCH SIDES AND REPEAT ACTIONS 1 AND 2.

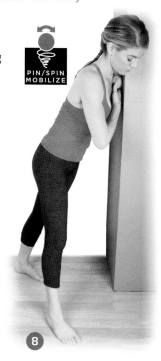

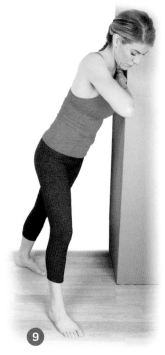

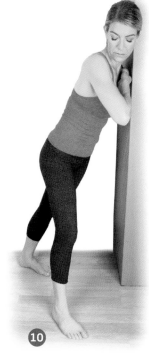

ReCheck: Shoulder Flossing

ReCheck your shoulder mobility by tracking your shoulders through their range of motion again. Notice if your shoulders glide more freely than before.

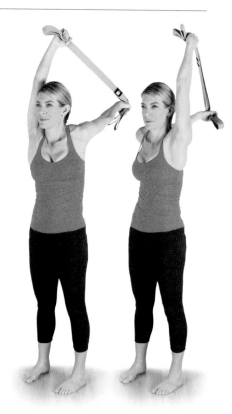

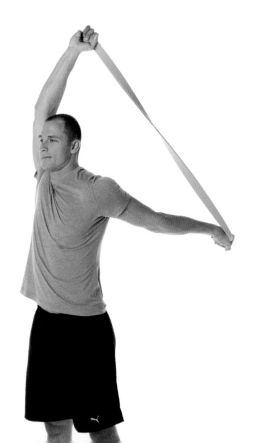

Reflect

1. Look in the mirror. Are your shoulders even? Are they lower or higher than normal?

2. Try walking your fingers and hands up the back of your body as if you were scratching an itch. How high do they climb?

3. Finish this statement: I feel _____.

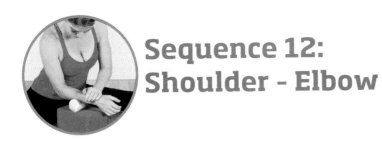

Sequence 12: Shoulder - Elbow

Setup

Roll Model Balls: Original YTU, PLUS, or ALPHA Twins in tote

Mat

Block

Wall corner or doorway

EmbodyMap

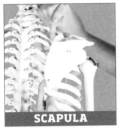

SCAPULA

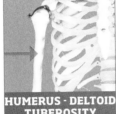

HUMERUS - DELTOID TUBEROSITY

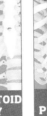

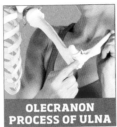

OLECRANON PROCESS OF ULNA

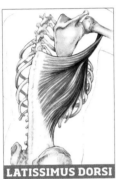

LATISSIMUS DORSI

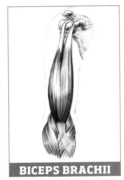

BICEPS BRACHII

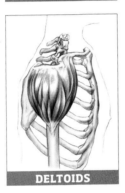

DELTOIDS

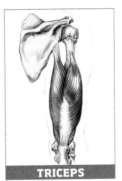

TRICEPS

Basic Ball Stops

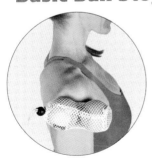

Deltoids

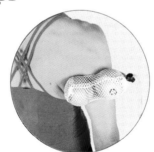

Triceps

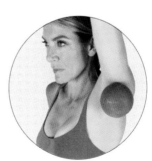

Latissimus start

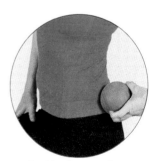

Latissimus stop

Check In:
Flexion & External Rotation of Shoulders

- (1) Stand with impeccable posture (see page 84) and spin your upper arms so that your palms are facing forward. Keep your abdominal and back muscles firm so that your spinal bones remain completely stable.

- (2-3) Sweep your arms upward toward the ceiling without letting your shoulders pivot inward. In other words, your palms should attempt to face the wall behind you. Note that your shoulder range in flexion might stop the movement before your arms are straight overhead. In that case, don't try to force your arms overhead; simply note where they stop.

- (4) Take 5 Abdominal-Thoracic Breaths, concentrating on maximizing your shoulders' end range of motion without letting your ribcage or spine change shape.

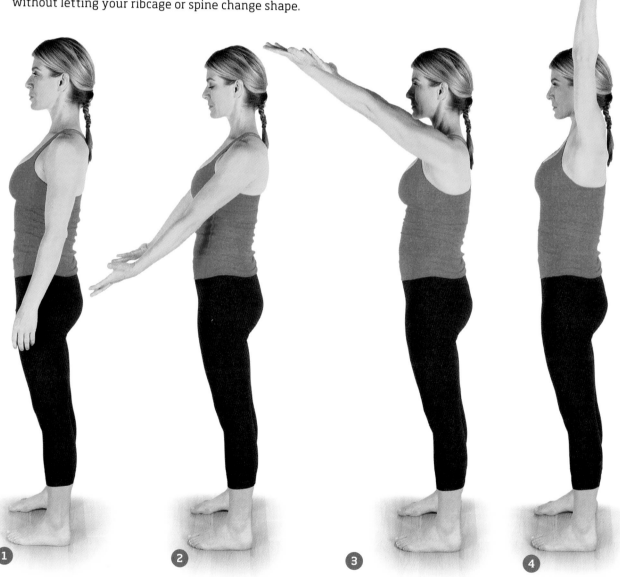

1   2   3   4

Roll Sequence
SHOULDER SHRINK-WRAP

Action 1:

(1) Lean into a wall with the toted balls on either side of your outer shoulder (medial deltoid). (2-4) Strip your deltoids by bending and straightening your knees.

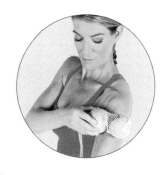

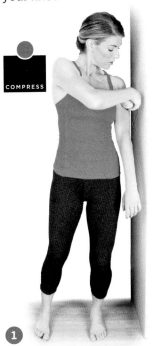

COMPRESS

STRIP

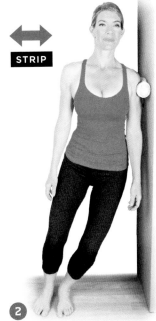

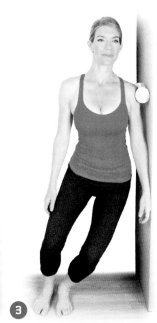

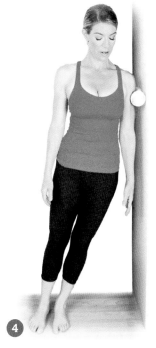

Action 2:

Actively contract your deltoids by pushing your hand into the wall, hold for a few seconds, then release. Repeat 5 to 8 times.

CONTRACT
RELAX

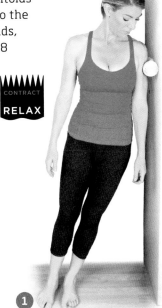

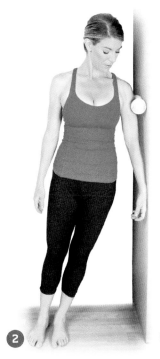

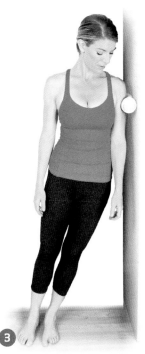

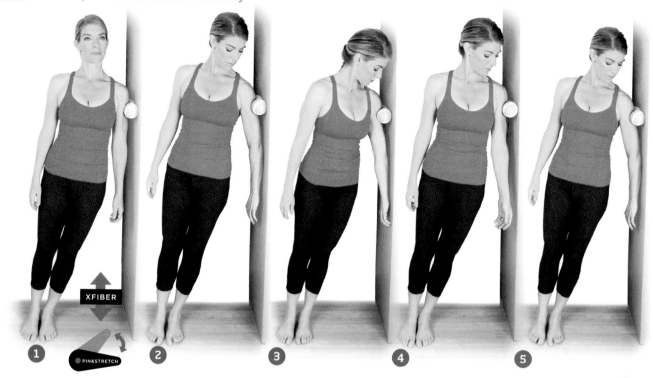

Action 3:

(1) Explore several CrossFiber and pin & stretch options by rotating your left shoulder in every possible way. (2-3) Externally rotate your shoulder as if you were hitchhiking. (4-5) Then internally rotate your shoulder and (6) bring the back of your hand to your low back. Keep constant pressure on the toted balls.

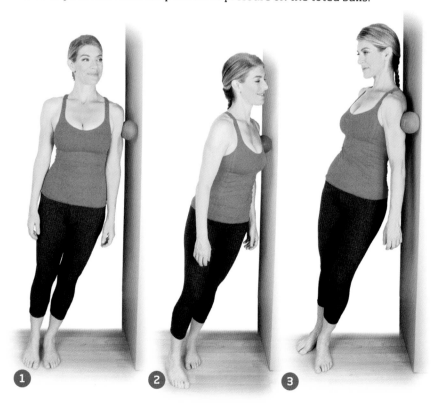

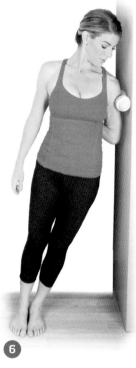

(1-3) This can be done with a single ALPHA Ball as well.

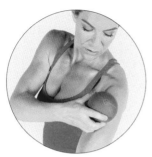

Action 4:

(1-2) Grab an Original YTU or ALPHA Ball and pin/spin & mobilize as many sections of deltoid tissue as you can. (3) Move your shoulder and arm in every direction, then deepen the coil of your spin. Reverse the direction of your spin and try new moves.

SWITCH SIDES AND REPEAT ACTIONS 1-4.

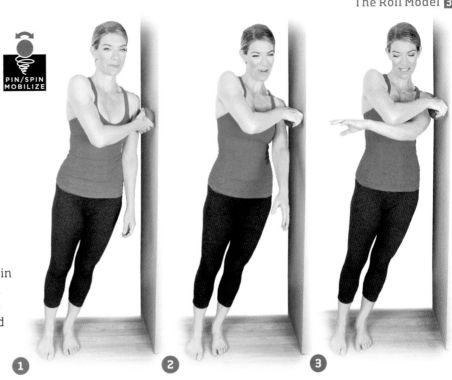

TRICEPS TREATMENT

Action 1:

(1) Tuck your toted balls on either side of the back of your upper shoulder (humerus). One ball will nuzzle into your lateral scapula. (2) Lean into the wall and take a few deep breaths. (3-4) Then strip your triceps by bending and straightening your knees. Do 8 to 12 stripping motions.

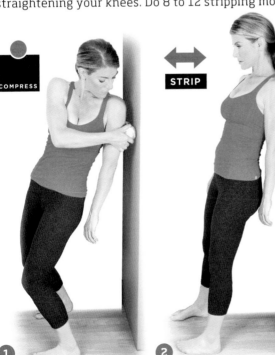

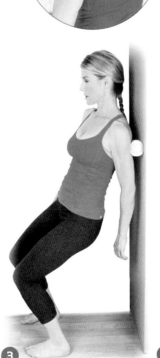

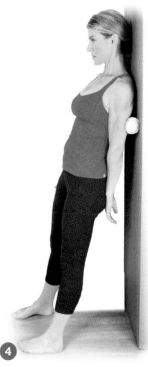

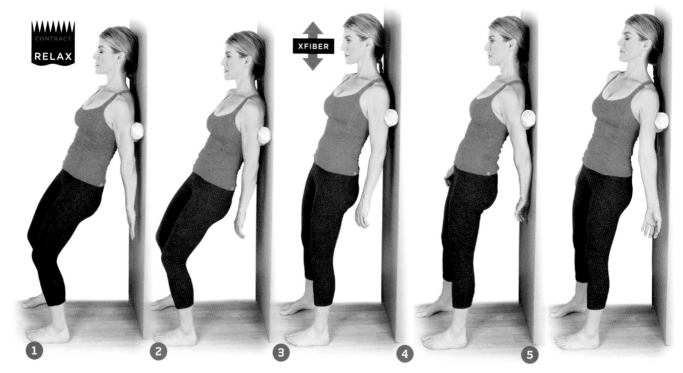

Action 2:

- (1-2) Activate your triceps by pushing your left palm into the wall. Hold the pressure for a few seconds, then release. Contract/relax your triceps 5 times.

- (3-5) CrossFiber those same tissues by spinning your shoulder in, then out. This tracks the mass of your triceps between the toted balls and massages across its line of pull.

Action 3:

Bend your elbow and maneuver the triceps junction just above your elbow into the balls. Depending on your angle, allow your forearm to press into the balls, too. You can also use your right hand to help drive more pressure into your left arm and the balls (not pictured).

SWITCH SIDES AND REPEAT ACTIONS 1-3.

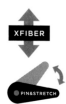

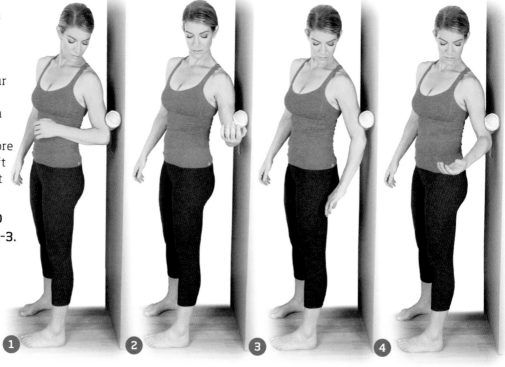

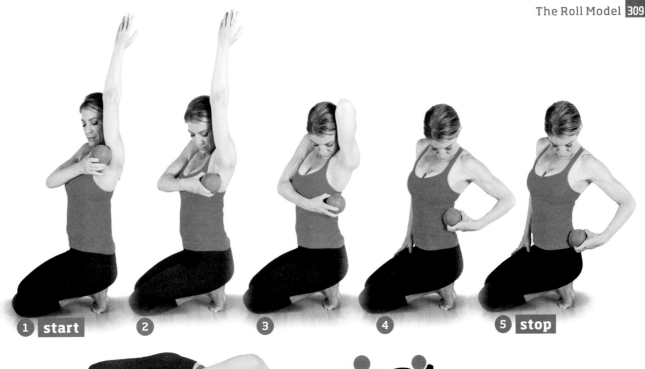

① start **②** **③** **④** **⑤ stop**

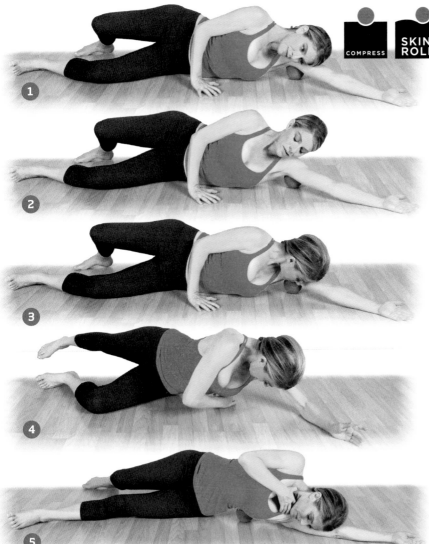

COMPRESS · **SKIN ROLL**

LAT SEAM

With the ALPHA, PLUS, or Original YTU Balls on the ground or against a wall:

- (1-5) To unstick your latissimus seam, navigate the span of the muscle between its "start" attachment on your humerus all the way to its "stop" in your low back. Intermix your Roll Model Balls, and use the floor or a wall, depending on your tolerance to the pressure. Utilize the different ball techniques in an attempt to resculpt more motion out of the interface of the latissimus and the tissues that lie beneath it (see images 1-14 on the next 2 pages).

- Spend 5 minutes on one side, then switch to the other side.

- Place a block or pillow under your head for comfort (not pictured).

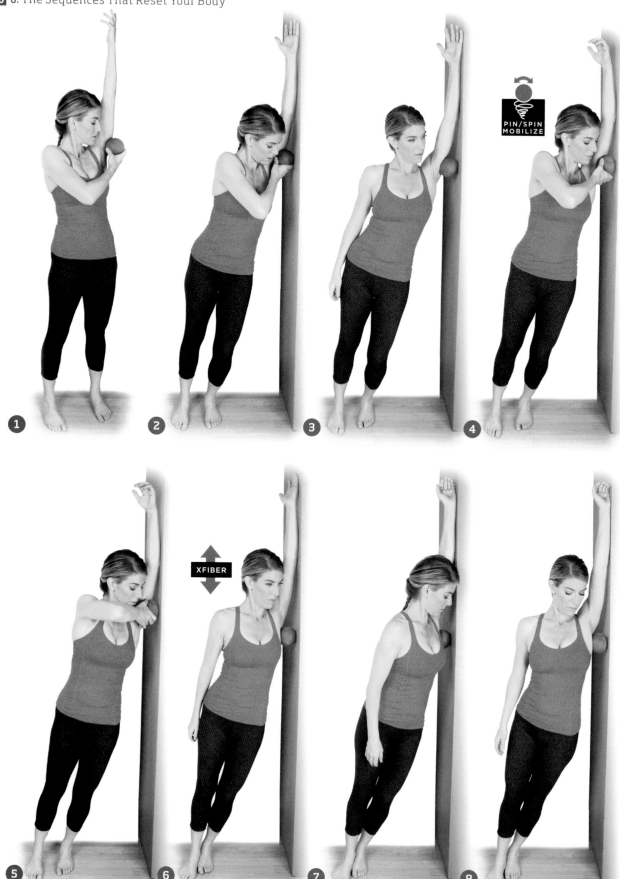

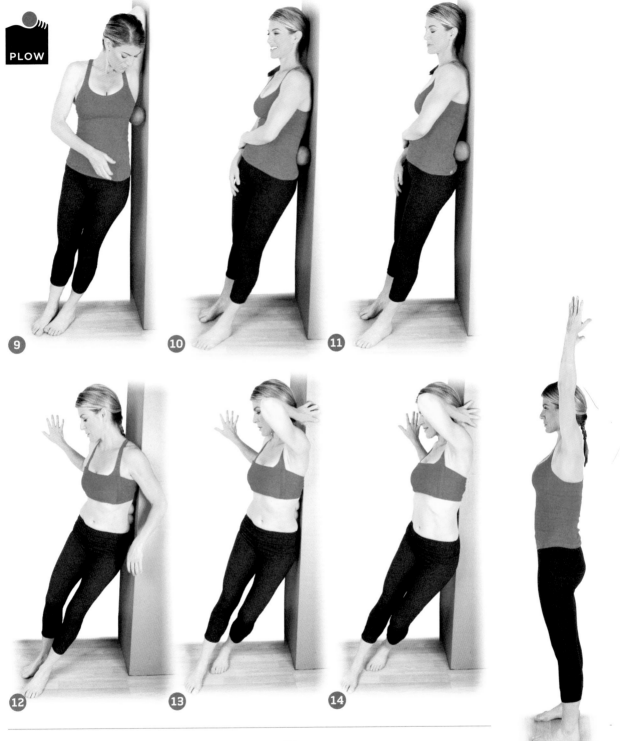

PLOW

9

10

11

12

13

14

ReCheck:
Flexion & External Rotation of Shoulders

Reset your shoulder position and notice if your range of motion has improved, and if you feel less resistance to the motion.

Reflect

1. Take some ribcage breaths and notice how that feels.

2. Give yourself a long, sustained bear hug and crawl your hands as far around you as possible. Can one hand go farther than the other?

3. Finish this statement: I feel _____.

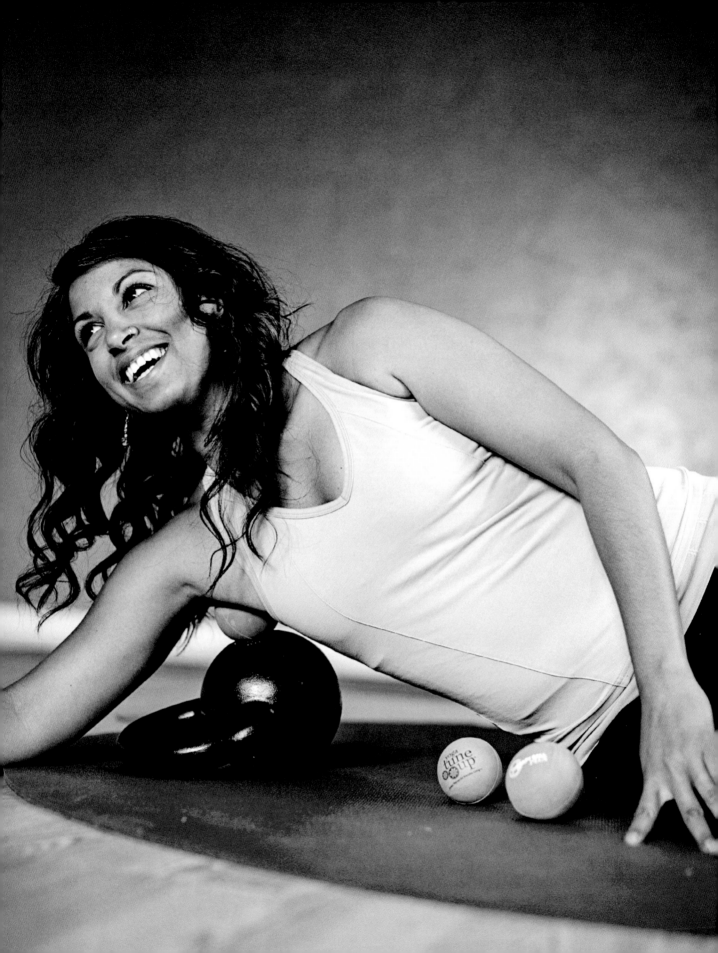

She Shoots, She Scores!
The Pain-Free Gold Medalist

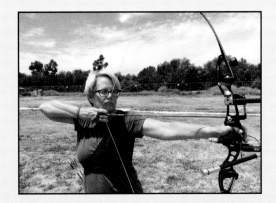

Karen Kroll, 63
Retired Graphic Designer
Los Angeles

Dear Jill,

I wanted to share this with you:

Six and a half years ago, I had two frozen shoulders and was just coming off of two years of really bad back trouble. I couldn't even straighten my arms all the way. As a surprise, my husband arranged for three archery lessons for my 57th birthday. I fell in love with it and haven't stopped since.

In addition to my day-to-day life, I have used the Roll Model Balls to roll away pre-competition stress, loosen up, and relieve pain. I have used them just prior to shooting a personal best. They were invaluable in rehabbing my shoulder after an impingement incident two weeks before the national competitions.

Last weekend I won a gold and a silver medal in the Masters division of the U.S. National Target Championships and the U.S. National Open. I am 63 and I'm not done yet.

Best,
Karen Kroll

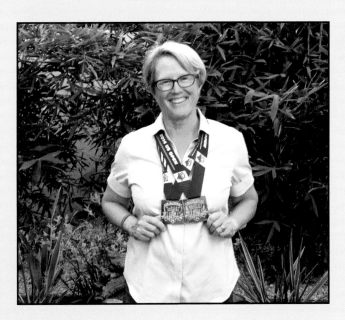

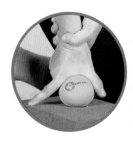

Sequence 13: Forearms, Fingers, Hands, & Wrists

Setup
Roll Model Balls:
Original YTU,
PLUS, or ALPHA
2 blocks

EmbodyMap

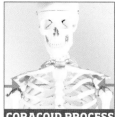
CORACOID PROCESS

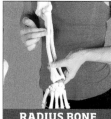
RADIUS BONE

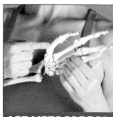
1ST METACARPAL

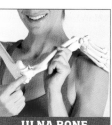
ULNA BONE

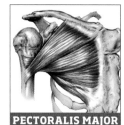
PECTORALIS MAJOR

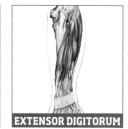
PECTORALIS MINOR

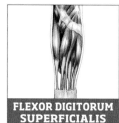
EXTENSOR DIGITORUM

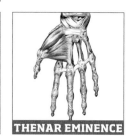
FLEXOR DIGITORUM SUPERFICIALIS

THENAR EMINENCE

Basic Ball Stops

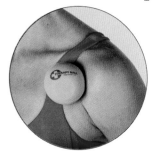
Pectoralis minor/
coracoid process

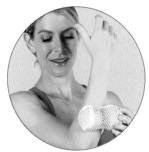
Forearm bones

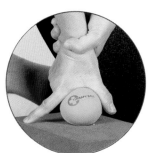

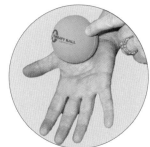
Thumb

Check In: Double Wrist Extension

- Place both palms on a flat surface (the floor, a table, or a chair) so that your thumbs are on the outside and your pinkies are on the inside. Adjust the pressure and angle so that your whole palm is in contact with the surface. (Your wrists may not have the steep angle that mine display.)

- Exaggerate the spread of your fingers and attempt to migrate your forearms and elbows toward your body to increase the stretch for 5 Abdominal Breaths.

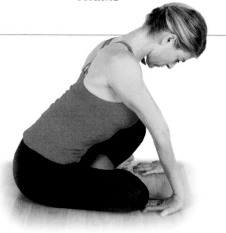

Roll Sequence

PEC, PEC, PEC

Action 1:

- (1) Place 2 Original YTU or PLUS Balls on top of 2 blocks (or use 2 ALPHAs on the floor), positioned for each coracoid process/pectoralis minor tendon, and lay your chest on the balls. (2) Rest your forehead on the floor or a folded towel. Breathe into the balls while you remain still and passively compress for 1 to 2 minutes.

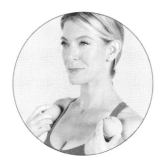

- (3-4) Initiate a pin & stretch matched with a breath rhythm: inhale and raise your palms toward the ceiling (shoulder extension), then exhale and guide them back to the ground.

- Repeat this breath action 8 to 15 times.

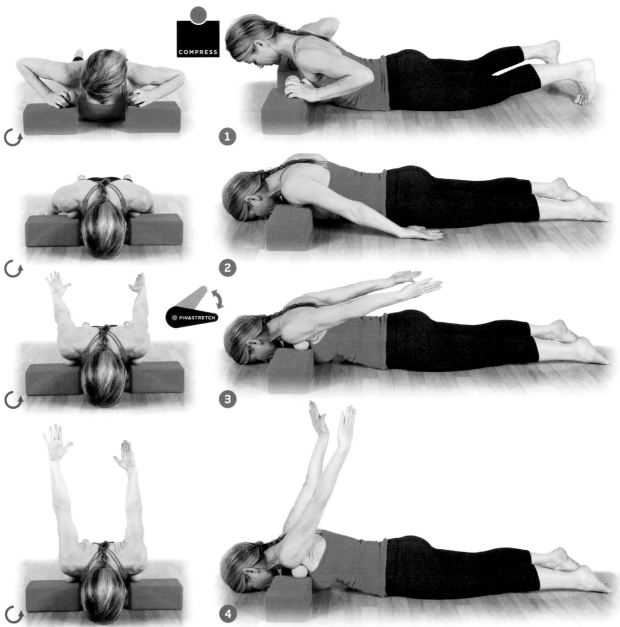

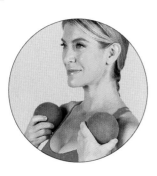

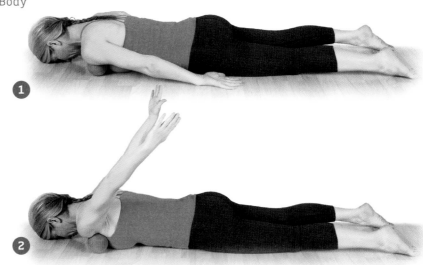

(1-2) You can also use 2 ALPHA Balls directly on the floor.

Action 2:

- (1) Let your shoulders and arms imitate the action of a swimmer doing the butterfly stroke. (2) Sweep your arms into a full range of extension, then (3-4) rotate them externally so that they can continue to reach out to your sides and finally (5) land on the ground overhead with your palms facing up.

- (6-8) Slowly reverse the motion while breathing deeply.

- Do 8 to 12 butterfly strokes.

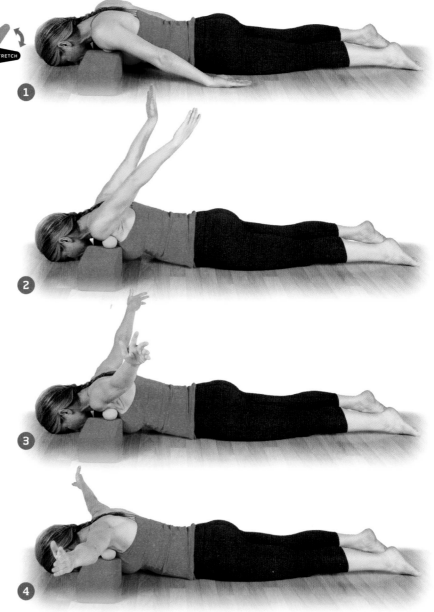

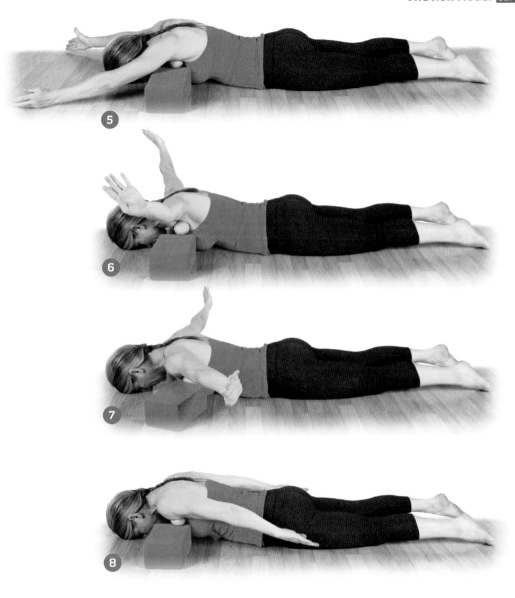

Action 3:

- (1) Initiate the full swimmer's breaststroke. Start with your arms alongside you, palms facing up. (2) Bend your elbows and drag the backs of your hands along the floor, then...

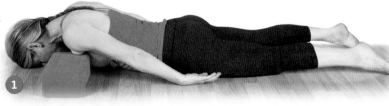

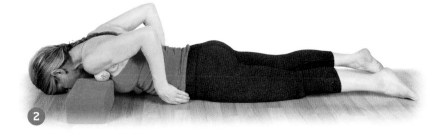

- **(3)** Track them over the blocks until **(4-5)** your palms touch above your head. **(6-9)** Broadly sweep your arms up and out to the sides and back down to the start position as if you were swimming. Coordinate this stroke with your own breath rhythm.

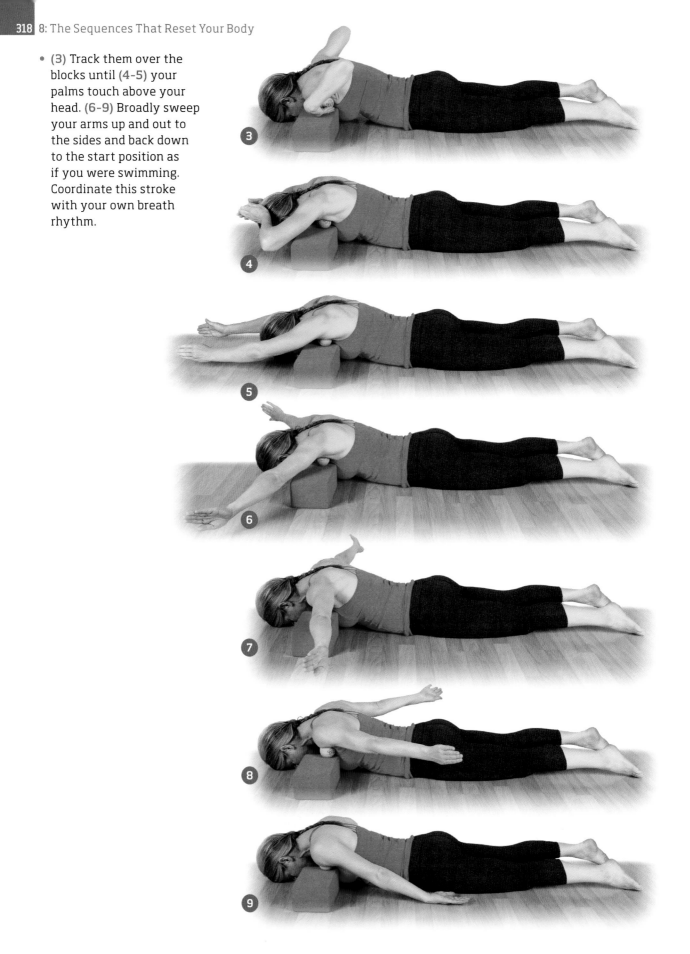

FOREARM MELTDOWN

Action 1:

- (1-2) Lock your right forearm between toted balls. This can be done at your desk, at the kitchen table, or on the floor with a block. Strip the top of your forearm (extensors) by (3-4) tracking your forearm up and down the balls as if sharpening a knife.

- (5) Use your left hand to pin the balls close to the tendon mass near your elbow (olecranon process of ulna). (6-8) Then contract/relax your wrist through a range of extension and flexion or by making circles.

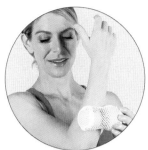

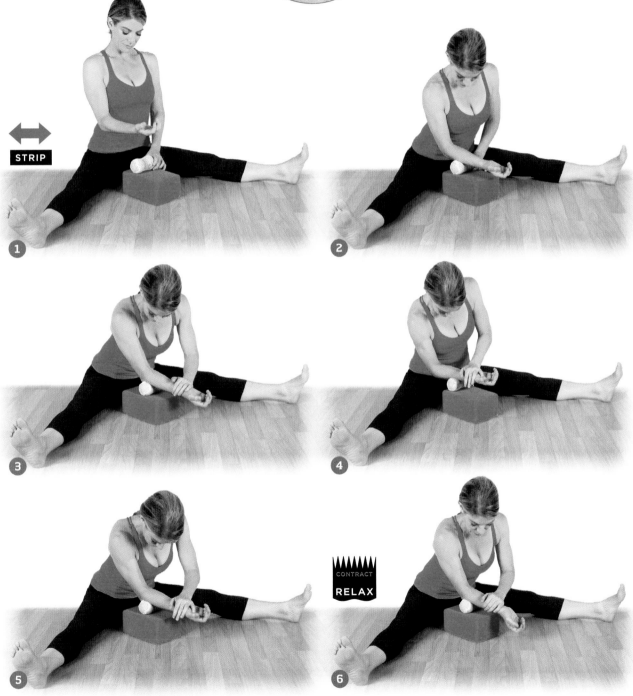

Action 2:

- **(1)** Flip your forearm over and strip the flexors. When rolling the underside of your forearm (flexors), **(2)** make sure that your wrist goes slack, and lighten up on your pressure a bit.

- **(3)** Pivot your wrist and forearm to favor the pinky (ulna) side in a karate chop angle. **(4)** Use your left hand to encourage more pressure into these tissues as you **(5-7)** migrate the balls into the different tissues and tendons all along your forearm bone.

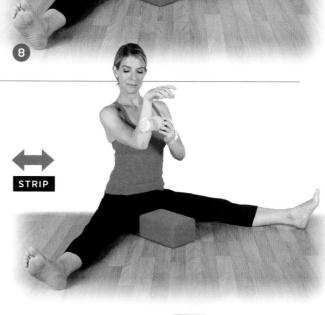

←→ STRIP

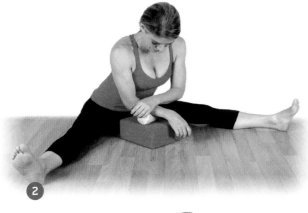

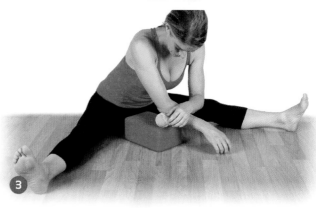

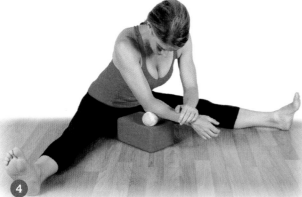

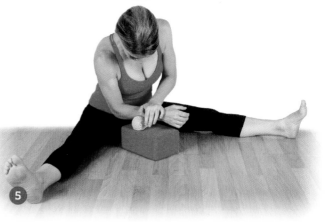

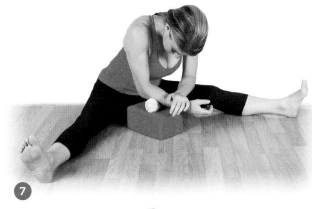

6

7

Action 3:

- Use your left hand to actively plow your forearm tissues as you flip your forearm from a palm-up (supine) to a palm-down (prone) position. Catch as many fascia layers as possible and stir up heat in your forearms.

- Remove one ball and pin/spin & mobilize any area of your forearm, winding up either the flexors or the extensors, followed by moving your wrist and fingers (not pictured).

SWITCH SIDES AND REPEAT ACTIONS 1-3.

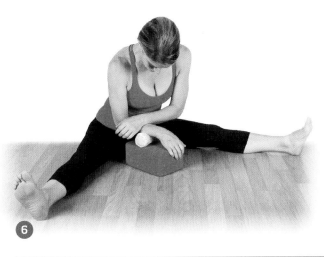

PLOW

SKIN ROLL

1

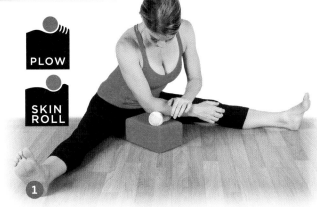

2

3

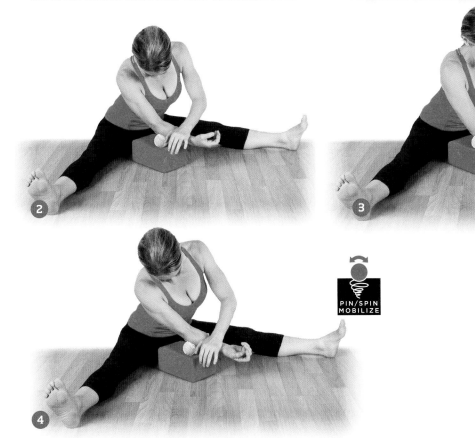

PIN/SPIN MOBILIZE

4

THUMB SPLITS

Action 1:

(1) Spread your right thumb and index finger on one ball to perform "thumb splits." (2) Compress for 20 to 30 seconds to feel the stretch. (3) Then contract your thumb and index finger into the ball, (4) followed by another 20 to 30 seconds of relaxed stretch with deep breathing.

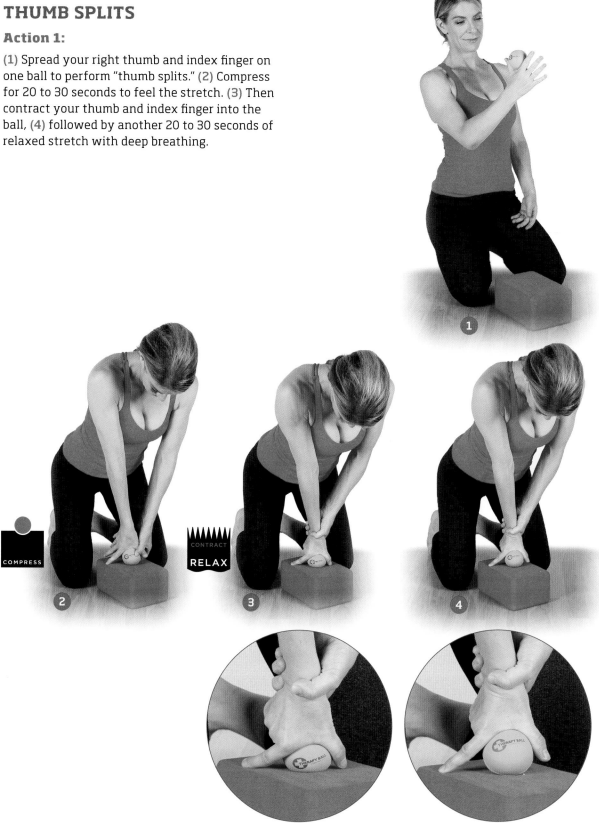

COMPRESS

CONTRACT
RELAX

Action 2:

Interpret all the techniques over the thumb-pad area. Create massive skin-rolling and shear friction. Plow the thenar group (the pad of muscles at the base of your thumb) by using your left hand to control a plow action across your thumb joint (at the first metacarpal). Pin/spin & mobilize the area by squashing the ball as if you were making orange juice out of it. Then repeat throughout the rest of your palm. Have a ball!

SWITCH SIDES AND REPEAT ACTIONS 1 AND 2.

SKIN ROLL · XFIBER · PLOW · PIN/SPIN MOBILIZE

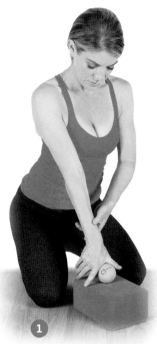
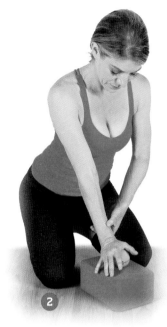

1 · 2

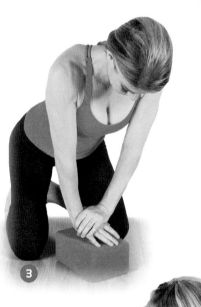
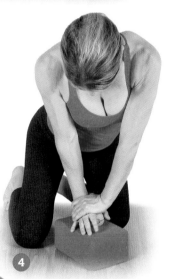

3 · 4 · 5

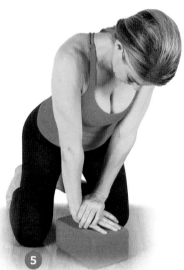

ReCheck: Double Wrist Extension

Reset your stretch and notice if the same limitations and sensations are there, or if anything has changed.

Reflect

1. Look for redness or rosiness in certain areas of your hands from the increased circulation.

2. Grasp a thick object (or an ALPHA Ball) and notice if your grasp is stronger.

3. Finish this statement: I feel _____.

Pushing Past the Breaking Point: A Hockey Scout Scours Out His Own Pain

Lee Callans, 41
Scouting Operations
Coordinator
Los Angeles

Lee always knew that there was something wrong with his neck. His head looked crooked in pictures from the time he was a baby. That didn't stop his zeal for hockey. He played throughout his southern California childhood and learned to work around his misalignment. Operating under the "if it ain't broke, don't fix it" principle, his parents were unconcerned that he was always uncomfortable and had trouble sleeping. They finally took him to a series of doctors and specialists, and after getting no definitive answers, they resigned themselves that "this is the way it is" and that Lee would "learn to live with it and tough it out." So Lee adopted his own version of this philosophy: when the going gets tough, toughen up.

Lee has a vague recollection of the doctors' diagnoses: "scoliosis, or reverse curvature...but I didn't trust any of the doctors. I kind of got that from my parents." He didn't let his neck get in the way of his beloved hockey. Missing the ability to turn his head fully like the other kids, he learned to turn by twisting from his waist. At age 41, he knows now that "I trained the wrong muscles to do the moves I wanted to do. I compensated."

Even though everyone could see that his neck was "off," it didn't cause him searing local pain in his neck during his childhood and early teens, just constant general discomfort. His agony would manifest at night. Lee could never find a comfortable position to sleep. Lying on his back, his head did not nestle comfortably into the pillow, and lying on his side would trigger shoulder pain. Sometimes he had to sleep sitting up. If he had worked out particularly hard or been struck in a game, sleep would be restless and troubled for days on end. His insomnia became the litmus test for whether things were "really bad." But instead of talking about his hurt and lack of sleep with a professional, Lee believed that he could work his way through it and block out the pain so that he could continue to play.

Toward the end of high school, he realized that his weight and skills (and neck) were not going to be enough to guide him toward a professional hockey career or his "other dream of being an astronaut," but he still played recreationally in college. In college the pain expanded and became insurmountable, his sleep was horrific, and he began seeing a chiropractor. "The adjustment would help for two hours or so, but then I was right back where I started. I was giving away money for Band-Aids, and none of the chiros I saw could lay out a long-term strategy, so I just went back to living with it. It wasn't worth the money."

Lee graduated with a communications degree that led him to work in television, and he spent several years laying cable for sound. Eventually, he worked his way up to boom operator. A boom operator's duties include holding a heavy microphone attached to a long broomstick-like handle above the heads of the actors while they are taping a scene. The boom must be held high enough that it does not dip into the view of the camera, and it needs to be perfectly steady.

For someone with chronic neck pain, holding a boom overhead for hours a day is probably the absolute worst job. Lee remembers beads of sweat dripping down his face while he held the boom. He recalls his unsteadiness and the onset of uncontrollable tremors from holding the boom in awkward positions in take after take. The fact that he lasted nearly three years is a testament to his "tough it out at all costs" mentality and pure grit. At one point on a non-union show, Lee remembers that his job performance was particularly shaky. The director took him aside and told him that if his dream was to make it in Hollywood as a sound guy, Lee was "not going to be able to cut it, son."

Angry and frustrated, Lee sought refuge in his beloved hockey in order to burn off steam. He religiously practiced his hockey shots in his driveway

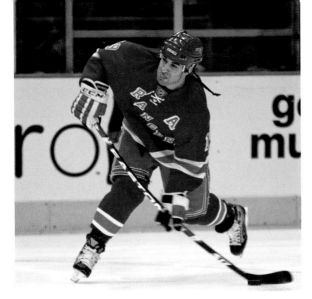

A classic slapshot.

or on the ice, shooting 300 to 400 slapshots a day with massive force that began to take a toll.

"When you strike a puck, you don't just swing at the puck; you aim the stick to hit the ground about an inch behind the puck in order to leverage the stick to flex before it swipes the puck. The stick grabs a lot of ground or ice. This was into my concrete driveway or ice hundreds of times a day, and I lost feeling in my hand and could no longer grab. I had searing pain traveling from my hand up my arm to my shoulder to my neck." He had destroyed the flexor tendons in his hand and wrist, inflaming and damaging the tissues that allowed his thumb to grip a hockey stick. Each spell of pain would last several days (cue the unbearable insomnia), and then he would attack the pucks again. Eventually, he literally could no longer grip a hockey stick or boom with his right hand, and he quit his job in August 1997.

During this hand pain, Lee never saw a doctor or therapist. He also refused to take pills, except an occasional Advil. He had no insurance and no money. He would just wait it out—"tough it out," as his parents had advised. His bad experiences with doctors left him with a deep mistrust in both conventional and alternative therapies. "They were just chasing symptoms. My shoulder would hurt, and they would give me shoulder exercises for a few weeks, but nothing ever changed permanently." He also believes that his "athletic mentality" allowed him to create an air of invincibility and "tough guy-ness" in order to get it done and win

the game—even though the "game" he was playing was destroying him. Hockey was his one pure emotional outlet, but the pain and sleeplessness were spiraling out of control.

With Hollywood behind him, Lee turned his energy toward building a career that brought him closer to his beloved game. His determination landed him a job with an NHL team in 2000, working in the public relations department. This gave his body much needed rest, and eventually he was hired as a scout by the team. He excelled, and after a few short years, in June 2006, he ended up securing a dream job: Scouting Operations Coordinator and Assistant to the General Manager. Working in professional athletics has its perks; Lee's offices include a world-class training facility, and he is surrounded by top-notch athletes and is privy to cutting-edge strength, conditioning, and therapeutic geniuses.

As a scout, he continued to suffer occasional bouts of horrific pain in his hand, neck, and shoulder, as well as insomnia. Much of it was triggered by stress related to travel for his job. New pains in his back and hips popped up from time to time. Nonetheless, he continued a workout regimen that involved running and weightlifting, but put his hockey stick down. Unfortunately, he could not outrun his injuries, and they finally caught up with him. His right shoulder succumbed to tears in his rotator cuff, likely stemming from the combined dysfunctions of his neck and hand. He could no longer tough it out; his tissues required surgery in July 2012, when Lee was 38. But even after the surgery and rehab, his pains and sleep troubles continued.

In July 2013, Lee attended a weeklong Yoga Tune Up retreat with me. Lee is not the "yoga type" and had never heard of Yoga Tune Up, but he was open to trying anything to de-stress during the off-season. In the first class he took, I introduced the students to a neck and shoulder sequence with the Roll Model Balls. Within a few minutes of rolling, his pain changed, and he knew that he had finally found a solution to his chronic problems. "They have changed me every day since," he states. Lee walked into the retreat's retail shop, bought every ball and video of mine that they sold, went back to his room, and continued to roll. He was in awe of the before-and-after sensations that the balls unrolled for him. Lee is an all-or-nothing type of man and immediately became disciplined about using the balls for self-care. He came to my classes every day, positioned himself in the front row, and soaked up as many techniques as he could.

On his last day, I taught a hand sequence (find it beginning on page 314). We spent about three minutes on the thumb, and I glanced over at Lee. Suddenly his head jerked up, and his eyes grew mega-wide and fastened in on me. When the class ended, he walked up to me and said, "The reason I quit playing hockey is because I lost my ability to grip the stick 15 years ago. It felt as though there was always a clamp pressing down between my palm and thumb." Doing the simple thumb sequence with the Roll Model Balls immediately loosened that clamp. He describes that it "almost felt as though my thumb had been soldered into my palm, and the ball sequence untethered the two." That single session was a turning point for his wide-grip issue.

Back at home, Lee noticed immediate changes if he skipped a day of using the balls. "I started to recognize what normal and aligned felt like. The balls gave me reference points for my body, and I could feel what was 'off.' I just wouldn't feel right. As soon as I used the balls, I could slip back into normal." Lee was talking about a "new normal," though. He created his own intuitive workout based on his live lessons with me and some of the stretch routines from my exercise videos. Within one month of solid practice, Lee remembers having this thought: I can't believe I even had pain.

"I spend about 30 to 45 minutes rolling at the beginning of my workout. It's my meditation, using the balls on my back, up into my neck and shoulders, then into my chest, hand, and wrist. I have a set at home, keep a pair in my travel bag, and have others in my desk at work. I change it up and use the different sizes."

Lee's workouts used to be full of pops and clicks, but he no longer has them. His gait is noticeably longer when he runs; his workout partner recently asked him how he had "changed his gait." He wasn't trying to improve his gait with his new regimen, but he realizes now that all his body knew was compensation. His soft tissues were so imbalanced that they had created

tread to avoid all his problems. "Your body will find a way to do it, but that's not always the right way," he says. Now his body falls more correctly into place because he's given it options for improvement and an environment that will host and adapt to these positive changes in performance. When he trains, he feels healthier and can be much more active. His favorite pastime sport is riding race motorcycles on a track. His newfound flexibility allows him to ride in ways that he never could before.

Travel is a massive part of Lee's job; he averages 30 to 40 flights per year. "I always travel with the PLUS," he says. He positions them along his spine in his seat, traveling them up and down his back throughout his flights. In the past, he remembers never knowing if his back would seize up once the plane had parked at the gate. He would watch other passengers spring out of their seats while he cautiously clawed his way out of his seat like a man old before his time. "I think these balls should be in every plane, in every seat pocket on every flight all over the world. These are the real 'life-vests.'"

But perhaps the most profound change for Lee is that "I sleep like a baby now. Like a baby!" He no longer notices pain when he wakes, and he can get to the coffeemaker faster than ever before. Lee wishes someone had introduced the Roll Model Balls to him 15 or 20 years ago: "It's the first thing I've found that loosened me up and made positive change," he says. He's learned more about his body through using them than from all his years of working in professional sports and exposure to the best of the best. He's been exposed to every self-care tool, treatment modality, training regimen, and "of the moment" gimmick, but he never experienced lasting change until now.

Lee is convinced that the Roll Model Method will soon explode onto the athletic scene and be used by every club out there. "Fads come and go, but this has to stay. You'd have to be crazy not to use it. It's a game-changer." Lee is living proof that pain, insomnia, and suffering do not have to be normal conditions. Wear-and-tear caused by pushing yourself beyond the brink in your sport can be erased. You can improve your game and your life by devoting time and discipline to self-care that works.

Neck and Head Sequences

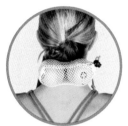

Sequence 14: Neck Gnar

Setup

Roll Model Balls: Original YTU, PLUS, or ALPHA Twins in tote

Mat

Wall corner or doorway

EmbodyMap

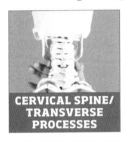

CERVICAL SPINE/ TRANSVERSE PROCESSES

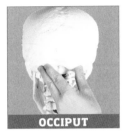

OCCIPUT

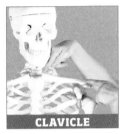

CLAVICLE

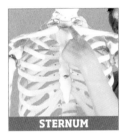

STERNUM

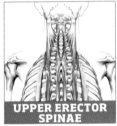

UPPER ERECTOR SPINAE

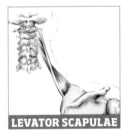

LEVATOR SCAPULAE

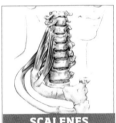

SCALENES

Basic Ball Stops

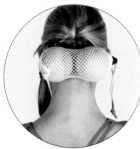

Base of skull/ suboccipitals

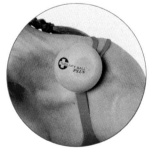

Supraclavicle area

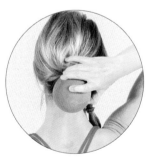

Nuchal ligament

Check In: Rotate Neck, Then Tuck Chin to Collarbone

- **(1)** Either sitting or standing, align your best posture (see pages 84-86), then **(2)** rotate your head fully to the right.

- **(3)** Drop your chin down toward your collarbone without letting your left shoulder shift or move. Take 2 to 4 Abdominal-Thoracic Breaths.

(4-6) SWITCH SIDES AND REPEAT.

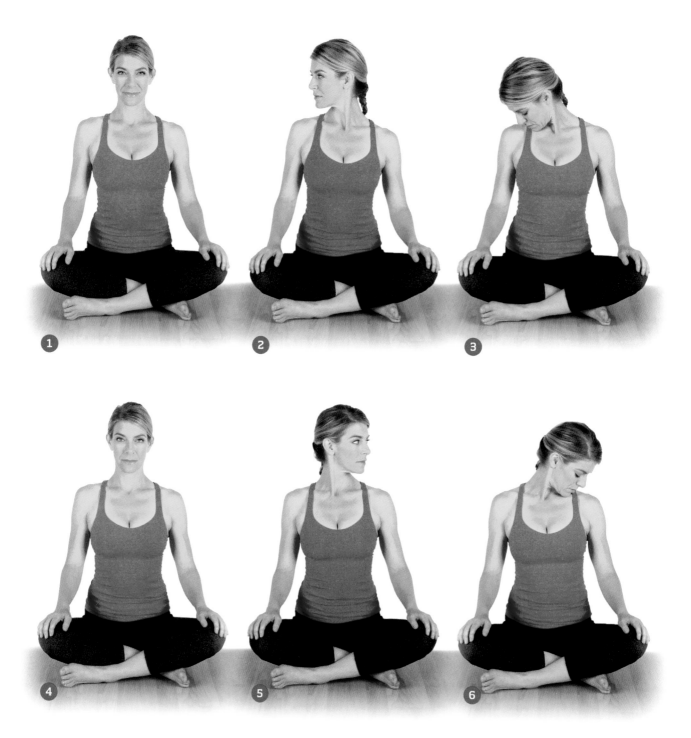

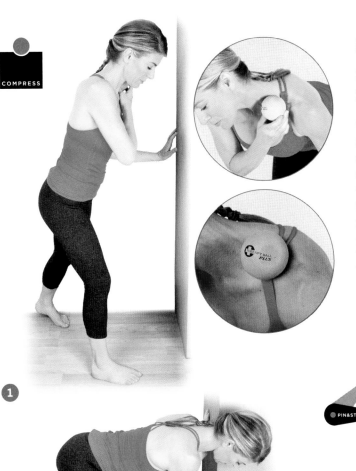

COMPRESS

Roll Sequence
SUPRACLAVICLE SCRUB-OUT

Action 1:

(1) Pin yourself against a wall corner or doorway. Place one ball above your clavicle and rest it directly on the scalenes, the soft tissues between the front of your shoulder blade and collarbone. (2) Hinge at your hips in order to pin the ball to the wall, making sure that your head is clear of the wall. Take several Thoracic Breaths, then (3-6) begin a variety of pin & stretch moves that travel your left arm and shoulder behind your back, around the doorjamb/corner. (7-8) Keep the ball pinned in place and stretch your neck by turning it to the right and looking up or down.

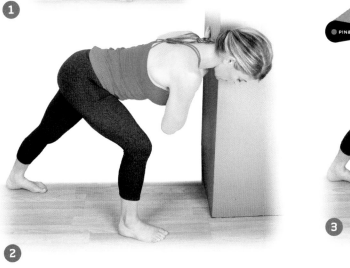

1

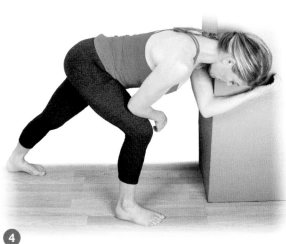

2

PIN&STRETCH

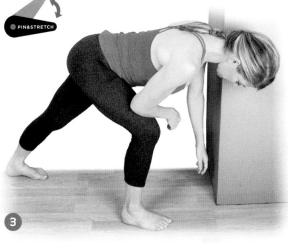

3

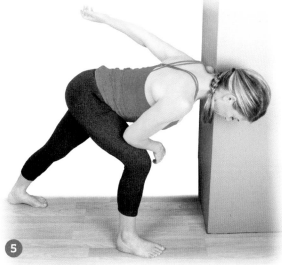

4

5

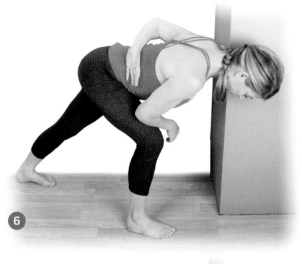

6

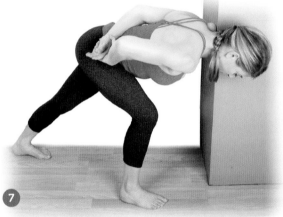

7

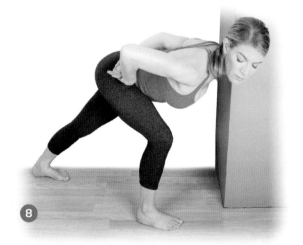

8

Action 2:

Use your right hand to pin & spin the ball while you remobilize your left shoulder, neck, and first rib. Continue to scroll the ball into the supraclavicle area, foraging for areas of tension. Then wind it in the opposite direction.

SWITCH SIDES AND REPEAT ACTIONS 1 AND 2.

PIN/SPIN
MOBILIZE

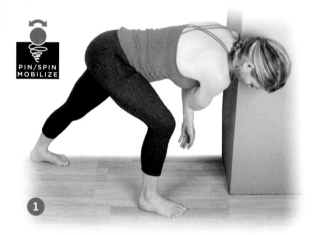

1

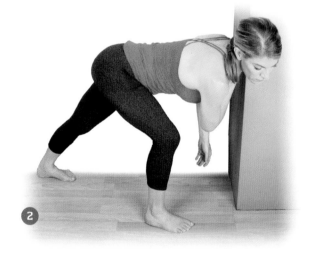

2

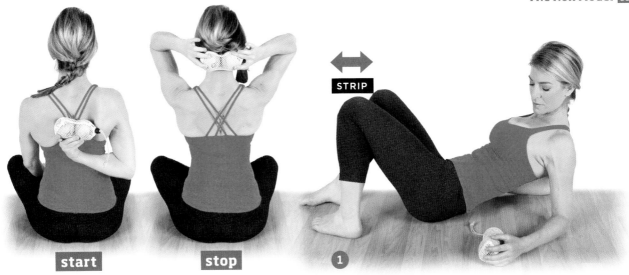

start   stop

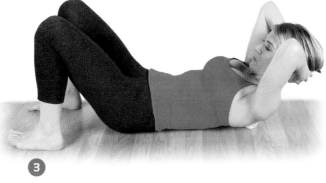

STRIP

1

STEM OF THE NECK

(1-2) Use your toted Original YTU, PLUS, or ALPHA Balls and lie on your back. Strip the balls up and down in a continuous roll from the upper thoracic to the suboccipitals. **(3-4)** Cradle your head in your hands and raise your pelvis a few inches off the floor in order to use the toted balls like a soft-tissue rolling pin.

TIP: If you have a difficult time propelling the balls between your upper back and neck, walk your feet in toward your body in tiny steps, which will move the balls down your back. Walk your feet away from your body to push the balls back up your spine.

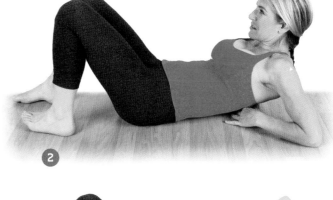

2

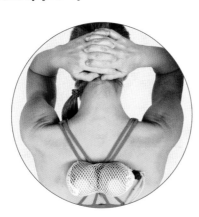

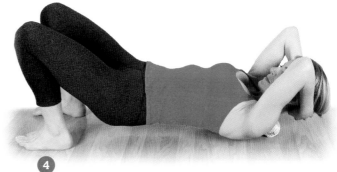

3

4

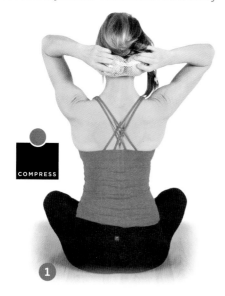

COMPRESS

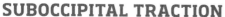

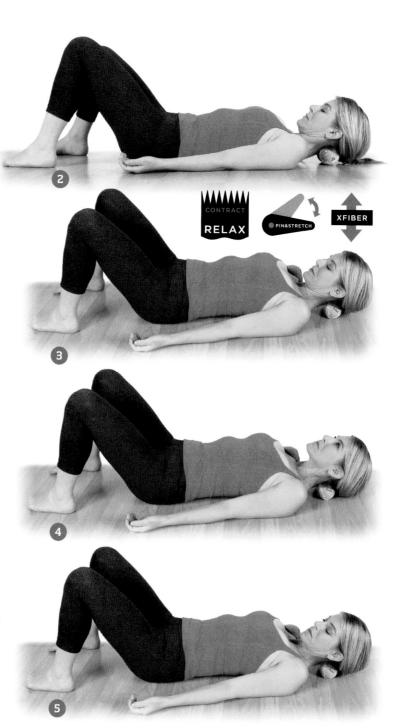

CONTRACT RELAX · PIN&STRETCH XFIBER

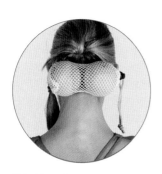

SUBOCCIPITAL TRACTION

- **(1-2)** Place your toted balls just below your occiput. Your head should be in the "bottom of a nod" position, with your chin angled down toward your chest. Compress here in stillness for 10 Abdominal-Thoracic Breaths.

- **(3-5)** Slowly activate a contract/relax and pin & stretch by creating a mini-nod action, hinging this small motion of your skull over the balls.

- **(6-7)** CrossFiber the back of your neck with a "say no" action, slowly moving your head in a small range from side to side.

- **(8)** Increase your range of motion so that your neck balances on one ball. Once you've rotated all the way to the side in a full "no" position, place your hand on your head for added compression, then nod "yes" again.

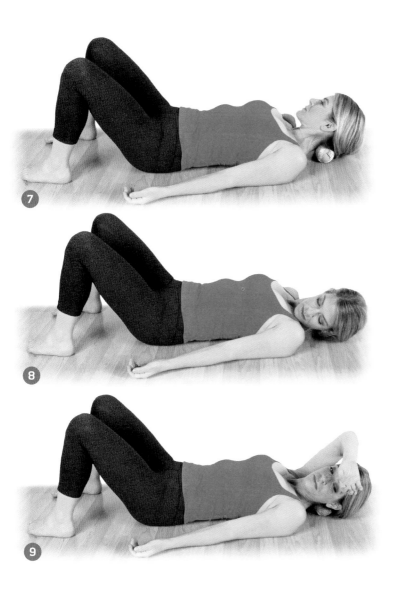

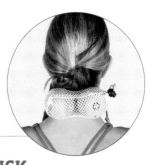

MID-NECK UNGUCK

• (1-2) Roll the balls down 1 or 2 inches to find some new territory in the middle of your neck. Rest with the balls centered on either side of your neck for 10 Abdominal-Thoracic Breaths.

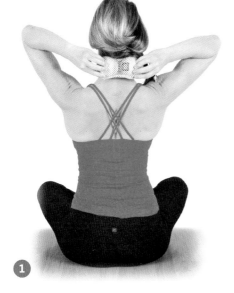

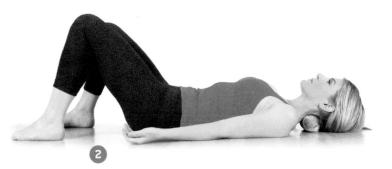

- Then repeat all the actions as outlined below:

(3-4) Slowly activate a contract/ relax and pin & stretch by creating a mini-nod action, hinging this small motion of your skull over the balls.

(5-6) CrossFiber the back of your neck with a "say no" action, slowly moving your head in a small range from side to side.

(7-9) Increase your range of motion so that your neck balances on one ball. Once you've rotated all the way to the side in a full "no" position, place your hand on your head for added compression, then nod "yes" again.

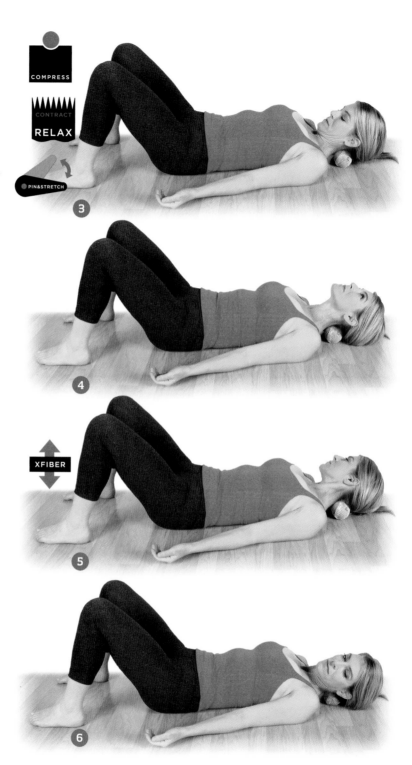

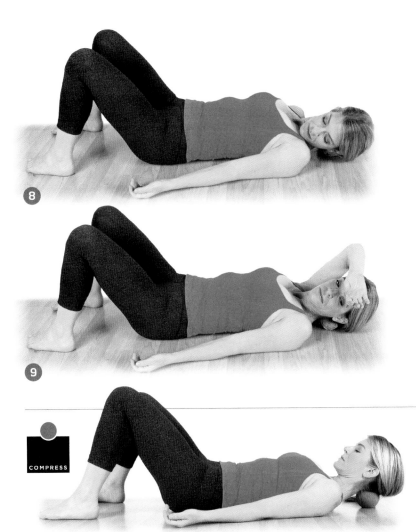

NUCHAL TRACTION

Place an ALPHA Ball on the nuchal ligament, where your neck meets your skull. Your chin will angle down toward your chest as at the bottom of a nod. Close your eyes and rest with passive traction on your neck. Breathe completely, slowly, and deeply for 2 to 3 minutes.

ReCheck: Rotate Neck, Then Tuck Chin to Collarbone

Reset your neck rotation with your chin tucked. Do you have more range of motion? Less restriction or compensation at the end range?

Reflect

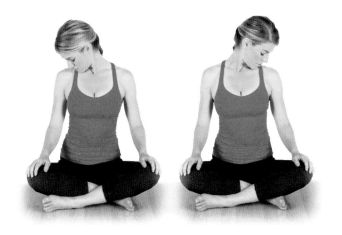

1. Can you breathe into the top of your ribs without recruiting your shoulders?

2. Do you feel clear-headed and focused, or a bit drowsy?

3. Finish this statement: I feel _____.

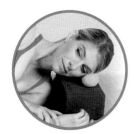

Sequence 15: Head, Face, & Jaw

EmbodyMap

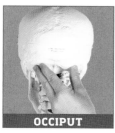
OCCIPUT

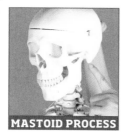
MASTOID PROCESS

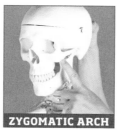
ZYGOMATIC ARCH

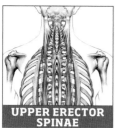
UPPER ERECTOR SPINAE

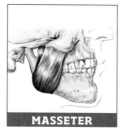
MASSETER

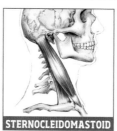
STERNOCLEIDOMASTOID

Basic Ball Stops

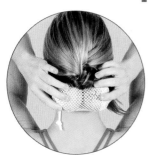

Suboccipitals

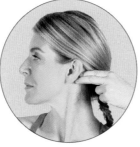
Mastoid process (bony earlobe)

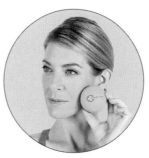
Jaw muscle (masseter)

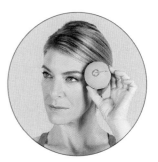
Temple (temporalis)

Check In: Neck Side Bend & Open/Close Jaw

- (1) Either sitting or standing, align your best posture (see pages 84-86). Connect your right hand to your left ear and gently bend your neck to the right. (Do not force the stretch at the end range of motion; let your neck find its natural stopping point.)

- (2) After taking 2 or 3 Abdominal-Thoracic Breaths, open your jaw as wide as you can and take another 2 breaths.

- (3-4) Slowly switch sides.

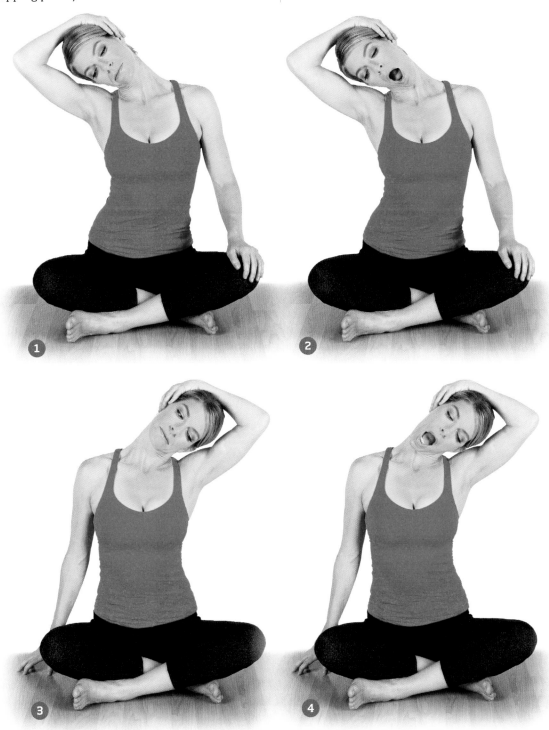

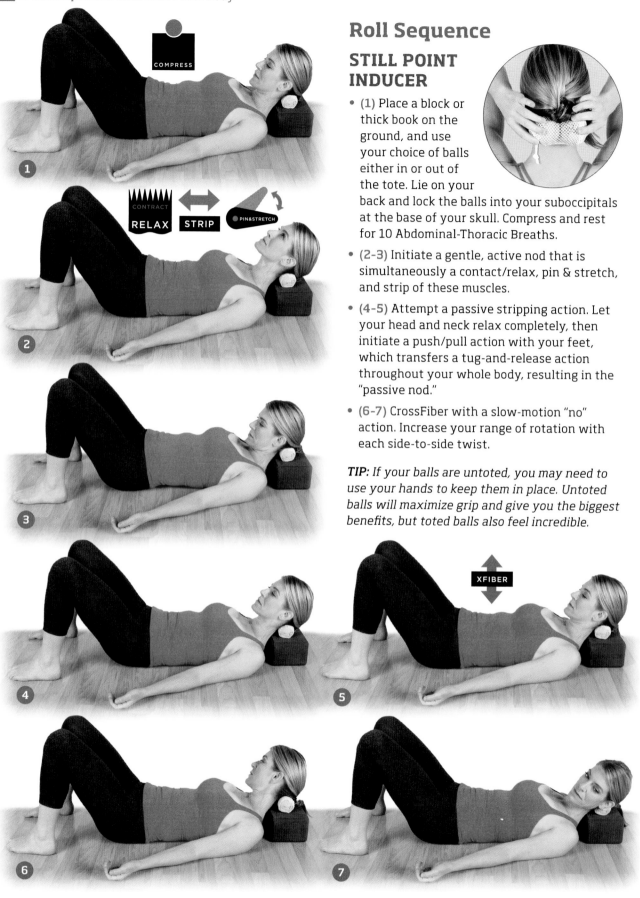

COMPRESS

CONTRACT
RELAX **STRIP** **PIN&STRETCH**

Roll Sequence

STILL POINT INDUCER

- **(1)** Place a block or thick book on the ground, and use your choice of balls either in or out of the tote. Lie on your back and lock the balls into your suboccipitals at the base of your skull. Compress and rest for 10 Abdominal-Thoracic Breaths.

- **(2-3)** Initiate a gentle, active nod that is simultaneously a contact/relax, pin & stretch, and strip of these muscles.

- **(4-5)** Attempt a passive stripping action. Let your head and neck relax completely, then initiate a push/pull action with your feet, which transfers a tug-and-release action throughout your whole body, resulting in the "passive nod."

- **(6-7)** CrossFiber with a slow-motion "no" action. Increase your range of rotation with each side-to-side twist.

TIP: If your balls are untoted, you may need to use your hands to keep them in place. Untoted balls will maximize grip and give you the biggest benefits, but toted balls also feel incredible.

XFIBER

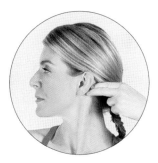

HEADACHE NO MORE

- **(1-2)** Using only one ball, twist your neck to the left and place the ball directly on the left mastoid process. **(3-4)** Your head will balance in compression on this point. Rest and breathe fully for 5 breaths.

- **(5-7)** Strip with a gentle nod "yes."

- **(8-10)** CrossFiber with a "no" action.

- **(11-13)** Pin/spin & mobilize by making tiny circles. Use your hand to twist the ball even deeper into the fascial interface of your scalenes and sternocleidomastoid (not pictured).

SWITCH SIDES AND REPEAT.

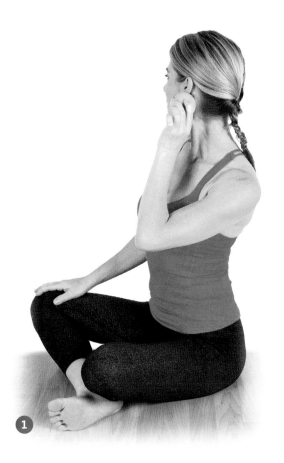

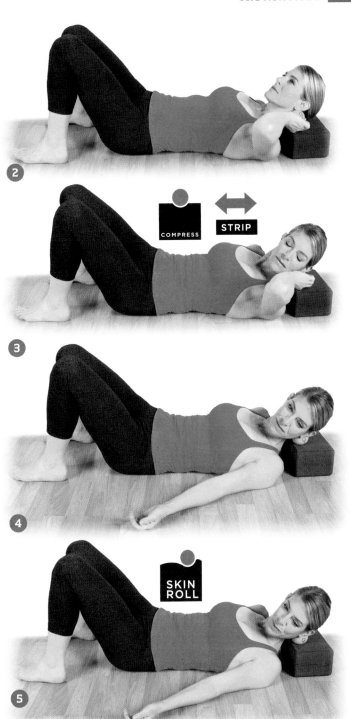

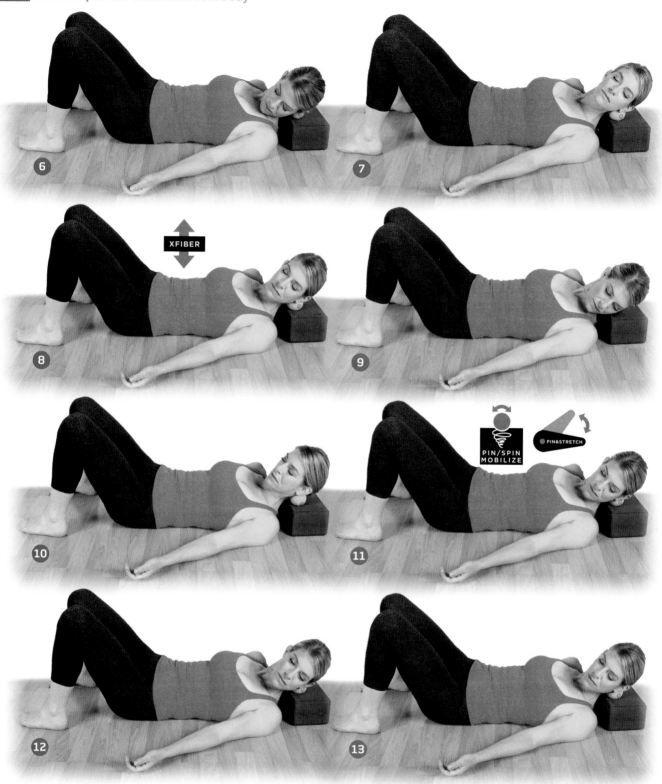

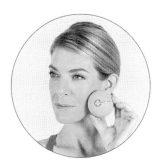

JAW JOINT

Action 1:

(1-2) Roll onto your left side and place one ball between your cheekbone and jawbone, directly on your chewing muscle (the masseter). Pause here for several Abdominal-Thoracic Breaths. (3-4) Contract/ relax by clenching and unclenching your teeth, followed by slowly opening and closing your jaw.

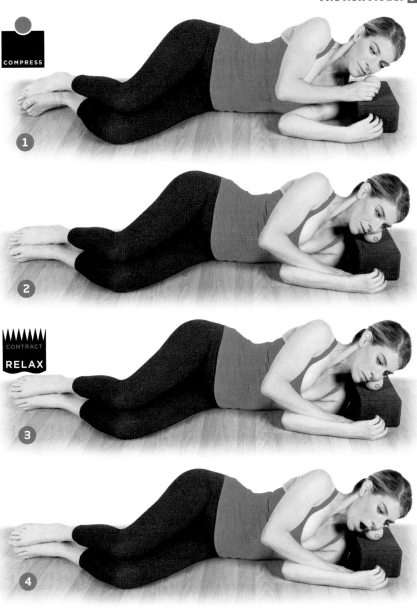

Action 2:

- (1-2) Begin to nod and strip your masseter along its line of pull, up and down.

- (3-4) CrossFiber by slowly moving your head in a "no" motion.

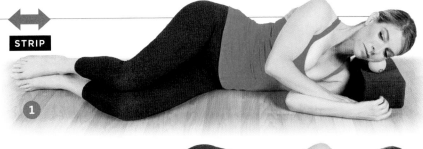

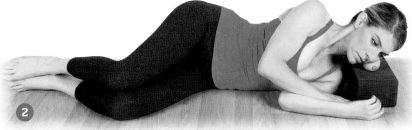

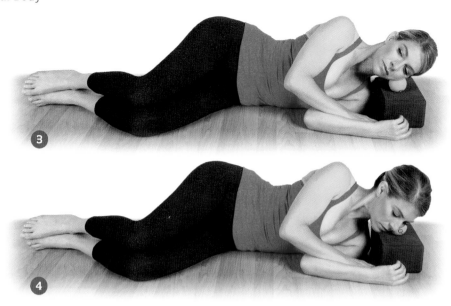

Action 3:

Combine CrossFiber and pin & stretch by opening and closing your jaw while moving your head in a "no" motion. You can also do the "no" motion with your jaw closed if having it open is too uncomfortable.

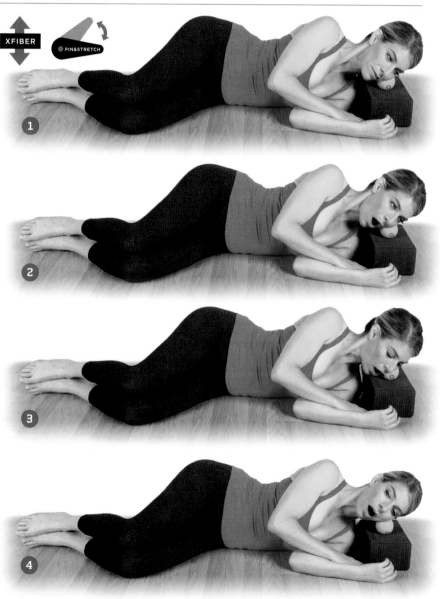

Action 4:

(1–2) Pin/spin & mobilize by twisting the ball into your jaw muscles (not pictured) while (3–4) making circles with your head and circling your chin and jaw like a cow chewing grass.

SWITCH SIDES AND REPEAT ACTIONS 1–4.

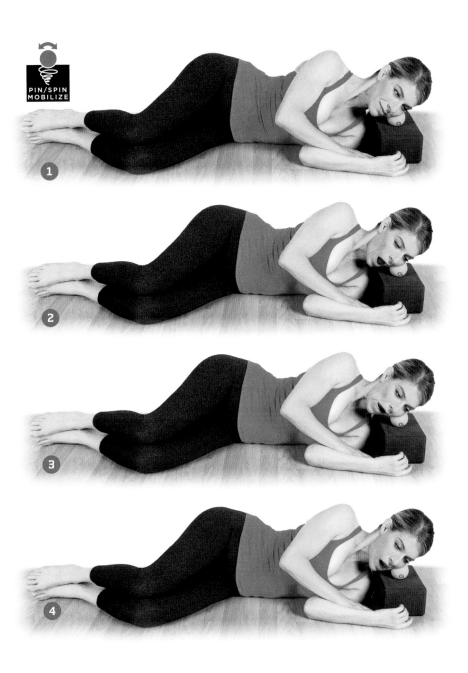

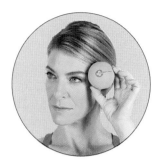

TEMPLE TAMER

Action 1:

- (1-2) Move the ball up to your left temple (temporalis) above your zygomatic arch and rest with compression for several deep breaths.

- (3-5) Strip with a gentle nod "yes."

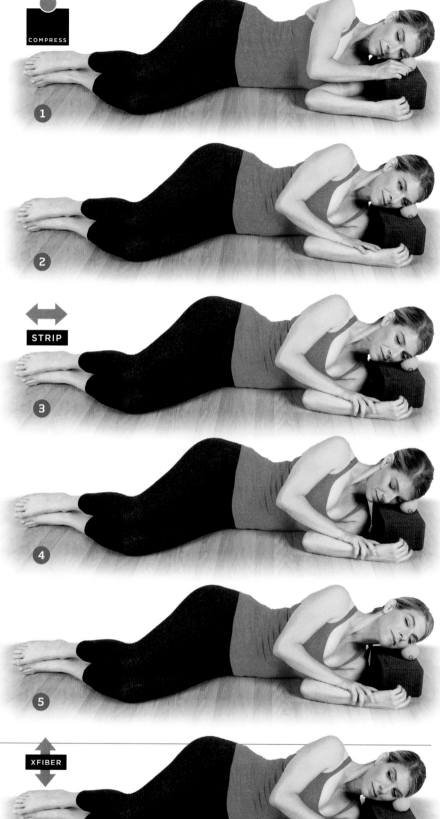

Action 2:

- (1-2) CrossFiber your temple by twisting your head in a slow "no" motion.

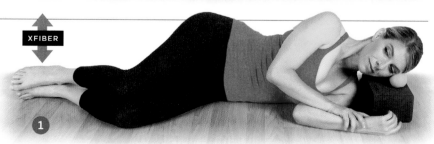

- (3–4) Make tiny circles to pin/spin & mobilize. Grab the other ball with your right hand and simultaneously spin the ball into your right temple to build a ball stack (not pictured) coupled with pin/spin & mobilizing. Move your head gently in every possible direction.

SWITCH SIDES AND REPEAT.

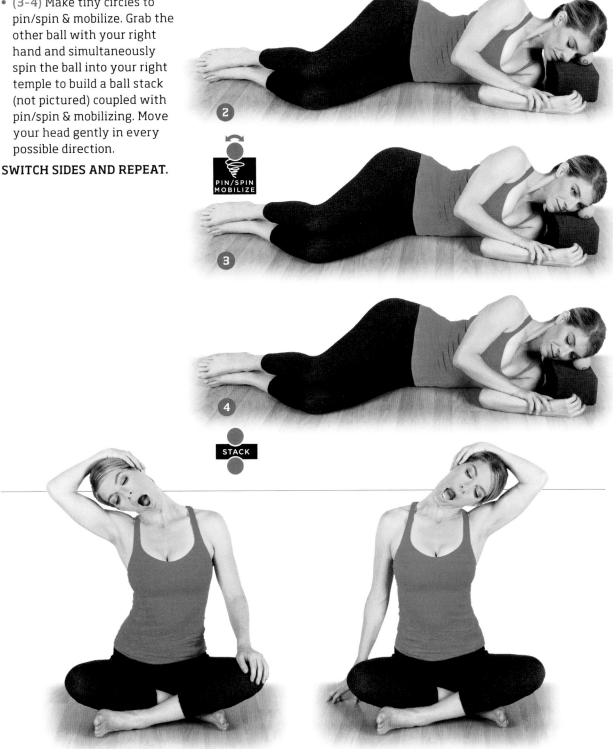

ReCheck: Neck Side Bend & Open/Close Jaw

ReCheck the range of motion in your jaw and neck and assess whether any change has occurred in your side-bending or in the looseness of your jaw.

Reflect

1. Do you feel revitalized or sleepy?

2. How is your breath different?

3. Finish this statement: I feel _____.

Staring Chronic Disease in the Face: Stalling Scleroderma

Amanda Joyce, 36
Corrective Exercise Specialist,
Movement Therapy for
Parkinson's Disease
Santa Monica, California

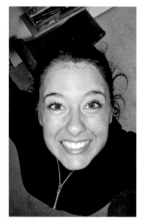
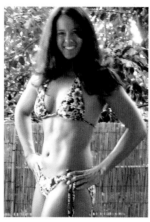

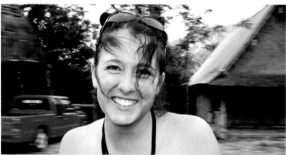

Amanda pre-diagnosis.

In 2006, Amanda Joyce woke up one morning to discover a waxy patch of skin on her left jaw, about the size of a quarter. At first she didn't give it much thought, but over the next few weeks it began to spread, even growing under her skin, so she finally went to a doctor. He was baffled by it, so she went to another doctor, who was equally nonplussed–it took the seventh doctor she went to, a dermatologist in Beverly Hills, to finally diagnose it as scleroderma. "By that point my husband and I were both convinced it was a tumor, because it was starting to make this weird indentation in my face, so we were incredibly relieved to find out it wasn't," Amanda says. Scleroderma is an autoimmune disease in which the body overproduces collagen, starting from the surface of the skin and down into the layers of muscle and connective tissue below, compacting the whole area into a hardened mass, and potentially even reaching down and fusing to the bone (in this case, Amanda's

jawbone). The effect was comparable to a third-degree burn on Amanda's face.

Amanda was diagnosed with linear scleroderma, which meant that it was limited to one area of her body, rather than systemic scleroderma, which attacks the internal organs and can lead to hardening of the lungs and heart and, ultimately, death. Though Amanda was relieved not to be getting a death sentence, the dermatologist told her that there was nothing they could do, the cause was unknown, and they had no idea what might cause it to spread or go into remission. A rheumatologist suggested chemotherapy as an experimental treatment, but Amanda didn't want to do something so potentially destructive to her body. She's a movement and exercise specialist with a southern California beach lifestyle and a daily yoga practice, and she wasn't about to subject her body to such an aggressive treatment when there was no conclusive benefit.

For the first four years after her diagnosis, Amanda wrestled with shame and anger. She thought she was a model of health, training her clients to get into shape or get out of pain, yet she was suffering from a disease that she didn't totally understand and could do nothing about. The scleroderma pulled on her jawbone so much that it began to change the bone's shape and decrease its mass. She would feel the disease move

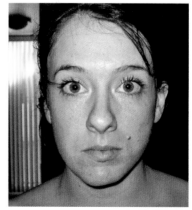

The lower left side of Amanda's face began to "shrink," and her skin started to harden in early 2006.

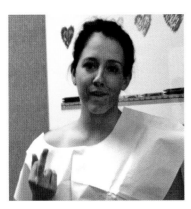

Amanda was repulsed by the treatment strategies she was offered.

through her cheek, painfully attacking muscles, creating tension and constriction down into her throat, making swallowing difficult, and up to her eye, causing tension and dryness. Her facial muscles continued to wither to such a degree that the loss of muscle volume (also known as microsomia) stopped her from being able to open her mouth wide, making brushing her teeth a massive challenge.

Additionally, her teeth would chatter, and she would constantly bite her tongue and mouth as she lost control of the muscles in her jaw. She had to wear a mouth guard to avoid biting herself. For someone who has to talk all day to cue clients in their movement, this effect was debilitating. As the disease crept up the left side of her face, it began to pull on her temple and part of her forehead (the temporalis muscle), causing massive charley horse spasms. Thin liquids were hard to swallow without choking, and she'd have to use a straw to drink anything. Chewing gum or sour foods that caused saliva overproduction was out of the question. And she had to learn to be extra careful while eating, especially the first bite of food, as her jaw muscles (masseter and pterygoids) would sometimes go into spasm and lock down, smashing her teeth into each other, with a mouthful of unchewed food she had to fight not to choke on, and no way to pry her jaw open again. Her only recourse was to relax, focus on her breathing, meditate, and wait for the muscles to release and her mouth to open again. The insides of her mouth are covered with scar tissue from biting herself repeatedly over the years.

At night it was hard to fall asleep, because as soon as she relaxed, her jaw would spasm. She learned to sleep with her head turned to the left,

the weight of her skull pressing down on the left side of her jaw, but this created problems in her neck. In fact, the entire left side of Amanda's body is noticeably tighter than her right. Her facial (and fascial) tension has literally impacted her all the way down to the tiny sesamoid bones in her left big toe. She even has been diagnosed with chronic sesamoiditis (inflammation around the small bones at the base of the big toe) from her leg's inner-thigh muscles and their downstream tightened fascias pulling on it.

Amanda's initial response to her condition was to "go full ostrich," she says ruefully. "After many years as a competitive athlete, I started my career as a movement educator because I felt deeply connected to its importance in a healthy lifestyle. However, as my disease progressed, I noticed that if my heart rate accelerated beyond 130, my jaw would completely lock down and spasm shut. This rocked my foundation because I could no longer participate in many of the styles of movement I was teaching to others, and to a degree it made me feel like a fraud." Amanda's husband, Jonathan, also a Master Level Personal Trainer with over two decades of experience, would suggest going to a support group or give her books or articles to read about the condition, but she was having none of it. "I wasn't trying to be brave–I was just blocking out what was happening," Amanda says. "I think I thought I was doing a better job of hiding it than I was." Though Amanda has a bachelor's degree in biology and has taken more than twenty certifications since 2000, she found it very difficult to navigate the unique challenges of this disease.

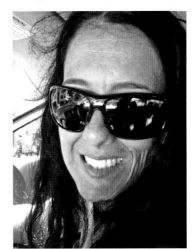

Finding photos in which Amanda allows the left side of her face to be seen is difficult. Here is a rare "sunglasses" shot from early 2012, a few months before we met.

After a while, it wasn't just her face—Amanda's spirit began to harden as well. Formerly a hippie chick, free spirit, painter, singer, and lover of art and movement, she now couldn't allow herself to be vulnerable or to relax, because as soon as she did her jaw would spasm. "My easy-peasy vibe was gone, because you only bite yourself so many times before it's like—enough," she says. Intimacy with Jonathan was hard, because she could never really let her body relax enough. She felt self-conscious in photographs, purposefully turning the right side of her face to the camera. After an exhaustingly painful day at work, Amanda would come home and isolate herself, tired of having to explain to other people through her frozen jaw why what looked like just a funny patch of skin was so debilitating to both her body and her spirit. Amanda felt that she should concentrate on being grateful that it wasn't systemic, but she was tired, short-tempered, and, to her horror, developing new symptoms of arthritis and Reynaud's syndrome (loss of circulation that causes aching) in her hands and feet.

After about three years of this, Amanda allowed a body worker to do some manual release work on her face, which was excruciating. "It was aggressive—he would come at it from inside my mouth and work on it for half an hour, which hurt like crazy, but would give me a day or two of relief," she says. She continued to see him once a month for about a year, but the relief was short-lived, and he was so expensive that it didn't seem worth it. She was hitting bottom psychologically, torturing herself with the idea that her whole world had been about health and fitness and now, "just walking through the world made my face freak out."

Amanda had been expanding her personal yoga practice to soothe her nervous system, and she thought it would make sense to explore becoming a yoga teacher again. In addition, she noticed that her client base had slowly shifted from wanting high-intensity training and needed something else. She began to specialize in working with clients suffering from Parkinson's disease, injuries, and other chronic conditions. It seemed that the universe was trying to tell her something: As her own chronic pain had increased, so had her natural sensitivity to suffering in others.

Amanda had trained to teach yoga over a decade before, but decided to take another training to brush up on her skills. Yoga Tune Up teacher Jillian Wintersteen Putney happened to be in the same yoga teacher training, and one day, when another trainee was complaining of back pain, Jillian pulled out the Therapy Balls and started talking about the Roll Model Method. Amanda had seen tons of myofascial release work done with a slew of different balls, rollers, sticks, and bars, but something about the way Jillian talked about the Roll Model Balls just clicked. Jillian convinced Amanda and Jonathan to take a day-long training with me in December 2012.

Even after years of practicing various forms of myofascial release, Jonathan was immediately sold when he felt how the anatomical accuracy of the Therapy Balls increased his shoulders' range of motion. However, Amanda's breakthrough came during the last sequence of the workshop, laying her jaw on a ball with a yoga block underneath and using the grippy balls to roll out her stiff temporomandibular joint (TMJ). She and Jonathan were facing each other, and the moment she put her aching jaw on the Therapy Ball and felt instant relief, she thought, "With all my training, why hadn't I thought of this?" and began to cry.

The training day ended shortly thereafter, and Amanda walked over to me to talk. I had noticed the scar on her face earlier in the day, but thought it was an old burn. Amanda's eyes were on fire as she said to me, "I developed local scleroderma on the left side of my face over five years ago. I have been to every doctor, chiropractor, Rolfer, and therapist under the sun, and nothing helped my jaw. Until now. I can move it now for the first time, I can open my mouth wide from the left side of my jaw and tell you this." We were both crying.

Her shift was profound, and Amanda got a huge, overwhelming rush from the empowerment she felt for the first time with her disease. In one moment, with one simple tool, she took control of her pain, immobility, and hopelessness, and her jaw became hers again. The intense grippy shear created by the Roll Model Balls toggled her tissues in just the right way (learn this technique on page 144).

She went home that day and rolled her jaw for another half-hour. In her thrill to finally have the tools she needed to take care of herself, she admits she went a little overboard at first. After three days straight of rolling for an hour a day on her jaw, it began to lock down again, so she backed off, recognizing that she would have to temper her enthusiasm and allow the years of immobile tissue to slowly release. She would roll on the Therapy Ball maybe once or twice a week, focusing a lot on the skin-rolling technique that the grippy balls were so good at, teasing apart the layers of connective tissue that had been stuck together for so long. She uses the PLUS and ALPHA Balls for the rest of her body, helping with the tightness throughout her left side and with her neck pain from years of sleeping with her face turned to one side.

The range of motion in her jaw has increased dramatically, and she has regained sensation in the area, able to feel her husband touch her cheek, and even "growing a little peach fuzz!" she says proudly. Swallowing is easier, and her pain and muscle spasms have been dialed down dramatically. While she's not necessarily able to control the spread of the disease, she's able to control the damage it does, and she uses the Roll Model Method throughout the day to roll her skin, promote circulation, and retain mobility in her jaw. "I am supremely confident that I now have powerful tools I've been searching for to combat the progress of my disease. I love the fact that I can choose for myself what I think I need at any moment–I can choose to 'go in deep' or maybe just keep it light–and I've found both approaches with the Therapy Balls to be awesome. This skin-rolling technique is so easy I literally do it zooming around Santa Monica in my Mini Cooper," she says. Previously, Amanda had to visit her dentist every three months for a cleaning since she couldn't reach the back of her mouth very well. Now she's brushing with much more ease, and she supplies Therapy Balls to her delighted dentist's office for patients with TMJ pain.

Amanda's psychological shift has also been radical. She's once again able to relax and allow her creativity to flow, and as a result is back to painting and singing. The Roll Model Balls allow her to feel what is happening instead of ignoring it, and in a lot of ways they reduce the drama of her condition, giving her some emotional relief from the anxiety of constantly being on guard. The self-discovery of the Roll Model Method helped her process not just her physical pain, but also how she had shut down for so many years. "I heard the doctor say there's nothing you can do, and I just embodied it. And now I am empowered by this little rubber ball that gives me permission to take all of my learning and use it on myself. It gave me permission to be broken in front of my clients–I could be a human being, I didn't have to be this model image of fitness. I was fixing damage that I thought I was just going to have to live with forever. And I really wanted to go back to that doctor and say, 'You know what? Maybe you need to say, "There's nothing I can do," rather than, "There's nothing you can do." Because there is something we all can do for ourselves, and you don't have to have a degree to do it. You just have to start."

Amanda knows what it's like to be in pain, and she empathizes with her clients who want to disconnect from the part of the body that is hurting, but she knows from her experience that connecting with and working through the emotional content of the pain gives her power back and ultimately allows her full, authentic self to shine through all aspects of her life. "This program has helped me feel less victimized by an illness that I have little control over. Now I can do something about the way my scleroderma affects my body–I can take back the reins and say, 'Not so fast.'"

On a side note, I have personally watched Amanda and Jonathan grow closer and more successful in love and in their training businesses. They both recently became certified Yoga Tune Up teachers and now share all of my self-care techniques with their clients.

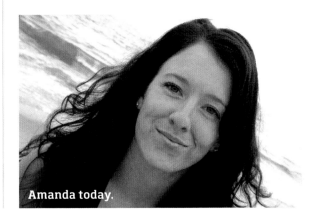

Amanda today.

Freestyle Exploration

*We shall not cease from exploration
And the end of all our exploring
Will be to arrive where we started
And know the place for the first time.*

–T.S. Eliot

These last three sequences are all about improvisation. There is no formula to follow other than to let your instincts be your guide. Quite often, this is how I roll out my own body. I'll start at a point on my front, back, or side and follow the needs of my body with the "kneads" of the various balls. My husband and I plunk down in front of the TV and freely style our own self-soothing sequences. This opens up a gateway to new moves and novel interpretations of old classics. Once you feel comfortable with the general map of your body, as well as the nine rolling techniques outlined in chapter 6, you are truly ready for some real jazz: freestyle. Play ball!

Use these silhouettes, suggestions, and photos as inspiration and intermix all the balls to carve paths of release and relief through your body.

Let the balls be your rubber scalpels for a 10-, 20-, or 45-minute "ball-et" designed by you. Greg Reid, the personal trainer and former bodybuilder featured on pages 36–39, told me that he unrolls his entire body from foot to head three times per week. His personal unlacing sessions that involve working through every possible contour and seam take about two hours. Whether you have two minutes or two hours, take the time to sneak in some self-care.

Working on one "seam" will truly help you feel the interconnectedness of the fascias associated with that aspect of your body. For example, working along any of the tissues along the back of your body should help all the tissues on the back of your body improve their slide & glide. Take each of these different "seams" through a progressive detangling, and feel the ease in your range of motion and pain reduction change after you roll. I offer you a general Check In and ReCheck in these sequences rather than a specific pose. Review the next section to refine your own ideas of how to create a "before" and "after" for your own freestyle routines.

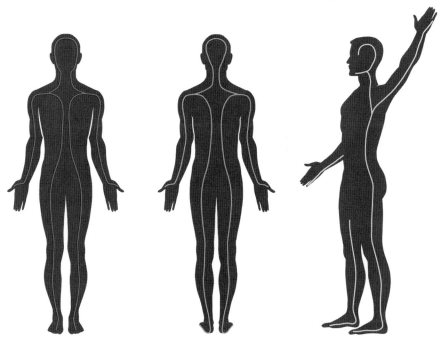

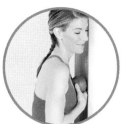

Sequence 16: Front Seam

Setup
Roll Model Balls: Original YTU, PLUS, ALPHA, Coregeous

Mat, block, wall, chair–ANYTHING

EmbodyMap/Basic Ball Stops

Anywhere on the front of your body.

Check In

Check In with any movement that stretches the front of your body, like a simple backbend that arches your whole body. Or mobilize in any way that stretches along the front of individual areas of your body.

Roll Sequence

- Start at any point along the front of your body and attempt to cover all the territory marked in red within the silhouette (see page 350).

- Incorporate all of the balls, or stick with just one type. When rolling out your abdomen, however, I recommend using only the Coregeous Ball.

- Intermix all 9 Roll Model techniques as you move.

- Remember to breathe. (See the breathing options on page 161.)

- Linger wherever you feel you need the most attention.

ReCheck

Arch your body in the same way you did during your Check In. Is there more movement? Less resistance? How does your breathing feel? How do you feel emotionally?

Reflect

1. Try to breathe exclusively into the front of your body. How is your breath's mobility?

2. Which areas are surprisingly tight? Which are the most open?

3. Finish this statement: I feel _____.

TIP: I am demonstrating an extreme range of motion here. Please do not try to force yourself into this shape. I use this image to make it obvious that this sequence aims to open the entire front of your body.

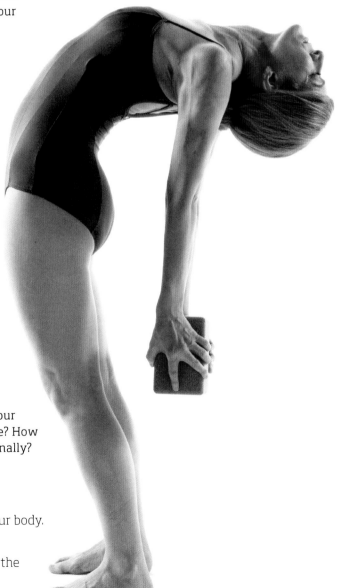

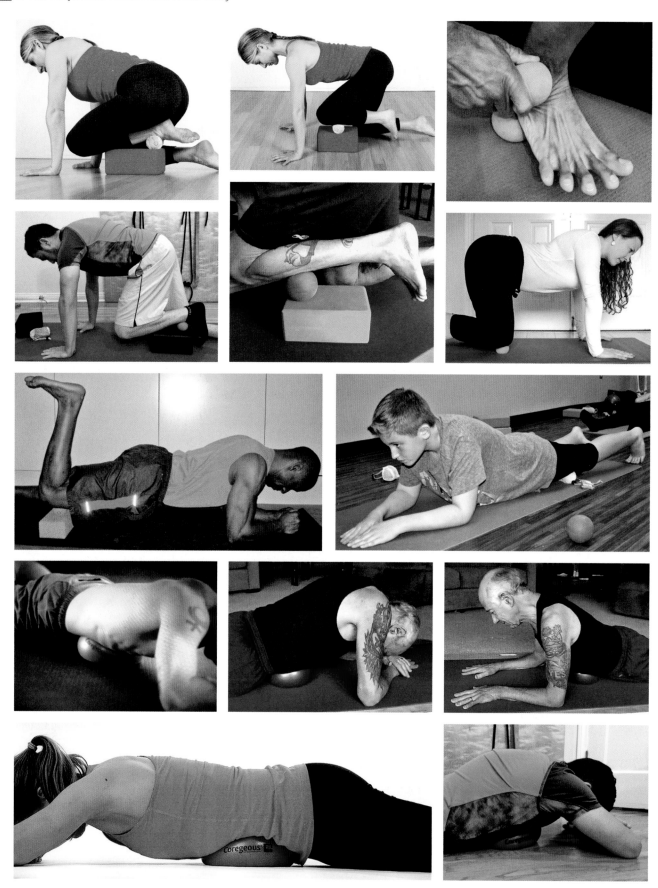

Use these images to inspire your front seam freestyle exploration.

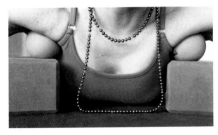

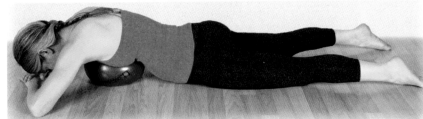

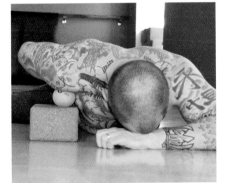

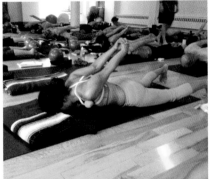

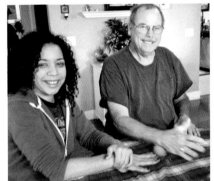

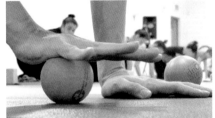

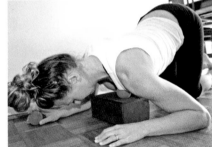

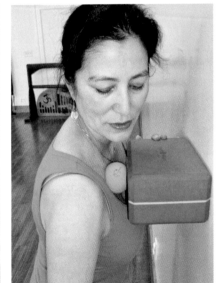

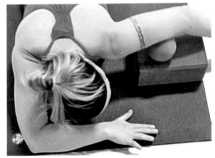

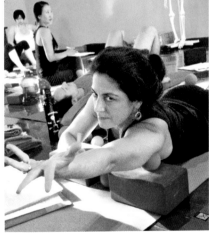

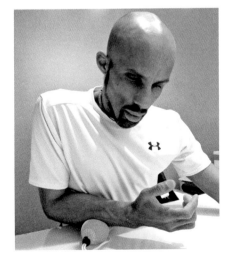

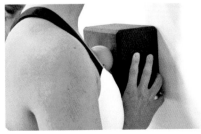

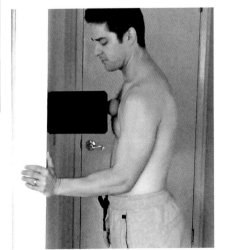

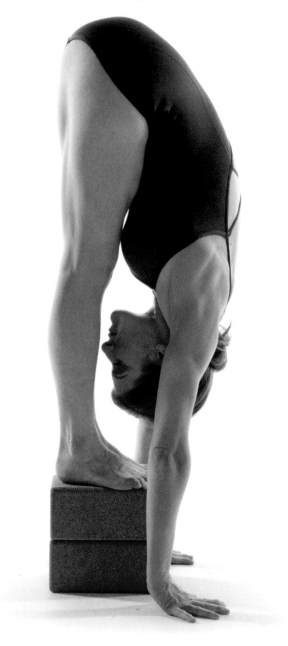

Sequence 17: Back Seam

Setup
Roll Model Balls: Original YTU, PLUS, ALPHA, Coregeous
Mat, block, wall, chair–ANYTHING

EmbodyMap/Basic Ball Stops

Anywhere on the back of your body.

Check In

Sample any movement that stretches the back of your body, like a simple forward bend. Do any motion that creates a stretch in any part of the back of your body, or a grand whole-body back stretch.

TIP: I am demonstrating a fairly extreme range of motion in this forward bend. Please do not try to force yourself into this shape. I use this image to make it obvious that this sequence aims to open the entire back of your body.

Roll Sequence

- Start at any point along the back of your body and attempt to cover all the territory marked in blue within the silhouette (see page 350). It's also fun to start on the sole of one foot, work your way up one entire back side of your body until you roll into the back of your head, and then reverse the pattern on the second side. In other words, foot to crown, then crown to foot.
- Incorporate all of the balls, or stick with just one type.
- Intermix all 9 Roll Model techniques as you move.
- Remember to breathe. (See the breathing options on page 161.)
- Linger wherever you feel you need the most attention.

ReCheck

Stretch your body in the same way you did during your Check In. Is there more movement? Less resistance? How does your breathing feel? How do you feel emotionally?

Reflect

1. Spend 3 solid minutes lying on your back consciously breathing. Where do you feel most open? Where would you like to spend more time?

2. Stand up and check your upright posture. What does it feel like?

3. Finish this statement: I feel _____.

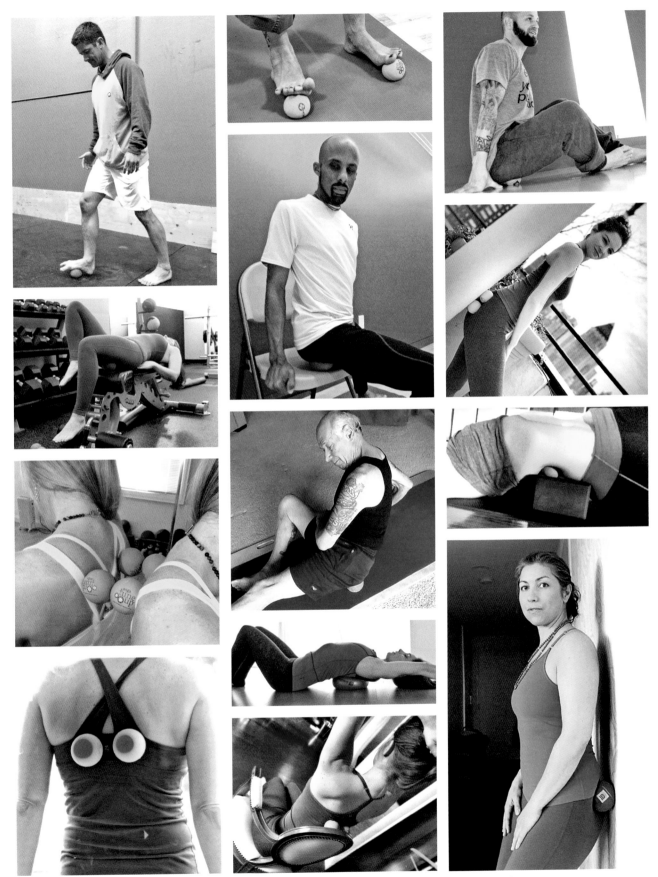

Use these images to inspire your back seam freestyle exploration.

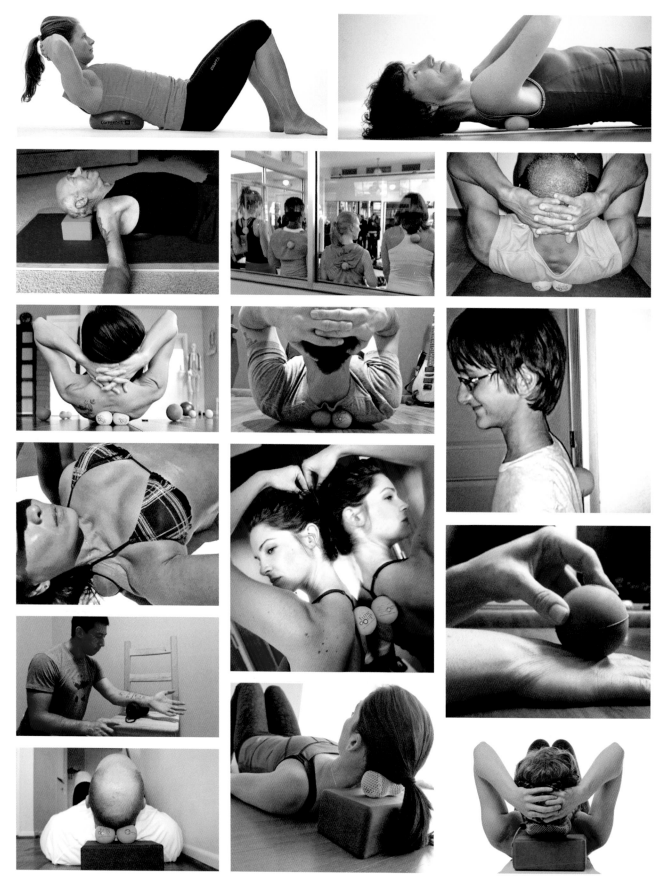

More back seam freestyle exploration.

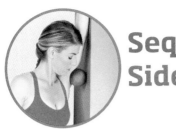

Sequence 18: Side Seam

Setup

Roll Model Balls: Original YTU, PLUS, ALPHA, Coregeous

Mat, block, wall, chair–ANYTHING

The side seam can be a bit trickier. Use your imagination with the nine techniques, and make use of your balls inside the tote to gain maximum access to your inner and outer thighs and your inner and outer arms.

EmbodyMap/Basic Ball Stops

Anywhere on the right or left side of your body, including the insides and outsides of your limbs.

Check In

Perform any movement that stretches the side of your body, like a simple sideways bend. Try any move that creates a stretch in any part of your side, or a grand whole-body side stretch.

Roll Sequence

- Start at any point along the side of your body and attempt to cover all the territory marked in yellow within the silhouette (see page 350). It's also fun to start on the side of one foot and ankle and zigzag your way up the entire outside of your leg and thigh while simultaneously using a ball stack to roll out your inner thighs.

- I recommend switching to the Coregeous Ball on the side of your abdomen, or position yourself with the ALPHA while leaning against a wall to scrub the sides of your abdomen and ribcage.

- Try using the wall with a ball stack (keeping the balls in the tote) to roll out both sides of your arms at once.

- Incorporate all of the balls, or stick with just one type.

- Intermix all 9 Roll Model techniques as you move.

- Remember to breathe. (See the breathing options on page 161.)

- Linger wherever you feel you need the most attention.

ReCheck

Stretch your body the same way you did during your Check In. Is there more movement? Less resistance? How does your breathing feel? How do you feel emotionally?

Reflect

1. Take 15 breaths that balloon the sides of your abdomen and ribs outward. How is your access?

2. Take a slow "dance break" and move your body like a snake. How is the quality of your motion?

3. Finish this statement: I feel _____.

TIP: *I am demonstrating an extreme range of motion in this twisted side bend. Please do not try to force yourself into this shape. I use this image to make it obvious that this sequence targets the sides of your body.*

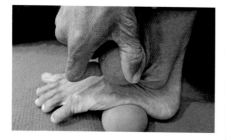
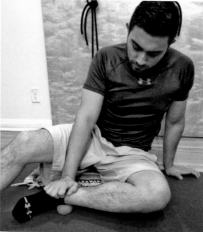
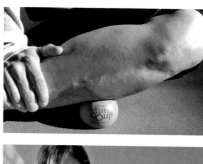
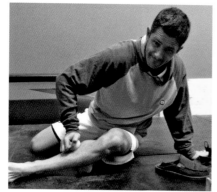
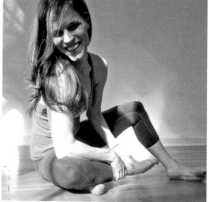
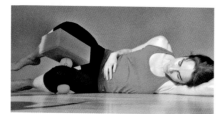
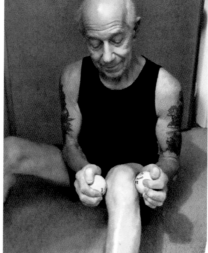
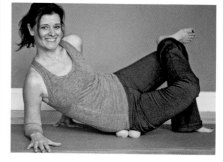
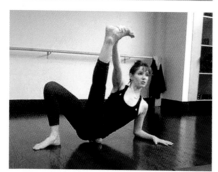
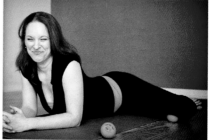
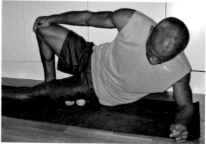
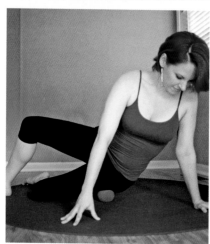
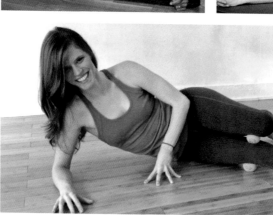

Use these images to inspire your side seam freestyle exploration.

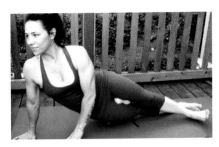
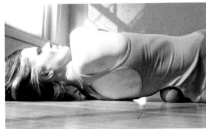
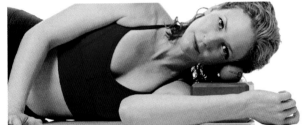
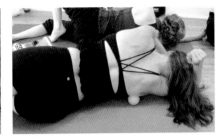
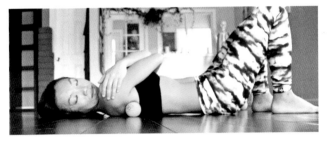
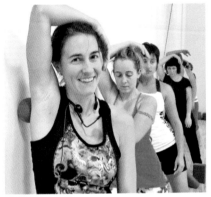
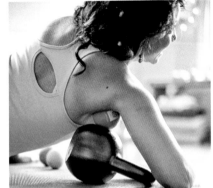
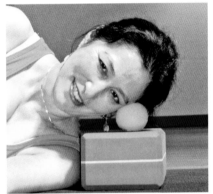
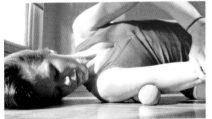
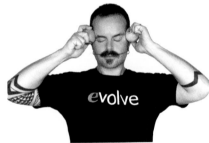
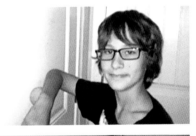
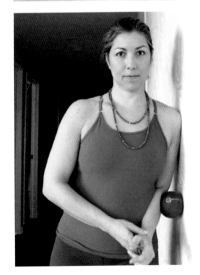
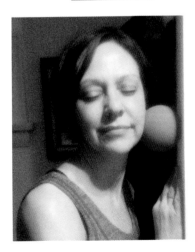
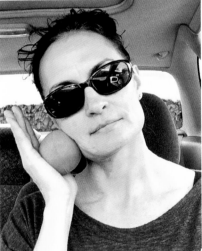

9 The "Roll" of Relaxation

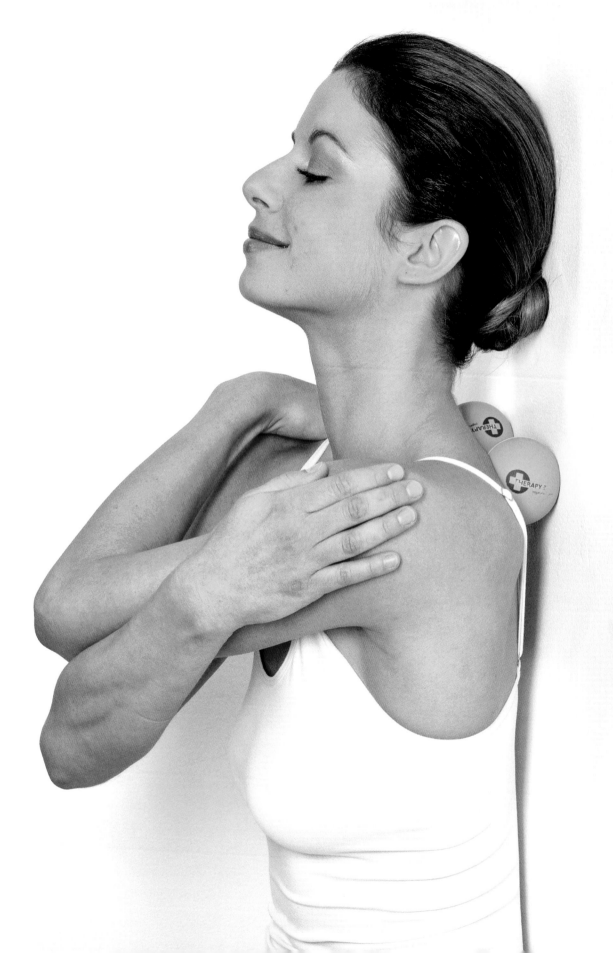

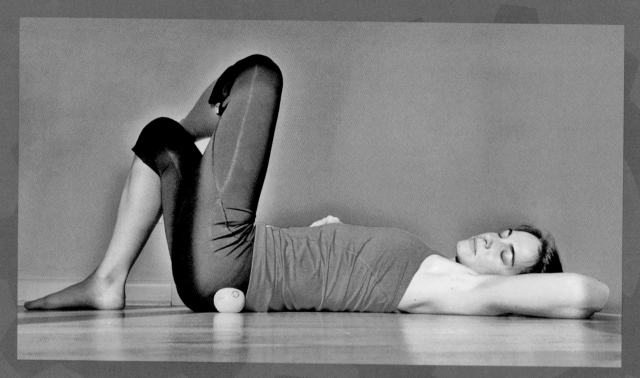

The Roll Model Method can be boiled down to the simplest of instructions: *get down and roll!* And just like that, the Therapy Balls will certainly help you, even if you are "mindlessly" rolling while watching *The Real Housewives of Beverly Hills*, sitting on them during an overseas flight, or standing on top of them at your standing desk or while doing the dishes.

To truly reap the benefits of your time on the balls, add in a few other steps to maximize their effects on every system of your body. Just as my teacher Glenn Black told me to make my practice into "orange juice concentrate" in order to magnify my "movement vitamin intake," you can enhance the balls' effectiveness by concentrating your relaxation efforts.

By bringing your body, mind, and heart to your sessions, you create a deeply relaxed internal environment that will compound the benefits of the Roll Model Method.

A Brief Tour of Your Nervous System

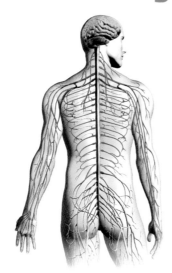

Your nervous system is divided into three main branches: the somatic, the autonomic, and the more recently discovered enteric.*

The somatic branch innervates skeletal muscle and receives sensory information. You consciously use the somatic system all the time to move your body through space, react to input from your environment, or act on your thoughts.

The autonomic branch controls your internal organs and functions autonomously, meaning that you cannot will it to do things. It is comprised of sympathetic and parasympathetic components, which seem to have a "mind" of their own. The sympathetic nervous system gears up your internal organs and musculoskeletal system for the fight-or-flight response. It is your **arousal** state, your own personal "on switch." When you break into a panic, blame the sympathetic response. The parasympathetic nervous system supports the day-to-day functioning of your internal organs and is often called the "rest, digest, and recovery" response. It is your **drousal** state, your "off switch." When you slip into relaxation, thank your parasympathetic nerves.

* The enteric nervous system governs digestion and behaves autonomically. For more information, see Dr. Michael Gershon's book *The Second Brain* (Harper Perennial, 1999).

Because the autonomic branch is not within your conscious grasp, you must employ a sort of trickery in order to create optimal conditions for it to function well and help the organs and systems it regulates to flourish. With the Roll Model Therapy Ball work, you use the mastery of your muscles and somatic control to directly impact the states of arousal or drousal in your autonomic system. With practice, you can learn to *bring your mind into your muscles.*

The conscious link toward helping your autonomic nervous system function optimally is total care of your health through diet, exercise, sleep, breathing, and relaxation.

When you relax by systematically addressing the muscles that are within your conscious control (somatic nervous system), you can manipulate your excitable self into states of sedation. Luckily, there are several accessible methods that you can use to down-regulate your nervous system and lull yourself into parasympathetic dominance.

Developing a practice of relaxation takes some discipline and dedication because the lion's share of your brain is dedicated to being aroused and in sympathetic mode. Your brain has more neurons dedicated to alertness than to relaxation. It's much easier for your nervous system to accelerate from 0-60 than it is to slam on the brakes and decelerate from 60-0 without skidding off the road. Your parasympathetic system needs a lot of nurturing in order for down-regulation and sedation to occur. To maintain balance in your brain chemistry, restore your tissues, eradicate pain, and diminish the ravages of stress, you must learn how to turn *on* your off switch consciously.

Joanne Spence, 49

Executive Director, Yoga in Schools;
Yoga Therapist, Western Psychiatric Institute;
& Clinic Director, Yoga on the Square

Pittsburgh, Pennsylvania

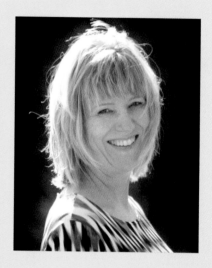

Dear Jill,

I recently added the Roll Model Balls to our weekly class with teens at the Rankin Promise Program, an alternative school in the Woodland Hills School District in Pittsburgh, Pennsylvania. Often, I have new kids each session who have little or no connection to their body. The main reasons students are referred to our school are for fighting and assaults on other students, chronic classroom or hallway/cafeteria disruptions, chronic defiance issues, and possession of a weapon or controlled substance on school grounds. They lack the ability to regulate themselves.

What I am finding is that the refreshment the kids are experiencing with the Roll Model Balls is immediate. The fact that they even want to try them is still amazing to me. Some of the stress I can see in their bodies just melts away. Their interior worlds are so chaotic, yet simple tools and techniques like sustained compression give immediate and visible relief. My favorite part is seeing unsmiling, distracted faces break into smiles as they float back to class. "I feel so much better." "Amazing, I didn't think it was possible to feel better." "I could go to sleep now." "My body has never felt so relaxed." "Thank you, Miss, can you come back tomorrow?"

The students who use them more than once know exactly what they want to do for a repeat experience. I see bodies visibly relaxing. I see kids who have a hard time letting go of anything being able to let go of tension once they realize that they can.

I feel that the Roll Model Balls have the potential to offset immense stress for kids in school, and this will lead to happier, more resilient kids who can actually learn better and weather the storms of adolescence and the tough challenges they are facing. I would recommend the Roll Model Balls to any educator who is at the end of their rope with attempts at classroom consensus and calm. If they work with the kids I am working with, they will work with any kids.

Thank you!
Joanne

The 5 Ps of the Parasympathetic Nervous System: Sedate Yourself

There are a handful of ways to turn on your off switch. The more your body meets and saturates itself in the conditions listed below, the more profound your relaxation response will be, and the better chance you'll have of thoroughly adapting to the positive changes that the Roll Model Method is attempting to effect.

1. Perspective–mindset
2. Place–peaceful
3. Pace of breath–emphasis on exhale
4. Position–reclined
5. Palpation–ball massage

This is not a fixed order; many of these conditions occur simultaneously. You'll want to meet as many of them as possible to have the best outcome.

Let's look at each one individually.

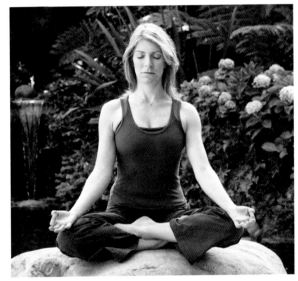

You don't need to sit in lotus position in the middle of paradise to convince yourself to relax, but at a minimum, you'll want to adopt an attitude that permits you to relax deeply.

Perspective

Perspective boils down to how you think about your actions. It's about the orientation of your attitude. To truly reap the benefits of conscious relaxation, you have to create a mental blanket of sorts that will protect your respite.

Say to yourself: "I allow myself to relax completely."

Give yourself permission for a time-out. Mentally frame your time administering self-care and line it with optimism. You are doing something very powerful by taking your health, healing, and transformation into your own hands. So take the time to acknowledge it, and create bookends around your self-treatment endeavors.

You have permission to relax completely.

Don't you feel better already?

Now let's make sure that your environment also gives you that permission.

Place

I have rolled on my Therapy Balls in airport terminals, in public restrooms, on the floor of my office, on the seat of my car, at rock concerts, at the movies, and in every other imaginable place. The balls will work their magic as long as you position them to help. But there are more ideal environments that make the best practice arenas if time and space permit.

Find a quiet, peaceful room that is not too cold. Ideally you want a clean surface, whether it's a wood floor, an industrial carpet, a linoleum floor, or a wall. The balls roll best on a firm surface; thick carpeting tends to absorb part of the ball's size and can also lead to rug burns on your skin (trust me on this one!). If you have an exercise mat or a yoga mat, place that on top of your carpet to help minimize rug burn. My father, the doctor, likes to use the Therapy Balls in bed to help his hip pains and to help him fall asleep at night (much better

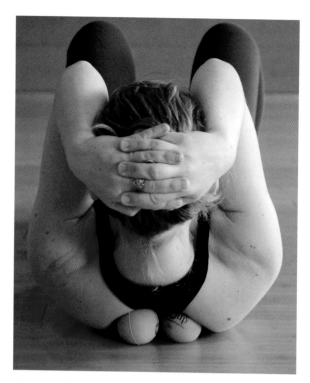

Your environment does not have to be a soundproof sanctuary, but it does help to minimize physical and sensory obstacles.

than sleeping pills!). Using them in bed can be tricky, though, if you have an extra-soft mattress or lots of bedding.

What is most important is that you find a place where you can feel peaceful and relaxed to do the unwinding you want to do.

If your goal is maximum relaxation, then dim the lights as well to decrease optic nerve stimulation.

There are times when you may not be able to meet the ideal conditions for "Place." For example, you may want to use the balls at the gym before exercising to prepare your tissues for your workout. I certainly do. The gym's bright lights, noise, and other distractions do not create the most tranquil space, but you can minimize the sensory overload by closing your eyes and concentrating on what you're feeling, connecting to your "perspective," and modulating your breathing.

Pace of Breath

Your breath is a great internal barometer that constantly gives you feedback about your state of mind. Rapid, shallow breathing indicates sympathetic overload, and slow, deep breathing signifies parasympathetic quietude. Master your observation and manipulation of your breath, and you will be able to control your body's physiology.

Every breath you take can be divided into four parts:

1. **The inhale**
2. **The pause after inhale, before exhale**
3. **The exhale**
4. **The pause after exhale, before inhale**

The duration of each of these parts differs depending on the physical or internal stresses you are experiencing.

When you are under high stress, your body spends more time inhaling and holding your breath in, like a balloon being filled to its taut capacity. For example, consider being startled: you gasp (a quick, gigantic inhale) and hold your breath until the danger passes. You won't find yourself yawning or sighing until after the fear is gone. This is the arousal/sympathetic state.

When you are under low stress, your body seems to deflate like an emptying balloon. Consider yawning, a prolonged exhale, often accompanied by a moan, followed by not breathing in again. In fact, when you finally do take your next inhale, you may be surprised to realize that you haven't breathed in for quite some time. This is the drousal/parasympathetic state.

FOUR-PART BREATH CYCLE

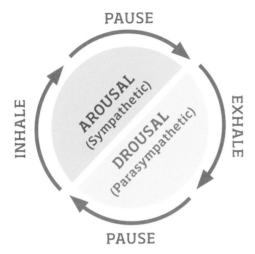

The ideal for relaxation is to spend more time exhaling than inhaling. When your body begins to surrender and let go, you will find yourself spontaneously letting out great volumes of air. You'll hear your own involuntary sighs when you tap into places that give you deep relief. This is an excellent sign that you are entering deeper into sedation.

Dig deeper into remodeling your breathing in chapter 7, then kick back, relax, and find a position of comfort.

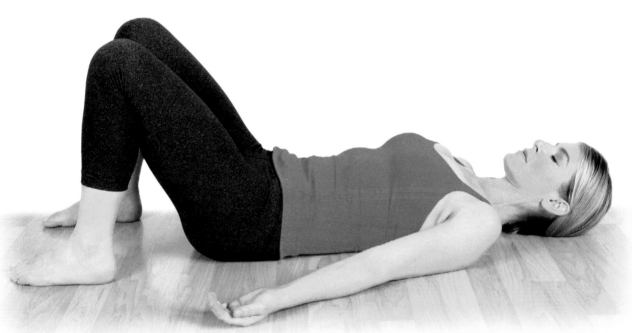

Position

Lie back and take a load off.

One of the easiest ways to induce the relaxation response is to recline. How many times have you flopped out on your bed or couch and felt the weight of the world fly away from your shoulders? Ever notice that within a few moments of lying down, you let out a prolonged involuntary exhalation? As soon as you recline, your off switch turns on.

When you lie down, the muscles and tissues that were supporting your upright spinal bones no longer have to be sympathetically firing to hold you up. There is less structural stress on your diaphragm and heart, so everything can slow... way...down.... Gravity acts differently on you, too, helping all your muscles stretch downward toward the Earth. (This is making me want to take a nap right now.) It's no mistake that we sleep best while we are reclined. If you've ever found yourself dozing off while seated, you don't typically wake up feeling as refreshed. Overseas flight in coach? Not the most relaxing way to dream.

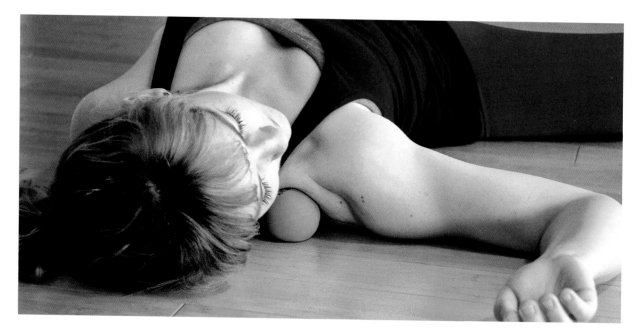

A reclined position is the ideal arrangement for rolling on your Therapy Balls because it minimizes extraneous stress on all the tissues of your body. The challenge for some people initially is that the weight of the whole slackened body may be too much to bear when rolling. Reclined positions maximize your full mass plus gravity's compounding effect onto the projectile touch of the ball. If the pressure is intolerable and you are unable to relax and breathe, you'll have to modify the placement of the ball and the position of your body. You may need to lean into a wall instead of driving your full relaxed body weight toward the floor.

There is one level deeper than reclining, and that is *inverting*. When you invert by raising your pelvis higher than your heart or your heart higher than your head, your body automatically shuts down sympathetic activity. It is the equivalent of pressing the off button on your computer. Folders and windows close, and your brain becomes a bit clearer and calmer. The inversion angle needed to plug into this relaxation response is very mild–you don't have to pop up into a headstand or shoulder stand. You can lift your pelvis on a pillow, some thick books, or a yoga block, or let your ribcage arc across the Coregeous Ball to induce the inversion response.

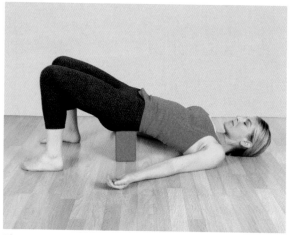

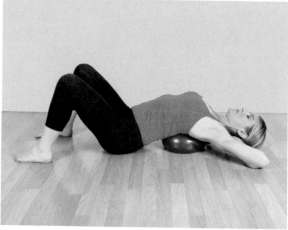

Elevating your pelvis on a yoga block or pillow or letting your ribcage arc across the Coregeous Ball can swiftly deepen your level of relaxation.

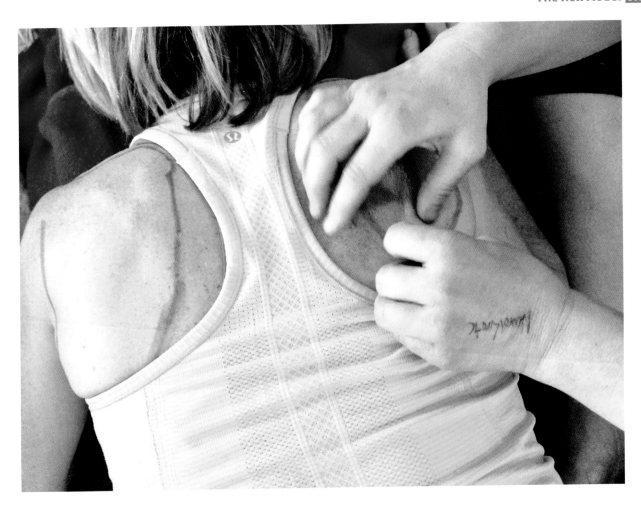

Palpation

Finally, it's time to get touchy-feely.

To palpate is to touch. Touch is vital for life and health. Children who are not held or given affection have a number of physical, mental, and psychological deficits; their brains don't develop healthfully. Therapeutic self-palpation is at the heart of the Roll Model Method. Its power to heal what hurts is extraordinary. Many of your aches and pains will literally vanish with the self-massage sequences that you'll find in chapter 8.

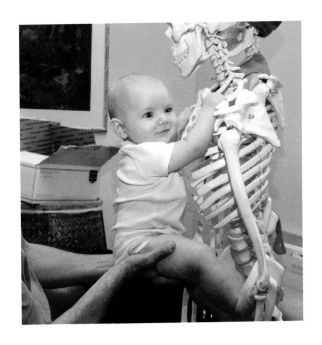

First, it's important to understand why holding any unresolved or unconscious tension in your body is at odds with true relaxation. Muscle tension is your mind's way of holding your body hostage to pain. Second, you need to understand how the Roll Model Method helps rid you of that tension and induce the relaxation response in your body.

Palpation–in this case, self-massage–leads to two primary *rollaxation* results:

1. It decreases sympathetic outflow by altering the resting tone of your muscles and their associated fascias.

2. It elevates your well-being chemistry, boosting endorphins, serotonin, oxytocin, and dopamine, a neurotransmitter cocktail that is naturally induced through therapeutic touch.*

* Sandy Fritz, *Mosby's Fundamentals of Therapeutic Massage,* Fifth Edition (Mosby, 2012).

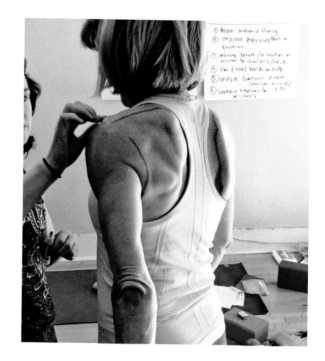

Resting Tone Is Not Always Restful

Resting tone refers to the level of resistance a muscle has to passive stretch while at rest. Even at rest, your muscles have a degree of contractile tension that the central nervous system relays to stretch receptors within your myofascia, called muscle spindles. These spindles contain specialized sensory nerve endings that communicate with your central nervous system about the stresses being placed on your muscles.

Your resting muscle tone can vary depending on your state of mind. An aroused mind exerts more pull on all the muscle spindles, and muscles are shortened, ready for action. Sometimes your mind will not let go, and certain muscle fibers remain in persistent contraction, resulting in the formation of trigger points. A calm, relaxed mind does not need to waste energy to signal muscle contraction other than when necessary.

The Roll Model Therapy Ball work can help you manually switch off unwanted and excessive contraction. The balls induce stretch motion into myofascia that dulls the signaling of those overactive muscle spindles and results in a "turning off" of the contraction. The balls can actually stop your mind from telling your muscles to stay short; they remind your mind to back off and let go.

Through deep touch, the Roll Model Balls induce a powerful change in the global nervous tone of your body. Muscles do not contract on their own; they require an impulse from the central nervous system to shorten. Often, chronic tension develops because your mind *thinks* that your body should *feel* a certain way. Your tissues are consistently being told to stay short (or long) because your mind has become hard-wired around a physical disposition or an emotional attitude. Your habitual level of tension or resting tone may be protecting an injury, or perhaps your body is not making full use of its tissues (sitting in a chair all day or walking with slouched posture, for example), so your mind recalculates how long or short certain tissues need to be for daily function (as opposed to optimal or ideal function). Your mind and body have an automatic relay about this until your greater awareness decides to consciously create change. Chronic pain is often the big motivator.

The Chemistry of Touch Induces Relaxation and Well-Being

Many published studies substantiate that physiological shifts in blood chemistry occur after therapeutic massage. Massage boosts your levels of serotonin, dopamine, and endorphins and decreases cortisol.* There are no formal studies specifically on self-massage, so the personal testimonials throughout this book, along with the thousands of others I've received over the years, will have to suffice as testimony to the power of this type of self-care healthcare. With

that, I say, do your own *self-study*. Get down and roll and let the process speak for itself. The entire point of this book is to take the power of healing and pain relief into your own hands and not let others tell you what or how you should be feeling.

Allow the kneading, rubbing, and shearing to have its effects on your body. Feel tight tissues transition into tranquility and cellular recovery.** Get down and roll and tell me how you feel.

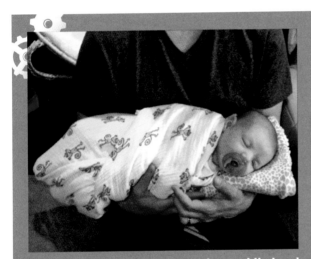

Five-week-old Lilah Iris is snugly swaddled and reclining with a hint of inversion in her father's arms. Babies aren't the only humans who enjoy the relaxing effects of a swaddle.

SWADDLING

There is one subset of palpation that you may have left behind you as a child. If you are a parent, you are probably familiar with swaddling. Firmly wrapping an infant can calm her or him down in a flash. Add to that tipping the baby's head downward a bit—inversion—and baby becomes silent and sweet again. Wrapping yourself in blankets or towels so that your whole body is compressed is a great way to induce another level of relaxation. The *ball stacking* technique seen in some of the sequences, where you use multiple balls to surround an area, also aids in creating that compressive/swaddled feeling.

Time

The factor that ties all these relaxation buttons together is time. As I stated earlier, you cannot expect your human machine to decelerate as fast as it can accelerate—we are designed mostly for alertness, not tranquility. Be prepared to give yourself a minimum of two minutes to reap the relaxing effects of rolling. A twenty-minute session that combines all of the above off switches will leave you feeling calm, cool, and collected for hours...unless, of course, you fall asleep!

* M. Hernandez-Reif et al, "Cortisol decreases and serotonin and dopamine increase following massage therapy," *International Journal of Neuroscience* 115, no. 10 (2005): 1397-413. Accessed via www.ncbi.nlm.nih.gov/pubmed?term=Field T%5BAuthor%5D&cauthor=true&cauthor_uid=161624471

** Crain, Tarnopolsky, et al, "Massage therapy attenuates inflammatory signaling after exercise-induced muscle damage," *Scientific Translation Medicine* 4, no. 119 (2012).

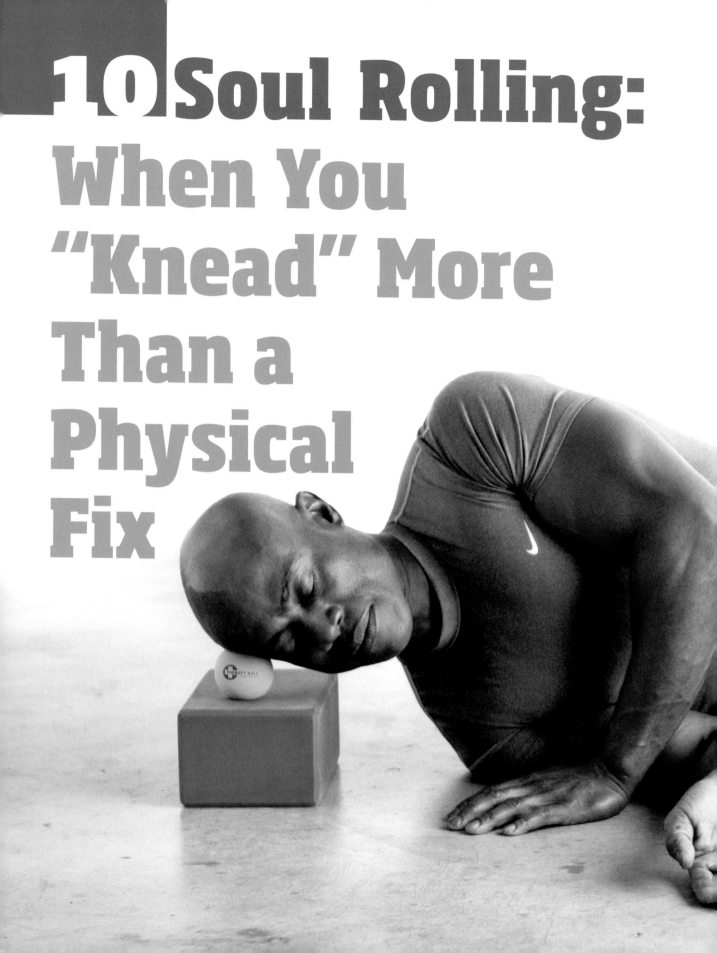

10 Soul Rolling: When You "Knead" More Than a Physical Fix

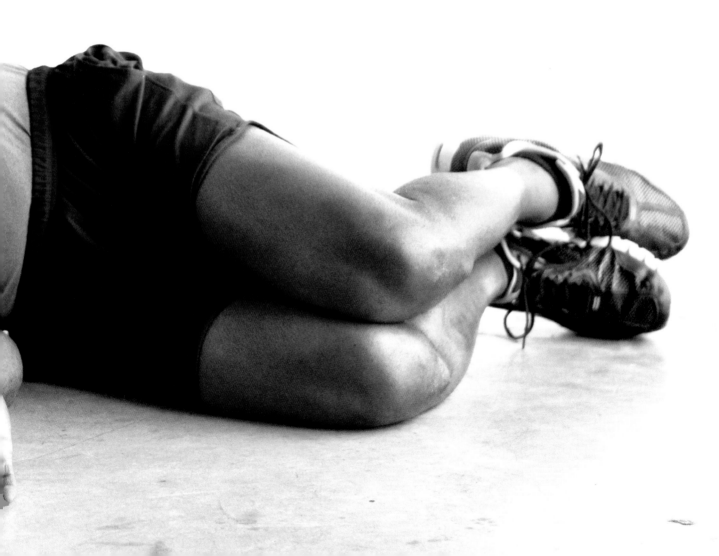

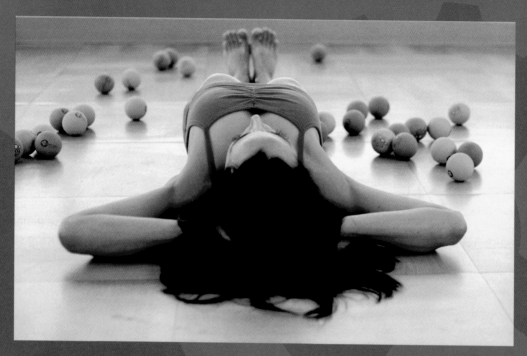

When I decided to write a book about the Roll Model Method, I reached out to thousands of students and Therapy Ball users and asked them to send in their stories of how they've used the balls to help themselves. To my astonishment, one of the largest "categories" was trauma. I received story after story of men and women who had lost faith, been abused, or lived through emotional catastrophe, assault, the death of a loved one, and more who used the Roll Model Method and the Therapy Balls to find peace of mind and spirit when nothing else could comfort them.

Your Emotional Roller Coaster: Smoothing Out Your Edge

Massage is known to release endorphins, dopamine, serotonin, and other "feel-good" chemicals in the body.* It also lowers levels of stress hormones such as cortisol and vasopressin.** There have been few studies to date to verify whether *self*-massage releases this same neurochemistry cocktail, but I'm willing to bet there is a significant difference in your body's chemistry before and after. Even in the absence of quantitative data, your own experimentation will enable you to sense the emotional satisfaction of releasing the stress stored in your tissues.

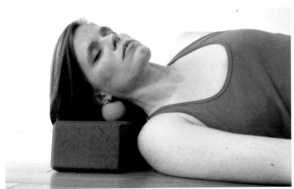

Laurel has used the Roll Model Therapy Balls to help her cope with the loss of her mother. She felt unable to fully grieve until she tapped into her emotions while rolling in the privacy of her home.

Many of the stories you will read in this chapter are accounts of grief, anger, fear, and trauma that were once trapped inside. Unprocessed emotion festers and seethes inside your mind and heart and can alter your behavior. I have had this experience many times over. Talking with friends, family, loved ones, and therapists was not always terribly effective for me. I often could gain mental clarity only in the privacy of my own rolling practice.

Unassimilated emotion finds a way of expressing itself in your body as well. It becomes physical tension. Though you may not have specific hip, neck, or back pain, the inner congestion caused

by hiding your feelings from yourself and others is on display in the general tone of your body. In the psychiatric world, many anxiety disorders list muscle tension, trembling, twitching, aching, and soreness as part of the profile.*** Your emotionally beaten body is harboring these generalized aches partly because it is experiencing stress overload (an overtaxed sympathetic nervous system—see page 363), and you cannot unwind and let go.

The balls will find your tension *and* your emotion. Your suffering will no longer stay hidden. As the balls touch your tissues, they also touch the nerves that tunnel from the surface of your body into the emotional centers of your brain. These emotional centers may cue you to cry, laugh, or reexperience anger or other unexpressed sentiments that remain lodged in your tissues.

The emotions you may feel while rolling are normal, natural, healthy, and necessary. The balls provide discretion and privacy—a wonderful service. Using the Roll Model Method gives you a chance to get in touch with yourself on your own. Self-soothing with the balls is empowering and beneficial. As you start to identify the pain within you, you may start to emerge from the state of darkness you were in and experience lightness. When this happens, I highly recommend that you seek a loving friend or skilled therapist to talk through some of the challenges you are facing as a way to further work through the feelings you are harboring.

* M. Hernandez-Reif et al, "Breast cancer patients have improved immune and neuroendocrine functions following massage therapy," *Journal of Psychosomatic Research* 57, no. 1 (2004): 45-52. Accessed via www.ncbi.nlm.nih.gov/pubmed/15256294
** Sandy Fritz, *Sports & Exercise Massage: Comprehensive Care for Athletics, Fitness, & Rehabilitation*, 2nd Edition (Elsevier, 2013).
*** www.nytimes.com/health/guides/disease/post-traumatic-stress-disorder/print.html

May this self-care practice help you truly get "in touch" with all of the multifaceted layers of yourself. May you find peace.

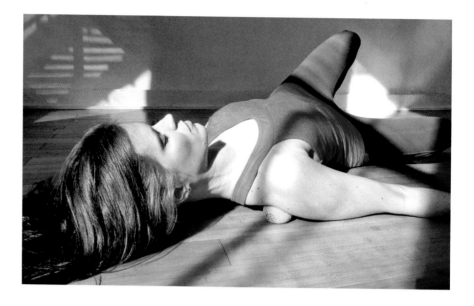

Rape, Recovery, and Reclaiming Center

Emily Sonnenberg, 25
Assistant Group Fitness Director at the Athletic Club
Waterloo, Ontario, Canada

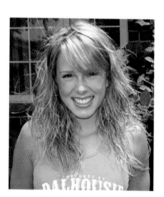

At 16, Emily Sonnenberg was the kind of daughter any parent would be proud of. She got good grades in her university prep classes, was on the track team, swam, rode horses, had tons of friends, and was one of those bright shiny people who could light up any room or situation. Her boyfriend, "Brian" (not his real name), had recently left for college in Alabama, so Emily spent the summer between her junior and senior years of high school planning their future, figuring out which colleges had the right kind of sociology and psychology programs so that she could become a teacher.

She missed Brian, but she was having a great time as a camp counselor for 5- to 7-year-olds, making good money and hanging out with "Chad" (not his real name), the 22-year-old co-worker she had been paired with. Together they would take the kids to the park and play storytelling games

with them. Over time, Emily began hanging out more with Chad and his older friends. She had made it clear to Chad that she wasn't interested in him romantically, even making sure that Brian knew it was harmless. "But Chad was grooming me for drinking," she says. "I mean, I drank occasionally with friends, because it was a small town and that's what everyone did. But he got me drinking more—he would talk about how he would go home on his lunch break and have a beer, and he made it sound cool, so I started to emulate him."

One night toward the end of the summer, Chad had a going-away party before he returned to college in the fall. Emily's friend dropped her off at his house, and Chad began to ply her with drinks. Emily is a petite 5'2", so it didn't take long before she was drunk. "There's a video of me sitting on the edge of his bed, singing a drunken song, but I don't remember it. A lot of that night is very mixed up in my head," she says.

What Emily does remember is that for the next four hours, Chad raped her. She surfaced in and out of consciousness during the relentless assault, with brief moments of awareness that would then plunge her back into confusion and darkness. She knows that at one point the much larger Chad had her pinned down in his bathroom, and then, with no memory of how she got there, he violated her again outside on the steps of a nearby school classroom. In a last, horrifying moment of lucidity, she recalls him being on top of her in the living room, with other people drinking beer and watching idly. In her confused, barely conscious state, she reasoned that since the others weren't stopping him, what he was doing must be okay. Emily was sick, dizzy, and exhausted and could not fight him away. The attack caused a deep split of her body from her mind–a break that would take years to repair.

Eventually, at around 4 o'clock in the morning, she regained clarity. "I woke up and it was still going–I was lying on my back on his bed and Chad was standing over me," she says. She realized she had to get home, somehow finding her clothes and making it outside. "I found a cab to take me to my father's house. The cab picked up another couple on the way, and I felt so unsafe, but I couldn't do anything about it. I just kept telling the driver I needed to get home."

At her father's house, Emily made her way inside without waking her dad or sister and went to bed. She woke up the next morning feeling completely battered, like her body had been hit by a truck. But she didn't tell her dad what had happened. "He has non-Hodgkin's lymphoma, and I didn't want to break his heart. I didn't tell anyone. I treated it like I had done something bad. I blamed myself." It is not uncommon for date rape victims to feel that they are at fault for "letting it happen." Emily eventually told her best friend that she "had sex with someone who wasn't Brian," but that was it. Neither her parents nor her sister had any idea what had happened to her, and she shuttered this secret from them for months.

Some of the other people at the party had younger siblings who attended Emily's school, so it wasn't long before her classmates found out about the incident. But the story going around was that Emily had cheated on her boyfriend. Nobody asked her what really happened, and Emily sank into a deep depression, convinced that she was to blame. The guilt and shame were overwhelming, especially with no one to talk to. Her 16-year-old mind constructed a self-victimizing story to protect her from the trauma of that night. And with her own heart lying to itself, she withdrew deeper and deeper inside, away from other people and away from reality. The weight of her secret cloaked her in a thick, painful despondency, leaving her numb, disembodied, and barely able to function. Emily systematically withdrew from every part of her life. She stopped riding and swimming, quit the track team and all her school committees, and pulled back from her friends. "I was just existing," she says. "I did not know how to keep going. I started to plan out how I was going to kill myself."

She ran into Chad a few months after the rape, and he admitted to her that he had planned the whole thing. In a horrible ironic twist, her attacker, the one person who knew the truth of that night, was the only person she felt she could talk to. She told him how much pain she was in, how depressed and withdrawn she had become. While he seemed to feel sorry for her, Chad never admitted that it had been anything other than two drunk people fooling around and having a good time. In the end, talking to him did nothing to take away Emily's self-blame and self-loathing.

A few months later, Emily finally told Brian about the rape. He was horrified and terribly upset for her. For the first time, it crossed Emily's mind that maybe it wasn't her fault–"but accepting that is hard, even to this day," she admits. Even with the relief of finally telling someone, Emily was still in a very dark place. Her mom was going crazy trying to figure out why her daughter had suddenly changed into this unrecognizable shell of a person. "My mom was desperate–she didn't know I was suicidal, but she knew I was in a really bad way, and so finally one day she said, 'That's it! We're going to see your godmother.'" Emily's godmother was a world-renowned life coach. "She had me sit in a chair, and it took me an hour of just sitting with the energy and the pain before I wrote on a piece of paper: 'I was raped.'"

That second, Emily felt a moment of lightness and freedom, like she could suddenly see in color again. Her mom collapsed in her lap and sobbed, finally understanding why the bright, sunny daughter she knew had disappeared overnight.

Emily's recovery began that day. Even though her confession had eased some of her psychological burden, her body was still holding onto an immense amount of shock and stress. She slowly started to engage in her life again–she went to prom and got ready for college in the fall (she had been accepted to a prestigious teaching college), but had to change who she hung out with, since one of her friends had started dating Chad. Eventually she and Brian broke up, and, as is often the case with women who have been sexually assaulted, she began to date more casually and become intimate quickly with guys who weren't right for her. "I wanted to reclaim something that I had lost," she explains.

At college, Emily gained the infamous 'freshman fifteen,' and when the guy she was dating gave her a hard time, pinching her belly and saying, "You'd be so much hotter if you didn't have this," she hired a personal trainer, restricted her eating, and worked out all the time. She became incredibly ripped, turning her body into armor, a fiery ball of muscle "so I wouldn't break, so nothing else bad could happen to me," she says. She wanted to protect herself from the bad feelings, and she tried to rebuild her self-esteem from all the attention her new body was getting her.

But building a hard body was not helping her fractured psyche. "I was having a massive problem with letting go and allowing myself to be soft. I was anxious all the time–I was wound up so tight and constantly stressed. I would never let my body take a complete deep breath in and out. My breathing was very high up and desperate and panicked."

At the time, Emily didn't really know that it was a problem. She only knew that she was responding to what had happened to her, and as far as she could tell, this was the best amount of recovery that she would ever achieve. She was no longer constantly suicidal, but she still suffered PTSD symptoms that would be triggered by day-to-day occurrences. Once, a man asked her the time at the mall and she backed away in fear, her body tensing, her senses on overdrive. "There's nothing scarier than feeling so out of control of your body and your situation, but that's what trauma does to you. You're so disconnected from what's going on, you don't even feel your feet on the floor."

This kind of "managing" went on for several years. After college, Emily moved into the fitness industry and became the assistant group fitness director at the Athletic Club. One day, the director sent an email to employees about a master yoga teacher coming in to teach a class. Until then Emily had no particular connection to yoga, but something piqued her interest, and she decided to take the class.

Emily had no idea that Yoga Tune Up teacher Todd Lavictoire, the visiting teacher, would introduce her to the Roll Model Balls. As she rolled for the first time, she was blown away by the immediate relaxation she felt in her tight upper back and feet. Emily loved that the Therapy Balls gave her control over connecting with her body, because since her rape she had been unable to allow a massage therapist to touch her. "I didn't even know that was what I was looking for, but it was exactly what I needed," she says. The night after that first class with Todd, Emily purchased the Roll Model Balls and DVD for herself, convinced that this was going to be her path to healing.

The greatest catharsis came for Emily when she rolled her abdomen on the Coregeous Ball. As soon as she lay across it, she contacted the armor she had built through her core and diaphragm–all the tight layers of trauma that weren't allowing her to breathe. She began sobbing, releasing years of pent-up anger, sadness, and fear. Her core was like one big emotional trigger point that she hadn't been addressing, and over the years it had grown wider and tougher. Again and again she would roll her belly and allow the tears to come, letting herself soften and working through the pain so that she could begin to heal.

Soon after she began yoga teacher training with Todd, Emily began to see how constricted and tight she had allowed herself to become. The yogic breathing practices (pranayamas) she was learning would leave her in frustrated tears, as she had tightened her diaphragm and intercostal muscles so much that she was unable to take a deep breath. But she kept at it, and after a few years she has seen fantastic physical and emotional changes. "I can do uddiyana bandha now," she says proudly. (Uddiyana bandha is a deep stretch of the diaphragm that requires complete and utter

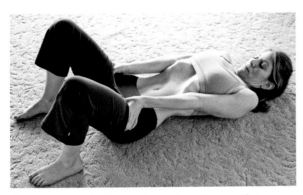

The only way to do uddiyana bandha, or the "diaphragm vacuum," is to completely relax all the layers of the abdomen after exhaling to create internal suction and stretch. Emily's tissues held onto their stress and refused to stretch until the balls finally helped her let go.

relaxation of the core muscles.) "I'm not a tight little ball of tension anymore. Situations that used to make me go into fight-or-flight mode–it was wild to see that they didn't bother me as often. I feel so much more connected to my body, like I have a whole new understanding of it."

Emily was inspired to continue her Yoga Tune Up training and was certified as a Yoga Tune Up teacher in 2012. She has also continued to peel away the old layers of what she calls "fake abs of steel" and build a strong and supple core that allows for both movement and stability in her yoga practice. "The core strength I have now is real–I'm starting to be able to hold a handstand," she says proudly. But the most profound change for Emily has been the rediscovery of herself underneath those layers of protection. In particular, working with me at

my Hips and Bliss Immersion brought Emily into contact with her sense of her own womanhood, since that path of growth and maturation had screeched to a halt after the attack on her teenage self. She barely knew who she was or wanted to be until this point in her life. The work on the balls allowed her to begin to eke out that connection. "The ability to make yourself feel good can completely change your life and send you on a trajectory that you didn't know existed because of the pain or loss of mobility or discomfort that's covering over your own potential. Now my strength comes from the inside–I'm embodying my own power, and I'm not pretending to be something I'm not anymore."

While she continues the work, she acknowledges that it isn't easy. Every step of the way, her body fights back, but she's grateful for the empathy that this experience has given her, and she is planning an online coaching business to work with women who have suffered traumas like hers. Her relationships with her family have deepened, and she is engaged to her long-term boyfriend, who has helped her reconnect with her spiritual self and recognize her own true power and capabilities. As a Yoga Tune Up teacher, Emily reports that her classes are jam-packed, and she loves being able to empower her students with a safe place that they can roll and feel better, helping them discover that they too deserve and are designed to feel good and don't have to live with pain, emotional or physical. Rolling her abdomen is a daily practice–like brushing her teeth– and Emily is excited about the future life that she can now, finally, both imagine and set in motion.

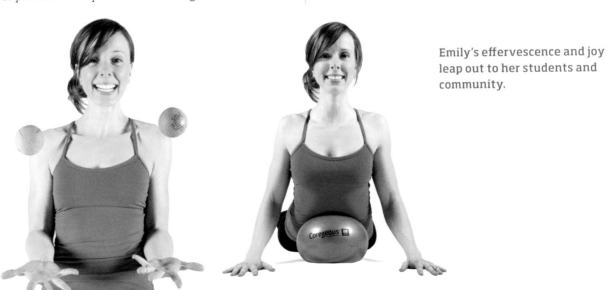

Emily's effervescence and joy leap out to her students and community.

Become Your Own Self-Care Therapist

During my classes and courses, I walk among my students as they roll, and I see their hidden worlds emerge as moans, sighs, cries, and laughter. Their "hard bodies" soften to the sensation of self-care. In group classes, I give them permission to feel whatever their bodies "knead" to feel, whether that means loosening a restricted chest muscle or processing an emotional wound. As I mentioned, not everyone is comfortable revealing their hurt in public. Based on the feedback I've received from Roll Models all over the globe, the majority of their soul-rolling happens on their own terms in private environments.

//My sanity and ability to cope with stress depend heavily on the magic pain-erasing Yoga Tune Up Balls. Exercise, sleep, and talking don't do as much for my emotional health as rolling does. It doesn't even have to be a specific area on my body; any part will do.//

–Alexandra Ellis, Burbank, California

How can you willfully get "in touch" with your feelings using the Therapy Balls? How can you support the full range of your *emotions*? Here are some helpful strategies and parameters to set in motion if you'd like to highlight and connect with your emotional body.

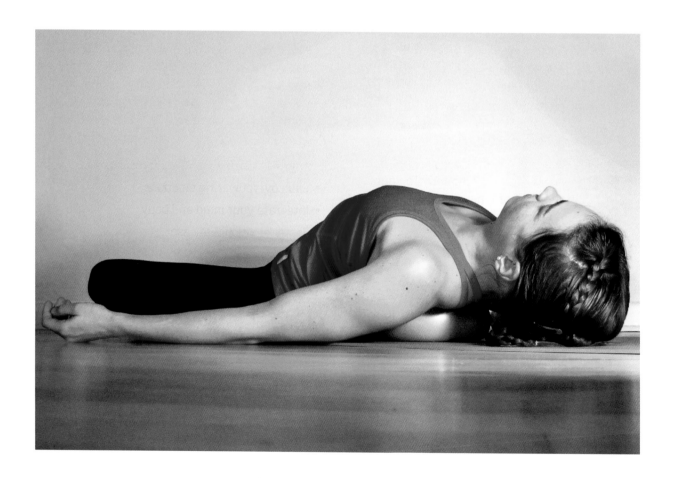

A 20-Minute Self-Care Soul-Rolling Session

1. Prime your body by activating a whole-body contract/relax (see page 148). Either standing or lying on the ground, inhale using Abdominal-Thoracic Breathing, and then hold your breath while simultaneously tightening every single muscle in your body, from the bottoms of your feet to your buttocks, shoulders, neck, and face. Clench everything for as long as you can hold your breath. Then exhale and release all that tension. Let it dissipate, allow your breath to normalize, and then repeat four more times for five complete rounds. This effort might leave you feeling fairly exhausted.

2. Lie down, set a timer for three minutes, and slowly take some Abdominal-Thoracic Breaths. Resist any urge to move, and observe your breath for the full three minutes. Notice what you feel during this time, make a mental note of any thoughts that come to your mind, and continue to breathe. Thoughts, feelings, and images may come up; observe them all as you breathe. As they arrive, welcome your thoughts, whether good or bad, with appreciation. Simply label them as "thinking" as you return your attention to your breath.

3. Give yourself permission to fully experience your feelings. Repeat to yourself three times slowly: "I am aware. I am aware. I am aware."

4. Let your awareness travel slowly from your feet all the way through your body to your head to get a sense of where your body craves touch (or you may already have a sense of where you'd like to roll). If a particular area is calling to you, start your ball-rolling there.

5. If you like a lot of structure, set your timer for ten to fifteen minutes (if you prefer less structure, don't use the timer) and begin rolling into the areas in need of contact.

   • As you roll, breathe slowly, consciously, and fully into those areas of your body.

   • As you breathe, visualize your breath helping to release tension within the specific areas you are rolling, as if your breath were simply blowing away tight areas, releasing all tension.

6. Continue to be aware of each thought and feeling that enters your heart and mind, and welcome them all with compassion and genuine appreciation.

7. Be willing to "roll" with whatever arises, and notice new sensations as they ebb and flow. There may be areas that seem numb or without sensation. Just notice where you have a lot of sensation and where you have little or none. If it feels safe, allow your attention to remain with that sensation or absence of sensation as you continue to breathe your awareness into those areas.

8. As you exhale, permit your feelings to be spoken aloud or expressed through sound. Allow the words, phrases, or sounds to percolate up and out of your mouth. If this seems a bit strange, simply make the sound of a large, deliberate, relaxed yawn at least eight times during your session.

9. End the session by giving yourself permission to feel genuinely grateful for the courage it takes to explore your inner spaces as much as your outer ones.

Soul-rolling–Your ultimate self-gift.

• Relax and gain perspective

• Release held tension

• Improve resiliency and ability to manage stress

• Calm overpowering emotions

• Integrate your mind and body

• Foster emotional release

• Shift your focus by changing your state

• Clear your mind to allow for new possibilities

As you learn what areas of your body retain the most emotional influence, you'll gain peace of mind knowing you have a go to program for managing stressful situations and emotional swings.

To explore further counseling to support your self-care endeavors with emotion and trauma, go to www.usabp.org, the United States Association for Body Psychotherapy.

A Lesser-Known Depression

Sarah Court, 39

*Doctoral Candidate in Physical Therapy
and Yoga Tune Up Teacher Trainer*

Los Angeles

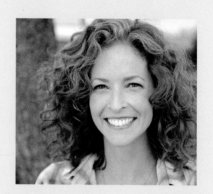

Dear Jill,

I wanted to share this story with you about a little-known depressive diagnosis that I experienced in recent years. *Adjustment disorder* is one of the many forms that depression can take, often occurring in the wake of a stressful life event.

According to most ads for antidepressants, a depressed person just feels extra sad and stares out into a rainy day. But when I became deeply depressed after a traumatic breakup, I wasn't sad: I had no feelings at all, even bad ones. I would have loved to feel sad. It would have been a welcome change from my complete and utter inability to care about anything. Myself, other people, school, eating—everything was covered in the same black tar. Even my work as a Yoga Tune Up teacher trainer that I adored became brittle and lifeless.

About 7 percent of Americans suffer from a form of depression at some point in their lives. Depression is characterized by a diminishment of emotion, energy, and self-worth and an increase in psychomotor impairment—a marked difficulty in performing mundane tasks. For me, the emotional stress had proved too overwhelming, so my brain split from any and all sensory input—and that included my body, previously a treasured wealth of feedback and proprioception. I'd spent years listening to everything my body told me, from pain to pleasure to intuition (aka "this person is giving me the willies"). Now all that feedback was gone—the dial was turned all the way down to zero.

So when a friend asked, "You are really disembodied right now. What are you doing to take care of yourself?" I couldn't even comprehend the question, because the effort it had taken to get dressed was exhausting. It took months for me to find the desire to feel again, and when I did, the Therapy Balls were like an old friend, waiting patiently for when I was ready to get back inside my skin. Rolling stimulated my comatose nervous system, gently reminding first my body and then my mind that feeling good was possible. I would roll and cry. Or laugh. Or sometimes, in a moment of pause, I would have an insight about what had happened, and some of the tar would begin to lift. Piece by piece, I put myself back together, my energy returned, and I came back to life. The tar is gone, but I keep rolling, and I'm determined to keep it at bay.

Love,
Sarah

A Public Defender Learns to Advocate for Herself

Carolyn Phillips, 57
Criminal Prosecutor, Public Interest Lawyer, and Homeless Advocate Manhattan Beach, California

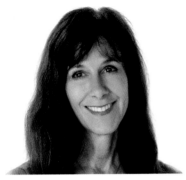

Carolyn has always been a voice for the voiceless and an advocate for society's downtrodden.

For twenty years, Carolyn Phillips prosecuted the worst kind of child sex abusers in northern California. During that time she tried more than fifty nerve-wracking cases, representing victimized children who had been abused by vicious criminals. She recalls a particularly horrific case in 1991, when she was five months pregnant with her daughter, in which she represented four children who had been sadistically tortured and abused, the oldest of whom was only 6 years old. Carolyn guided the boy through his painful, gut-wrenching testimony, which won him a bravery award from the attorney general's office and led to the offender's sentencing to 99 years in prison.

In contrast, Carolyn was raising her own family in idyllic Placerville, an enchantingly beautiful area full of vineyards, apple trees, and Christmas tree farms. But her bucolic surroundings weren't enough to soften the psychic onslaught of her work, and as the years went on, Carolyn ingested more and more of her clients' suffering. "The way I coped with this very intense and emotional work was basically to just disassociate–I would zoom out of the top of my head, even when I tried something like yoga," she says. She went to behavioral therapy sessions, attended a few different churches, and read Thomas Merton and C.S. Lewis, but trying to rationalize her way out of what she was dealing with made little difference to what the decades of grueling work were doing to her body and soul. She was several years away from discovering the Roll Model tools that would bring her back to her body and help her advocate for her own care.

She suffered from debilitating chronic migraines that meant days of missed work, weight gain that doubled her clothing size, and massive mood swings that caused her to lash out in anger at her family. "I was trying to take care of the victims in my cases, so I held on to their pain and suffering. I carried the weight of their abuses on my own shoulders. I was exhausted all the time, but I was doing such important work and I thought that it made me somehow special, that I could handle anything," she says. Carolyn remembers fights that ruined many Thanksgiving and Christmas dinners, and looking back, she feels guilty about how she treated her family, but at the time she couldn't understand why it was happening, unable to see how the emotional stress of her job was overwhelming her. She never allowed herself to hit bottom: in her mind, there was always another victimized child out there who needed her help, and stopping to look after herself was never an option. "So many women have confidence issues when we go into a public profession, and we overcompensate by never saying no, never stopping to breathe. I would have been much more balanced if I had ever allowed myself to be vulnerable."

Finally, after twenty years, everything in Carolyn's world shattered at once. She and her husband divorced, and in June 2002 she moved with her kids to southern California to be closer to her parents. A few months later, she lost her job at her criminal law firm, and her brother Tony died suddenly at age 38 from an undiagnosed heart condition. The day after his death, Carolyn fainted while in line at the bank. She was diagnosed with pneumonia. In addition, the onslaught of grief and anger weakened her so much that it ripped a small hole in her lungs.

Her life falling apart around her, Carolyn became child-like and vulnerable, no longer able to sustain a strong front. Trying to shepherd her children through the post-divorce period but unsure how she was going to pay the rent, she eventually found work at the public interest office in Korea-town, close to downtown Los Angeles. This time she was defending homeless hospital patients who were being dumped on LA's infamous Skid Row, left to fend for themselves among drug addicts and criminals. Even though it sounds otherwise, this work was far less overwhelming for Carolyn than her previous work with children.

Carolyn met me by total chance: she began to take my Yoga Tune Up and Core Integration classes at Swerve Studio in West Hollywood, which was on her way to work. On the weekends when her kids were with their dad, she'd stop at Swerve to take my class, in love with my "intelligent teaching and trusting that it would help heal the pneumo-nia." She also took long walks on the beach near her home, practicing breathing techniques, and slowly began to rebuild herself from the inside out.

Carolyn finally felt like she had found her equi-librium, and when she met the man who would become her second husband in 2005, she thought it was the fresh start that she longed for. She was so enamored of this idea that she glossed over mo-ments when he was verbally abusive and threaten-ing, choosing to once again disassociate from the truth. They married in 2009, but it wasn't until their honeymoon that reality finally came crashing in. "We were up in Big Sur–I mean, it's basically like being in heaven–and he started talking about how he thought I had been critical of his daughters at our wedding. I didn't know what he was talking about, and I began to drift off to sleep. He came around to my side of the bed, grabbed both of my wrists with one hand, and smashed his other hand up against my mouth, like he was going to shove it down my throat. It left bruises on my wrists and face."

Shocked and terrified, Carolyn began to suf-fer from debilitating migraines more frequently, brought on by her husband's bullying behavior. A few months after the wedding, after an emotional yoga class with Yoga Tune Up teacher Suzy Nece, Carolyn came home and confronted her new hus-band. "I'm crying, bawling in yoga class, and this is happening because of what you're doing to me, because I'm stuffing down the experience of being abused by you!" Her husband coolly replied that he

had no recollection of ever physically abusing her. Stunned, Carolyn heeded the advice of her friends, who were concerned for her safety, and moved her family out. They divorced shortly thereafter.

She took her youngest son, age 7 at the time, to therapy with her, determined to get to the bottom of why she would ignore all the warning signs and marry an abuser. She was ashamed that she had exposed her son to the chaotic environment of domestic violence, ironically similar to the situations her young abuse clients had been exposed to. This was a huge wake-up call, and Carolyn knew she had to reconnect with the work she had been do-ing with me. That year, she took my four-day Core Immersion and the seven-day Level 1 Yoga Tune Up teacher training. "I wanted to be the wise person my children and grandchildren could relate to, not the silly old fool who says meaningless things, and I knew I had to get to the root of my behavior, other-wise I would be doomed to repeat it," she says.

Her first experience with the Roll Model Method came in my Core Immersion. She was astounded by the "shock and awe" of the sensations that the Therapy Balls uncovered in her body, especially deep in her hips. She was immediately drawn to how the Therapy Balls allowed her to open up slowly, giving her a chance to experience the years of locked-in anger and grief without seiz-ing up or becoming fearful. She felt empowered to move through her psychic pain in a meaning-ful, purposeful way, to be in the moment and feel whatever thoughts and emotions bubbled up, breathe, and move through them. She knew right away that the Therapy Balls were going to rebuild her, and she felt deeply grateful that this tool was helping her transform her psyche. "I almost blew it with my kids, with this man that I wasted so much time and energy on. This felt like my chance for a comeback. Not to mention, I have so much more energy, and I don't need as much wine as I used to!" she says with a wink.

For Carolyn, the Roll Model Method is also an in-stant fix for the chronic migraines that have belea-guered her throughout her life, made worse during times of emotional stress. Though she enjoyed getting deep-tissue massages for her migraine symptoms, they were only temporarily useful, as the pain would migrate throughout her head, neck, and upper back, away from wherever the massage therapist worked. She hated spending the money to squeeze one more thing into her already packed schedule, when the pain often resurfaced in a new location even as she was driving home afterward. Most of the time her headaches come on at 3 or 4 a.m. Previously she would lie awake and suffer until morning, but now she crawls out of bed and lies down on the floor with the Therapy Balls, rolling around strategically to access the nooks and crannies of her pain until it has vanished and she can fall asleep again. She's a big fan of the Original Yoga Tune Up Balls; placing one right between her eyebrows feels like bliss.

In addition to erasing her migraines, Carolyn uses the balls to delve into her outer hips. They unlock the tightness and muscular holding in her piriformis and gluteus medius muscles, deepening her range of motion and making many of her beloved yoga poses more accessible and comfortable to get into.

As she allowed the balls to unroll the years of pent-up holding in her body, Carolyn felt the confidence that had been robbed from her return. She was no longer just coping—thanks to the Therapy Balls, she was finally thriving. She began carrying extra Therapy Balls in her bag to hand out to her stressed-out co-workers, her boss, even the courtroom bailiff. She would lie down on the floor and demonstrate for her colleagues what she had learned in the Yoga Tune Up teacher training, showing them how to roll the balls along the spine. "It was so easy for them to relate to, and when they tried it, they would all have these 'Ahhh!' moments," she says happily.

But one of her greatest joys has been sharing the Roll Model Method with her children, empowering them to take care of themselves and mirroring for them her own empowerment in the process. Her youngest son suffered from depression after her second marriage, and doctors suggested that he start taking antidepressants, but Carolyn knew that there was a powerful emotional component to the deep gut work she had learned in training with me and elected to try them out on her son. He didn't have a Coregeous Ball, so she had him roll his abdomen on a rolled-up towel as a substitute. It was such a powerful experience for

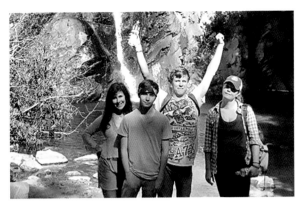

Carolyn regularly hikes with her kids. They have climbed through many of life's challenges together.

him that he didn't end up taking any medication. A little while later he contracted mononucleosis, and rolling the original Therapy Balls around his painful hip joints brought him a lot of relief.

Meanwhile, Carolyn's daughter was attending USC and was part of a high-profile singing group. Although she loved singing, the pressure was bringing on migraines, just like her mom's. Carolyn taught her the rolling techniques that bring her so much relief from her own migraine pain, and her daughter was able to regain the joy she found from singing. Finally, her oldest son had recently graduated college and moved to a new town for a new job, and the stress had brought on a lot of backaches and neck tension. Carolyn sent him a set of the Therapy Balls and the instructional DVD to follow. While her kids—like any kids—were a little resistant at first because it was Mom's idea, they eventually let her teach them, and they even come to the classes she teaches occasionally. Like a flannel nightgown and a bowl of chicken soup, the Therapy Balls have become an integral part of taking care of her kids.

Carolyn's greatest breakthrough has been learning that while she was undoubtedly put on this planet to take care of other people, it didn't need to come at the price she had paid with her body and soul for decades. She firmly believes that learning the Roll Model Method has been one of the most important elements in taking care of her own physical, emotional, and spiritual needs, and she is excited that she can empower her family, friends, and co-workers to take care of themselves in the same way.

My Own Experience with Soul-Rolling

As I mentioned earlier, I've experienced the emotional benefits of using the Roll Model Balls first-hand a multitude of times. I use the balls in lieu of other mood-altering options. I'd rather build a reservoir of positive side effects in my body than use medications that leave their chemical traces. When I was battling eating disorders in my early twenties, I tried a few different antidepressants. I took them reluctantly, and never for more than a few months. Interestingly, I was not able to put an end to my destructive eating habits while I was on medication, but thankfully, I ultimately healed on my own terms, unassisted by pills.

Looking back at that time, I can appreciate my doctor's concerns, as eating disorders have the highest mortality rate of any mental illness.* But my path led me to explore my emotional and body chemistry by other means. I was determined to uncover the root of my anguish and needed to be completely clear-headed to find my way.

The following story is my most recent trauma and triumph.

* Patrick F. Sullivan, *American Journal of Psychiatry* 152, no. 7 (1995): 1073-74.

Becoming a Mother: Coping with Loss and Finding My Way Back

In 2012 I became pregnant with my first child. I was 40, and once my husband and I decided that it was time, I got pregnant instantly. Given my age, I was encouraged by my doctor (and my own fears) to do a chorionic villus sampling (CVS) test, an invasive genetic test to determine the health of our baby at 13 weeks. The test did not go well. During the procedure, the doctor badly injured my membranes and uterus. I was placed on bed rest for the next two months in hopes that they would heal. They never did. In the middle of the night, while I was asleep, my membranes ruptured. My perfectly healthy boy lost his life during my twentieth week of pregnancy.

I was hospitalized for two days in the labor and delivery ward. I heard new babies cry in the rooms next door to mine while I suffered the most traumatic loss of my life.

My heartache knew no end. No words could console me, and no prayers washed my mind clean of the regret and the "what ifs" that I replayed again and again. I was furious, hopeless, helpless, and desperate. A terrible error by a doctor I had trusted filled me with unmitigated rage. But blaming my doctor would never bring my son back to me. I was in shock. I had spent three months full of hope, two months full of doubt, and now I was empty and missing a piece of myself and my future.

I looked for a "silver lining" and recognized that none existed. It was my own linings that had collapsed. The only way I could find a glimmer of hope was to create a healthy new lining and body for a new baby. I would have to rebuild my body as an environment that could become balanced again and could support a new pregnancy.

Throughout our ordeal, my husband remained loving, compassionate, and my constant advocate. He helped divert questions from friends and relatives. He took phone calls and paid hospital bills so I didn't have to be reminded and re-traumatized. During my bed rest, he reorganized our tech-free bedroom so that I could watch movies and have a bed rest "desk." He ran out to get food for me. He held me and we cried. He was, and still is, my rock and my anchor.

During my bed rest time, I was allowed to shower, go to the bathroom, and go up and down the stairs once per day. I felt caged and confined, but I followed my specialist's suggestions in order to minimize any further damage. I would bring my Roll Model Balls into bed with me and place them carefully on my neck, shoulders, jaw, thighs, and calves. I would move at a snail's pace or just maintain sustained compression. The balls gave me relief and helped me feel less sluggish.

After my loss, I needed to rediscover all the corners and edges of my body that had been neglected for the past few months. Oddly, though my heart was aching, my body did not have any persistent aches or pains. I did indeed feel weaker and a bit disconnected from myself, but I had no complaints in my joints or muscles. I felt very lucky that according to my new doctors, I should heal and be able to conceive again within a few months. I attribute my lack of physical pains to the years of self-care I've given myself with the Roll Model Balls and my approach to movement, fitness, and health. I had "banked" a lot of suppleness in my body, and the enforced downtime was ultimately not a setback to my overall health.

A day or two after being released from the hospital, I remember going to my practice room alone and lying down on a succession of the Roll Model Balls. I moved them gingerly into my tissues like old friends. They gently tucked into my weakened body, and I began to tremble and weep. I felt no pain, but my whole body had been holding onto a dream of motherhood for the past five months, my heart was raw, and I had not been able to express my pain through whole-body motion for months. My grief was pent up and locked deep inside me. The balls pressed release valves that allowed my tears to flow from every pore

and emotional sore. My body needed to be rocked and kneaded, and the balls gave me a private outlet in my own home and at my own pace. They soothed me while they salvaged me.

My desire to be a mother remained at the forefront of my heart and mind, and as soon as my uterus and tissues normalized, I was ready to try again. Any mother who has suffered the loss of a child and is trying to have another has likely felt a spectrum of emotions that beat different unsavory notes at different times. Our attempts to conceive again were often loaded with pain, distress, and untenable desperation. My husband and I grew alternately closer and further apart at different stages of this challenge, but we shared one unmet desire: to be loving parents. We were determined to build our family. I was 41, and he 47.

Over the months that followed, I rebuilt my strength, resumed my full teaching schedule, and committed to massive projects, such as writing this book, developing a new video called *Treat While You Train* with my friend Dr. Kelly Starrett, and mentoring my ever-growing teaching team. All these new projects served as distractions to help me heal and divert my attention in a positive direction. And then, in June 2013, while leading a certification training in San Francisco, I discovered that I was pregnant again, ten months after my loss. And I have written every page of this book with the embodied joy and thrill at this second chance to be a mom.

Thankfully, my second pregnancy was completely issue-free. In fact, the 1,000+ photos taken for the sequences in this book were shot during my eleventh week of pregnancy (my publishers at Victory Belt had no idea that I was expecting). I zigzagged across the globe maintaining a vigorous teaching schedule, all while writing this book. My body was filmed or photographed for stories on *Fox News, Good Morning America,* the Oprah Winfrey Network, *America Now,* and several more media outlets. I also created a webinar focused on healthy pregnancy with many of the friends who had given me hope during my darkest times. I wanted to share what I had learned in my first pregnancy, the processes I used to rebuild my health, and my overall

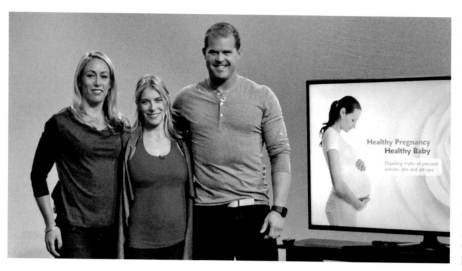

With two of my favorite role models and Roll Models, Juliet and Kelly Starrett.

* "Healthy Pregnancy, Healthy Baby: Dispelling Myths of Prenatal Exercise, Diet and Self-Care" webinar, www.creativelive.com/courses/healthy-pregnancy-healthy-baby-jill-miller

approach to prenatal health. The webinar allowed me to channel my grief and open my story to others. I crafted the two-day webinar with producers from CreativeLive, and we shot it for two consecutive days in San Francisco during my fifth month.

I called the course "Healthy Pregnancy, Healthy Baby: Dispelling Myths of Prenatal Exercise, Diet and Self-Care"* and welcomed my friends Katy Bowman, Kelly and Juliet Starrett, Esther Gokhale, Eden Fromberg, and Sarah Fragoso to share their wisdom. These experts offered a new paradigm for women to build trust in their bodies during pregnancy and beyond. I shared loads of Roll Model self-care techniques and my own story of empowerment from my pregnancies.

My daughter was born just over six hours after her due date. She has brought me indescribable joy and exposed my heart and soul to emotions that had never before seen the light of day. I am so grateful for the opportunity to be a mom and to join the legion of parenthood. All the nurses, my doctor, and my doula described my labor and delivery as more like those for a second or third child. The ease and speed of my labor and delivery, I can confidently say, has a lot to do with the structural environment I created for my daughter Lilah's birth. I truly believe that using the Roll Model Balls throughout my pregnancy and early labor was an asset to the ease of her birth.

My need for comfort and support throughout my pregnancies and loss was at an all-time high. Because one-third of my days and nights were spent traveling alone, I was unable to seek solace from my husband on a daily basis. I was grateful to always have the balls as a resource to feel better instantly. They helped pacify much of my stress, whether I used them for psychological coping, nipping aches and pains before they blew into larger problems, or prepping my body for a workout. They were my constant companions on my journey toward motherhood and continue to help me roll along in my new role.

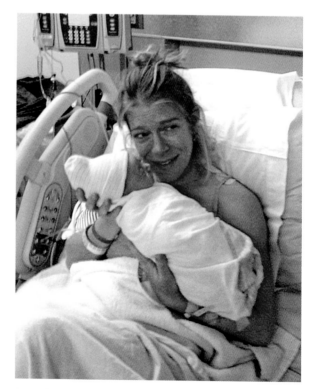

On February 27, 2014, at 6:32 a.m., after eleven hours of labor, Lilah Iris Faust entered the world.

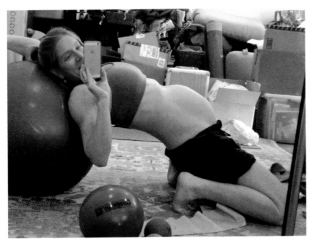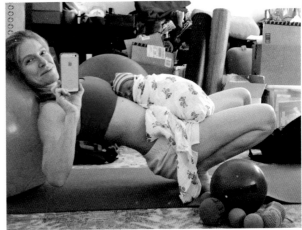

The photo on the left was taken just seven hours before my labor began. The Roll Model Balls were part of my self-care workout every day throughout my pregnancy. The photo on the right was taken seven days after Lilah's birth. Of course, I continued to roll my way through postnatal recovery.

I am not alone in discovering the psychological soothing that deep self-massage can bring to a heart that needs nurturing. Many of my students use the Roll Model Balls to calm themselves or to help them feel their feelings and get in touch with themselves without a middleman getting in the way.

The balls are a tangible way to give back to yourself and show yourself affection, tenderness, and care. They are tools for intimacy that are available at your beck and call whenever and wherever you "knead" them.

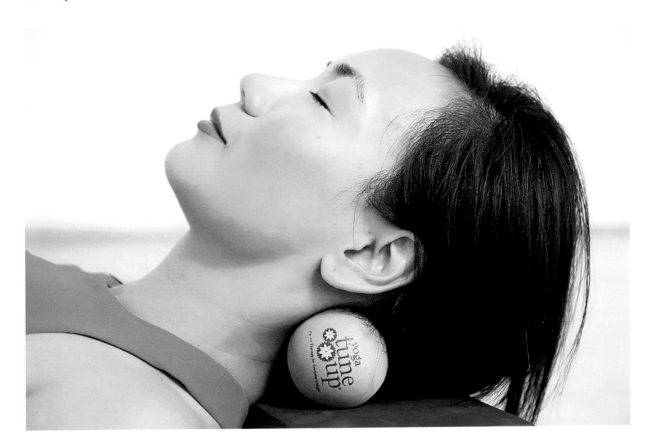

Lisa Highfield is a Yoga Tune Up teacher who works as a counselor for families who have adopted unwanted and neglected children. She helps transform chaotic homes into places of peace where children can thrive. In addition to her counseling skills, she employs all the methodologies outlined in this book. She recently told me about the positive changes she's seen using the Therapy Balls with children and teens who cut themselves. Cutting is a repetitive self-injury where a person deliberately cuts or picks at his or her skin, usually with a sharp object–an unhealthy way of coping with emotional pain, intense anger, and frustration. Typically, youths cut their wrists, arms, ankles, or thighs; it offers an emotional payoff or rush that makes them feel better temporarily. There is a momentary sense of calm, control, and distraction that releases their tension. Although it is normally followed by guilt, shame, and the return of painful emotions, it is an addictive habit. While it's not meant as a suicide attempt, the consequences can be fatal.

Lisa Highfield, 35

Child and Youth Counselor, CYC Founder, and Executive Director of Healing Hearts

London, Ontario, Canada

Dear Jill,

I have worked with children who cut for 15 years. I come across them often in the work I do with families who have endured some kind of trauma or have adopted neglected or abused children. These children are in crisis and have lived through unimaginable experiences. Their brains can't process or handle things like an adult, and they typically resort to unhealthy coping mechanisms such as cutting.

Cutting or any kind of self-harm is "acting out" behavior, which occurs because children don't have the language or awareness to express how they feel. Children who have experienced trauma and rejection in their life (i.e., divorce, abuse) can become numb to their pain and shut their feelings off completely. Some children disassociate at the time of their traumatic event to protect themselves, and many continue to hold their trauma within their body. It's terrifying to revisit trauma in order to process it. Thus, when children or teenagers cut, they are unconsciously expressing fear or anger without having to revisit the initial trauma. Children who have numbed pain simply need to feel something. For others, creating intense feelings in their body distracts them from their emotional pain.

Children who cut internalize things, blaming themselves or turning their anger on themselves. The kids I work with need to look within themselves, feel their pain, and see how amazing they are. When they learn to love themselves, they can release the anger and rejection from their physical body and move on.

In working with these children, I have discovered that the Yoga Tune Up Therapy Balls serve as a great tool in conjunction with appropriate counseling. The Therapy Balls are a safe touchstone that can help children open up their feelings. I can then work with the children on increasing their ability to communicate their feelings of low self-esteem, increase positive self-talk, as well as face the underlying feelings that cause them to abuse themselves. The Therapy Balls put them in touch with their body and what they are doing to themselves when cutting.

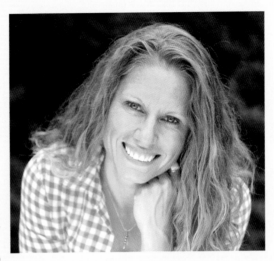

When children cut, it is to show people in a physical way the pain they cannot articulate. If children are taught to understand their pain and to express it, they can use the Yoga Tune Up Balls to connect safely to their hurt in a non-harming manner. When children who cut increase their feelings of self-worth, they will reach for the Therapy Balls instead of a razor, much like adults hit the gym or go for a run to release negative energy.

I worked with a 13-year-old girl who cut herself on her ankles, wrists, and arms. She had been relentlessly bullied emotionally, sexually, and physically for the entire time she attended elementary school. Working with her perception and increasing her self-esteem were essential in lessening her need to harm herself. When her buttons were pushed, instead of cutting, she was able to use the Therapy Balls to massage her tense muscles and fascia. She was able to redirect the pain she was feeling by using the balls to discharge her tension in a beneficial manner instead of hurting herself. She dug into the pain in her body and allowed it to release so she could move on and live a happier life.

When parents discover that their children cut, I advise them that the behavior is not about their capacity to parent, and not to take it personally. I urge these parents to seek a trained professional to support the children; in most cases a child will be more willing to talk to a third party. I also advocate that they find a Yoga Tune Up teacher to help their children in classes or in one-on-one sessions learn to connect to their body, unwind from stress, release their diaphragm, and calm their nervous system.

I tell these parents to encourage their children to use the Therapy Balls "when you notice they are angry, sad, or full of angst. Give them space and honor their feelings."

It is important to approach the whole situation from a holistic family perspective and encourage each family member to take responsibility for their actions. I remind these parents to "know you are a wonderful parent and remind yourself that you are doing the best you can and that is enough."

Thank you for introducing me to these tools,

Lisa

"If your compassion does not include yourself it is incomplete." —Buddha

11 What Next? Tune Up Fitness Corrective Exercise

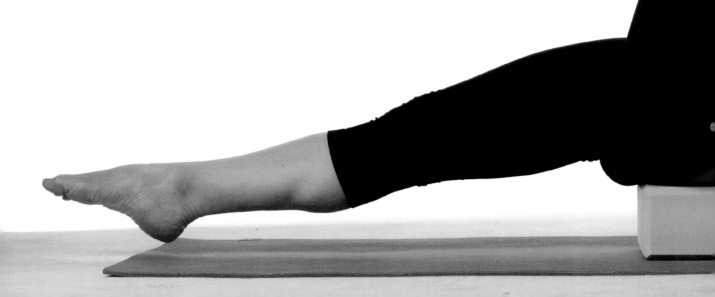

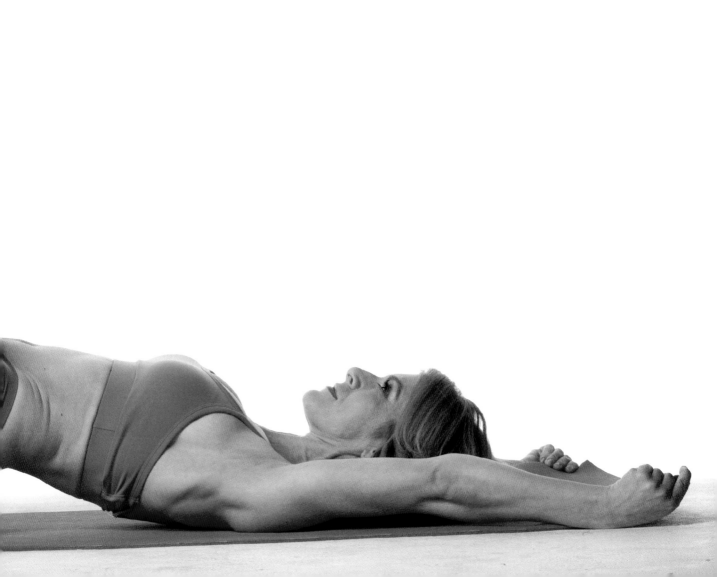

All the rolling, body blind spot healing, and self-locating that you've been practicing are forming a new foundation for your self-care hygiene. Once you start experiencing how much better your body feels with all this soft-tissue conditioning, there is no turning back. Can you imagine how you would feel if you suddenly stopped brushing and flossing your teeth for days? Weeks?

When you become a dedicated Roll Model, your body will begin to glisten from within, filled with *body bright spots*. It will demand that you care for its nooks and crannies on a regular basis. As your body adapts to its new state of being, you'll also likely begin to wonder how you ever allowed your body to become a habitat for pain and dysfunction. You'll want to learn more comprehensive self-care techniques that not only help relieve tension, pain, and anxiety but also strengthen and balance you physiologically. This is the organic process of a whole lifestyle makeover. You are no longer willing to settle for how things were, and are compelled to roll forward in your life with an open mind *and* an open body.

You have felt it for yourself. Soft-tissue self-care is a necessity for your health and movement "diet," but it is only one (significant) component of the inside-out makeover necessary to keep aches and pains from being a part of your daily story. **Rolling alone is not enough.** Spelling out the rest of the details for you is beyond the scope of this book, but I'd like to help hammer home this concept: **Everything in your body is interconnected.** Every move you make and every breath you take has a ripple effect on the rest of your structure and well-being. You are either making choices that build you up or making choices that break you down. Choose to nourish yourself and build better interconnections in your daily fitness and motion practices.

Beyond the Balls:
Training to Complement Rolling

The next step in the process, and the complement to all this rub-love, is to adopt a physical exercise practice and to reject unhealthy movement modes and body stagnation. There are many exercise and physical training programs to choose from (I've listed some later in this chapter), but naturally, I am most excited to share a bit about my other training programs. My company, Tune Up Fitness Worldwide, is built around not just teaching people how to roll around on balls, but also how to improve habits of mobility, conditioning, day-to-day positioning, and stress reduction.

Over the past twenty years, I have developed a number of fitness-based programs to complement the soft-tissue work you've learned in this book: Yoga Tune Up, Coregeous, Treat While You Train, the Rx Series at Equinox Fitness Clubs, the Roll Model Therapy Ball trainings, YTU Integrated Embodied Anatomy, and numerous corporate wellness programs. I highly recommend that you explore them, or find movement communities in your area that take human biomechanics very seriously and teach healthy movement skills as a basis for fitness programming.

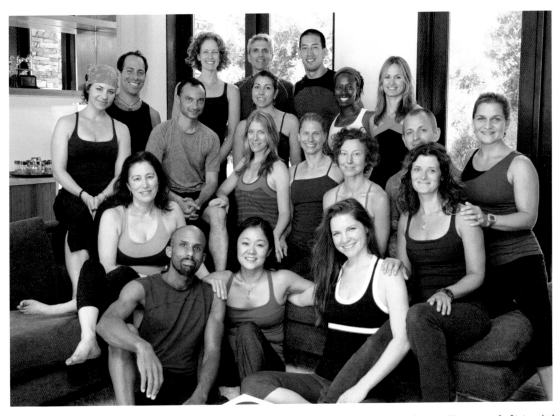

A gathering of some of the Tune Up Fitness Worldwide teaching team and trainers. Top row, left to right: Alex Iglecia, Sarah Court, Owen Grady, Keith Wittenstein. Second row: Maura Barclay-Creighton, Robert Faust, Dinneen Viggiano, Anietie Ukpe-Wallace, Trina Altman. Third row: Dawn Adams, Jill Miller, Kristin Marvin, Amanda Tripp, Todd Lavictoire, Sandy Byrne, Lillee Chandra. Bottom row: Louis Jackson, Kyoko Jasper, Ariel Kiley.

What Is Yoga Tune Up®?

My most widely known program is called Yoga Tune Up. Teachers certified under this label have passed my rigorous training program and are qualified to teach you my self-care healthcare methodology. For information about the other programs and trainings we offer, please see my website, **www.tuneupfitness.com**.

Yoga Tune Up helps with the three Ps: it erases *pain*, improves *posture*, and enhances *performance*. It is a way of working with the body using integrated embodied anatomy. It breaks down the nuts and bolts of human movement using anatomical awareness, conscious relaxation, and proper breathing techniques to bring you to an intimate understanding of your native architecture.

Yoga Tune Up can improve your overall strength, flexibility, and coordination no matter what style of movement discipline you practice or teach. The methodology helps you simplify your body into basic building blocks and identify where your mobility, coordination, or pain is stagnating your ease of movement. You learn to identify areas of your body that have been undetected and underused and are lacking awareness. You learn to locate your body's blind spots and inhabit your body joint by joint and breath by breath. The approach excavates unhealthy tension patterns to discover your "new normal" while moving back into physiological balance.

You are an architectural wonder: inside you are rotating columns, elastic cables, flowing rivers, and billowing archways loaded with potential. Attending a Yoga Tune Up class is like going on an archeological dig into the core of your being. I developed the Roll Model Method and its Therapy Ball tools to be used in conjunction with Yoga Tune Up to help you navigate each fascinating region of your body as both a pioneer and a soother of your own anatomy.

Yoga Tune Up is a conscious corrective exercise format that serves multiple pieces of the pie in the greater world of yoga, fitness, athletics, pain management, and more. It brings together best practices and provides innovative therapeutic movement medicine customized to each individual. While it draws from classical yoga, it is modernized and contemporized to help any person suffering from the physical imbalances of living in today's world. No prior yoga experience is necessary to benefit from Yoga Tune Up.

Yoga Tune Up teachers go beyond formulaic instruction and think creatively in the classroom. They employ a variety of novel techniques, including the Roll Model Method, to help their students discover their own biomechanics and physiology. Yoga Tune Up empowers every student to "be a student of your body" and customizes moves for each individual as an individual. This movement empowerment creates lasting structural change and is the basis for self-care healthcare.

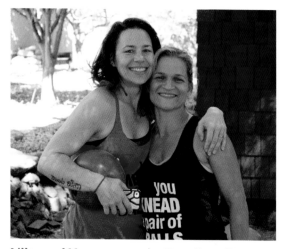

Lillee and Maura are senior Yoga Tune Up teacher trainers.

Going Beyond the Balls

Further education through Tune Up Fitness programs and Yoga Tune Up can help you develop new skills to help your body in a variety of ways. What are your postural habits? What are your repetitive stressors in life, mechanically, emotionally, and nutritionally? What old injuries or scars are you carrying? Where are your body blind spots? Yoga Tune Up teachers are able to comprehensively assess you and help you fully re-inhabit your body so that you can live better in your body.

THE MISTAKE OF YOGA AS A GENERIC RX

Yoga in a broad sense can help with posture, but it can also be a posture killer and a pain generator. Yoga poses are therapeutic only if you do them with attention to foundational posture (see chapter 3) and with the consciousness that each individual is a unique living ecosystem. Many yoga trainings pay little attention to the importance of anatomy and physiology as they relate to poses, movement, and each individual's structure at that point in time. While there is definitely a standard human "structure," the effects of daily living and each person's postural habits create body blind spots (points of weakness and imbalance), so not every pose is possible for every body. Many yoga poses are so extreme that they will pull the body out of alignment because the architecture of the pose is not suitable for the person attempting the pose. If a yoga teacher is not well educated enough to read the variance of the bodies in the room, his or her students will pay the price.*

Poses are not pills. If you do poses (or any exercise, for that matter) without knowing whether you should even be doing those particular poses, much less doing them with improper form and posture, you will eventually wear out your tissues and create pain. This is specifically why I developed Yoga Tune Up with its focus on anatomy, physiology, and human movement. Yoga Tune Up has a wide variety of exercises that isolate specific joints to assess their relationship to neighboring joints and connective tissues as well as to the body as a whole. This helps both the student and the teacher uncover these body blind spots within the context of different shapes and positions, both static and dynamic. It works to build strength and proprioception in these areas that have been overused or underused and bring them back to balance. Your body must be intelligently prepared for yoga or any other type of movement practice, which is why Yoga Tune Up helps students tune into their posture so that they can perform both their yoga poses and their daily postures more efficiently.

* For more on the dangers of yoga, check out William J. Broad's article "How Yoga Can Wreck Your Body," *The New York Times,* January 5, 2012, accessed via www.nytimes.com/2012/01/08/magazine/how-yoga-can-wreck-your-body.html?pagewanted=all&_r=0, and Matthew Remski's blog post "'I Was Addicted to Practice': A Senior Teacher Changes Her Path," June 5, 2014, accessed via http://matthewremski.com/wordpress/wawadia-update-6-i-was-addicted-to-practice-a-senior-teacher-changes-her-path/

Just because you *can* do a pose does not mean that you *should*. These are poses that I have retired from my repertoire. Retired. They made my hips, knees, and spine click and pop and are not suitable for my body. (See my Introduction for more.)

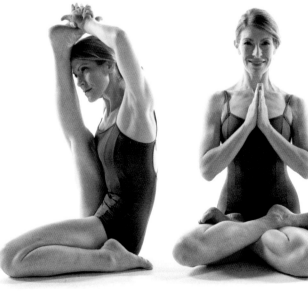
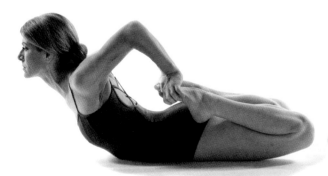

What if You Can't Find a Yoga Tune Up Teacher Where You Live?

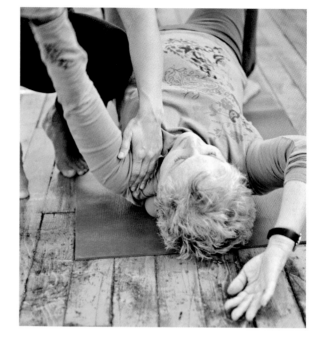

Find a skilled coach, teacher, or community that inspires you. Seek out people who support you on your journey and broaden your knowledge of self-treatment. Naturally, I encourage you to find a certified Yoga Tune Up teacher (find one near you at **www.yogatuneup.com**), but I also enthusiastically and wholeheartedly recommend the following movement educators, their trainers, and their programming:

1. **Glenn Black:**
   morethansound.net/shop/human-movement-yoga-nidra-box-set/#.VaZrzVxZFKM

2. **Katy Bowman:**
   nutritiousmovement.com/blog

3. **The Feldenkrais Method:**
   www.feldenkrais.com

4. **Esther Gokhale:**
   www.gokhalemethod.com

5. **Brian MacKenzie:**
   www.powerspeedendurance.com

6. **Kelly Starrett:**
   www.mobilitywod.com

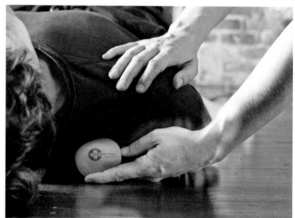

And we have many at-home programs and video products to ignite your journey. The library of Tune Up Fitness videos is a great start for helping you find your body blind spots. Learn more at www.yogatuneup.com.

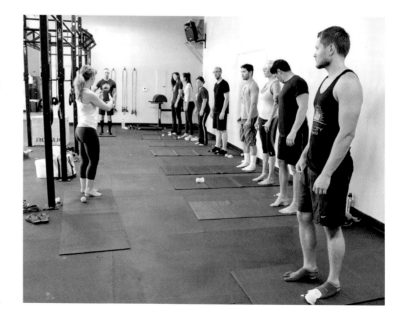

A skilled teacher provides an additional pair of eyes to help you find your body blind spots and more.

Reversing the Course of Obesity, Chronic Pain, and Diabetes: A Nurse Becomes a Patient of Self-Care and Movement as Medicine

Sharon Alkerstedt, 42
Outpatient Oncology Nurse
Shelton, Connecticut

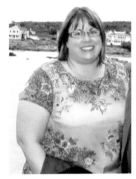

Sharon at 326 painful pounds.

From the time she was in nursing school, Sharon knew that she wanted to work with cancer patients. Though the excitement of working in the ER had originally piqued her interest, she quickly realized that it would be too stressful for her, and more important, there was less chance of bonding with her patients. Now 42, she has been working as an outpatient oncology nurse for fourteen years, administering kindness and compassion along with chemotherapy to patients who have all sorts of cancers. She builds relationships with patients and celebrates with those whose health improves, but she's challenged by those who don't make it. "People who don't understand oncology or aren't in nursing question how I could do this job, but the reality is that I'm here to treat patients and help them in their journey, whatever that length might be," she says simply.

Though overweight, Sharon had always been active, until one day in 1999 she fell while hiking and badly hurt her right knee. She went to physical therapy, but the combination of her injury and the externally rotated alignment of her right leg meant that it needed further attention. In 2002, she had an arthroscopic surgery to clear out her lateral meniscus, part of the cartilage on the outside of her right knee. While she tried to go back to exercising, her movement was limited. Over the years, her weight slowly increased, which put more pressure on her weakened knee, which made her knee hurt more and made her less able to exercise—a vicious cycle that fed on itself for the next eight years and resulted in a plethora of side effects related to weight gain, including high blood pressure and elevated blood sugar levels.

Eventually Sharon needed more knee surgery, this time a lateral patella release, since her patella was tracking too far to the right, as well as a second arthroscopy. Already out of shape, this second round of surgery in 2008 left her even more deconditioned, with weakened quadriceps on her right leg that made her rely too much on her left leg to get around. Another round of physical therapy didn't do much to help her regain strength, and in the following year Sharon's physical, mental, and emotional state went downhill rapidly.

As much as Sharon loves her work as a nurse, taking care of very sick patients is a grueling job. Long, stressful days of work would take all her energy, and when she came home at night with an aching knee, all she wanted to do was to sit on the couch. She didn't want to go out or socialize, and the less she exercised, the less she wanted to. No longer able to participate in the active lifestyle that her husband enjoyed, their time together grew limited, and both her declining health and her disinterest in doing anything about it put a strain on their marriage.

Sharon was now pre-diabetic and had to start taking metformin to manage her blood sugar levels. High blood pressure ran in her family, but her increasing weight made it worse, and her doctor put her on atenolol and hydrochlorothiazide to attempt to manage it. She lost so much cartilage in her knee that it became arthritic, so she tried Celebrex and every other anti-inflammatory out there for pain relief, but after a while they all stopped working. From the time she had her first surgery, Sharon had a jaw-dropping 18 injections in her knee: she tried Synvisc (for joint lubrication) three times and steroids (to reduce inflammation), but none of them gave her more than a few weeks of pain relief before her knee would begin to ache again. In 2004, Sharon had gone through a tough breakup, and her doctor put her on Lexapro for depression, anticipating that she would use it only short term. But Sharon never stopped taking it, attempting to manage her downward-spiraling mood that had plummeted along with her energy levels and her zest for life.

Her world became incredibly small. Locked in a body that hurt, with a plethora of health issues, she would go to work, come home, and collapse, rarely doing anything else. She looked to food for solace even though it was causing more weight gain and ill health. Troubled by poor sleep, she could never get physically comfortable. "It was incredibly isolating and lonely–I'm a naturally upbeat person, and I got to a place where I was just existing. I was in total denial–I tried to pretend it was just my knee and that there wasn't anything else going on, but obviously that wasn't true."

At 5'9", Sharon was clinically obese at 326 pounds, with a grade IV arthritic knee. She knew something had to change, and that need was highlighted by the cancer patients she treated, some of whom ironically were healthier than she was. "When I was in my 20s, I didn't really connect with the patients as much, but now a lot of them are in my age group, and they're getting sick and dying. There was one patient in particular who is exactly my same age, and she went through advanced esophageal cancer treatment, which meant chemo, radiation, and surgery. She was with us every day and required a huge amount of supportive care. She's doing well now, but it was touch and go for a while. All of my patients struggling so hard to combat an often fatal disease really made me take a look at my life, and I realized I needed to take better care of myself while I'm here, because I've only got a finite amount of time, and I had no excuses not to start. Maybe I can't beat my genetics, and I can't prevent some diseases that will happen to me, but I can change the external factors, and I needed to start focusing on that."

In January 2011, Sharon began her journey back to health. She started by looking at her diet and was shocked to realize that she was eating almost twice the amount her body needed. Having been on a diet since she was a teenager, she knew that a drastic change would ultimately fail, so she began by cutting back a few hundred calories a week for a month. She immediately began to lose weight, and after a month she began to look at the quality of the foods she was choosing, weeding out processed junk and choosing cleaner, whole foods with an emphasis on vegetables and protein. Since her aim was to create a better life for herself, and she knew that restricting her diet to the 1,500 calories a day that her doctor wanted would make her miserable, she made sure she ate mindfully without feeling like she was starving herself.

The real changes began when Sharon started exercising again, about a month after she changed her diet. A second round of physical therapy with a different therapist gave her much better movement tools, and she went back to the gym, working with a personal trainer twice a week to make sure that she took care of her arthritic knee. Sharon jokingly calls herself the "ADD child of exercise" because in those first few months, she tried everything out there: kickboxing, Zumba, Tabata, Pilates, yoga, spinning–it was an exercise buffet! She started to pay more attention to what her body, and in particular her knee, liked (yoga) and did not like (Zumba–"though I did like to shake it!"). Eventually she joined Tuff Girl Fitness, a gym that specializes in high intensity interval training, going four or five times a week, and her weight really began to come off. Not only that, but she continued to build impressive strength, able to lift 265 pounds on the trap bar deadlift.

As luck would have it, Tuff Girl Fitness had hired Yoga Tune Up teacher Brooke Thomas to teach a Roll Model Method class once a month. While Sharon had all kinds of exercise and massage tools in her home ("I could open a physical therapy office in my den!"), she had never experienced the Therapy Balls, and the gym's co-owner, Christa Doran, urged her to go, telling Sharon that the Therapy Balls were like nothing else out there and that she needed the Roll Model Method to balance out the assault on her body from all the training.

So Sharon agreed–she bought a pair of Therapy Balls, went to Brooke's class, and "Oh. My. God!" she exclaims. "It was exquisite pain. The Therapy Balls got into little nooks and crannies that other things couldn't. I call them my little nuggets of torture and happiness." Sharon had been a massage therapist a decade before, and she knew a good tool when she saw one. At the same time, when she laid the balls onto her IT band, upper thigh, and tensor fascia latae (TFL), she couldn't believe how much the side of her leg hurt, and that even with her massage background, she hadn't made the connection that some of her knee pain might be coming from a tight IT band. She gets a lot of quadriceps tendinitis because of her knee, and the Therapy Balls are the only thing she allows anywhere near it. She loves that she can control the depth and pressure in such a sensitive and chronically painful area.

She was immediately hooked. To complement her intense workout regimen, Sharon uses her Roll Model Balls every day, even when she doesn't work out, "because if I don't, I'll be a hot mess the next day–it's a preemptive measure against the soreness that comes from working out that much. For me to stay in the game, I have to be aware of my body and take care of it so that I can keep working out and stay healthy and strong." She uses all four sizes of the Therapy Balls all over her body, with the PLUS Balls getting more use on her quadriceps and TFL, the Original YTU Balls contouring to the smaller grooves of her neck and shoulders, and the mighty ALPHA to bring relief to her sore glutes. She loves the Coregeous Ball to soothe her psoas and bring her pelvis into a more neutral alignment. She doesn't limit herself to getting on the Therapy Balls at home–Sharon keeps a set of the Original YTU Balls at work and often rolls out her hips on a wall as her co-workers joke with her, "Do you have those balls on your butt again?"

Sharon's combined efforts of nutrition, exercise, and self-care have enabled her to lose more than 100 pounds and keep it off for over a year. In addition, her serum circulating insulin levels have

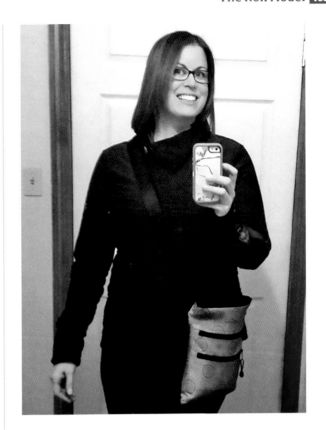

dropped considerably, and her blood pressure is lower, allowing her to significantly decrease her medications for blood pressure and blood sugar (and she's gradually taken herself completely off the antidepressants, realizing that she didn't need them at all). Even better, Sharon has come back to life with renewed enthusiasm, energy, and joy, excited about her future and feeling so much better in her body thanks in part to the Roll Model Method. "When I look at pictures of myself from my heaviest time, I'm really shocked–I don't think I realized how big I had gotten."

Sharon's marriage weathered the storm of her chronic pain and depression, and she and her husband have adapted to a new lifestyle that is healthy for their bodies, hearts, and relationship. They work out together now and recently completed a 5K obstacle course. Their shared passion for fitness has brought them closer together and introduced them to new ways to have fun. Her husband says that she inspired him to get active (he's training to do the grueling Tough Mudder course), though Sharon calls him "comically inflexible," so of course she's shared her Therapy Balls with him!

Sharon has also returned to school, working on a master's degree in nursing. She has no doubt that she wouldn't have the physical or mental stamina to do it without the energy she gets from the Roll Model Method. She plans to broaden her work in oncology by going into patient education, as she loves to empower her patients by helping them understand their diseases and manage their symptoms. She even recommended the Therapy Balls to a young patient who was frustrated by her inability to exercise and how tight and painful her body had become.

For Sharon, it's her patients who serve as a daily reminder of how far she has come. "Long-term patients who return for checkups every six months will walk into the clinic and say, 'Whoa! What happened? Did you have surgery?'" she laughs, "and I explain, no, I just worked really hard and kept at it." One patient in particular, a vivacious 50-year-old woman with breast cancer, lamented how her treatment left her fatigued and unable to exercise, so she loved living vicariously through Sharon and was always quick to offer a word of encouragement. She became Sharon's motivation: when Sharon has a rough day or is tired, she still pushes herself to exercise, calling to mind this vibrant patient to inspire her.

After a while, the loss of knee cartilage began to interfere with the intensity of her exercise and the speed of her recovery, and Sharon recently got a knee replacement, recognizing that biting the bullet and dealing with surgery while she's still young will help her remain active and keep up the lifestyle she now loves. Her Therapy Balls have been a tremendous help post-surgery to massage her angry quadriceps and gluteal muscles, and only two weeks post-surgery she was walking without assistance. "We have it in us to take care of ourselves–we just have to start it and to believe in it. I'm proof positive of that. I went from barely functioning to a much healthier version of myself that is not about numbers on a scale or a dress size, but about the quality of the journey of my life." She encourages those who feel discouraged by physical limitations not to give up. She stresses that they must reach and even roll toward their goals, just like she did.

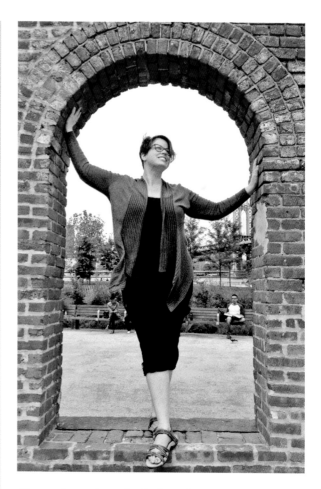

Sharon has taken the Roll Model tools along with movement medicine strategies and reversed her destiny. Allopathic medicine was simultaneously a savior and a crippling crutch for this medical professional. When she finally had the balls to take control of her own life, she unshackled herself from chronic pain and loss of self and avoided a deadly disease. Her integrated approach of diet, exercise, and the Roll Model Method is a long-term strategy that will continue to help her shed pounds, gain self-esteem, and contribute to the care of her family and patients. A true Roll Model.

Just before the book went to press, I received this update from Sharon. It speaks volumes about how self-care healthcare improves the environment of your body for healing and repair:

"Great news! I went to my surgeon for my two-week visit yesterday (to get my 35!! staples out), and he was more than thrilled at my progress–he and his physician's assistant both said that I have the flexion/extension and mobility/stability of someone they typically see at least three months post-op. Not bad for 15 days out!

The prognosis of getting full range of motion back are high, and I know it's because of all my hard work and tools. He even asked me to give a quick little pep talk to another (older) patient about to have the same knee replaced."

Sharon's speed of recovery is off the charts because she tended and tilled the soil of her own inner landscape, so that when she had surgery, her body was already primed to adapt and thrive. Your body always has the capability to improve its well-being. Your willingness to be there to serve yourself at every age and stage makes all the difference between a life of pain and a life of progress.

// *We have it in us to take care of ourselves–we just have to start it and to believe in it. I'm proof positive of that. I went from barely functioning to a much healthier version of myself that is not about numbers on a scale or a dress size, but about the quality of the journey of my life.* **//**

–Sharon Alkerstedt

Conclusion

I envision a world in which students enroll in physical education classes and learn basic self-care skills as common "body hygiene." These skills should be valued as highly as the fundamentals of kickball, basketball, football, and running.

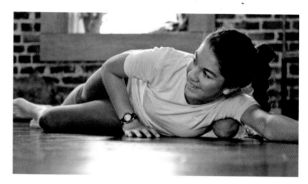

Kayla, age 12, takes Roll Model Method classes in Tennessee.

Hi Jill,

I wanted to send you a note thanking you for all you do. I stumbled onto your Yoga Tune Up program through Kelly Starrett, and you have changed my life. You and Kelly have changed how I approach my workouts, my job, and my recovery.

I'm a high school physical education teacher, and I have incorporated your Yoga Tune Up Balls into my classes. They have been a huge hit. My students now have a way to fix themselves when they are sore or hurt. For a majority of my students it has been a game-changer. Often I have students ask if they can borrow the Therapy Balls for the weekend.

I really think that what you and Kelly are doing is the future of physical education. I did some quick surveying with my students this year. 85 percent have some type of pain, and 95 percent have had back pain at some point in their life. Your therapy work is going to be really important.

Quick observation—at the end of each class we go into a relaxation pose (which of course is the students' favorite), but I also give them the option to roll during that time. Oftentimes 50 percent of the class is using the time to roll instead of relax. To me, that is solid proof that it works.

Discovering your program has been like learning a new language, and I feel like I am providing my students true physical education.

Thank you for everything. I really appreciate you.

(Name Withheld)

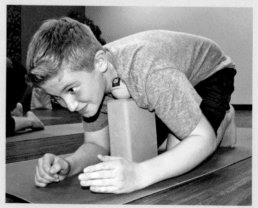

Blair is releasing his subclavius and pectoralis minor, areas that get tight and compressed from carrying around his heavy backpack.

It's hard to imagine that two little rubber balls could make such a difference for so many people on so many levels. When I first started using them, I knew that they were solving and preventing problems for me. Once I began to share them with my students, their benefits multiplied beyond my wildest imagination. Men, women, and children are using them to soothe their aches, pains, and ailments in a self-empowering and drug-free way.

Once you stop, drop, and roll, you will discover your own specific relief. But you must experience it for yourself. Your anatomy, agony, and pleasure live within your own body. It is your application of the suggestions I've made in these pages that will usher change into your tissues and your life. Get on the ball and feel what rolling can do for you.

And then please stay in touch. Let me know how you've used the Roll Model Method to help yourself. Share your story with me and the thousands of others who "knead" to know what you've discovered. Be a Roll Model.

Share your story here:

rollmodel@tuneupfitness.com

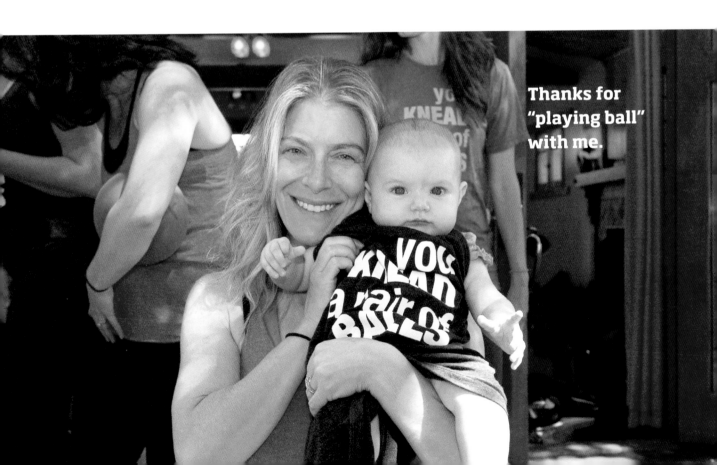

Thanks for "playing ball" with me.

Appendix

The Shortlist: Ball Benefits in Brief

1. You control the pressure; you control the pace.

2. You get a quick, convenient, on-the-go massage. The balls are ready anytime you need them.

3. The balls follow the contours of the bony structures of your body, making it easy to find (and learn) muscle origins, insertions, fascias, and every category of connective tissues.

4. Rolling refreshes, rejuvenates, and relaxes.

5. Using the balls increases circulation and overall hydration to your body's tissues.

6. The balls educate you about your own anatomy, helping you locate your tissues so you can improve proprioception and functionality.

7. With hands-off self-myofascial massage, your hands will never get tired.

8. These tools are economical; there's no need to "gamble" on an expensive and potentially disappointing or unsatisfactory massage.

9. The balls' grip mimics the hands of a skilled massage therapist.

10. There's no greasy oil to wipe up as there is after a conventional massage.

11. Rolling improves performance.

12. Rolling relieves stress.

13. Rolling increases your emotional resiliency.

14. Rolling loosens you up!

You know you knead them, and they knead you!

FAQ

The balls are painful— why does this hurt so much?

The ball work points out where in your body you already have pain. As a general rule, if you cannot take a full breath, you are either in too deep or you need to move the ball to an adjacent spot. If the pain worsens or persists when you move the ball from that spot, then this area may be in an acute phase of injury, in which case it is best to seek professional help. (*Never* use the balls directly on bruised tissue, broken skin, or fractured bones–see the warnings on pages 72-73.) However, if the pain you feel is on the borderline of wincing discomfort, then lighten your pressure a bit or move even farther from the "hotspot." Students often say that the balls are too hard, and at first they might be, but in reality, healthy muscle is yielding, springy, and buoyant, just like the rubber in these balls. If the balls feel hard, then it might be that the condition of your muscles is too "hard."

Imagine what it feels like to stretch an area of your body that has not been moved for days, weeks, or even years. When the balls penetrate to levels of your musculature that have been hidden from view, underutilized, and allowed to fall into poor condition, your myofascias and your mind will be unfamiliar with this new touch. You are exposing the aches and pains that already exist within the tissues to their own discomfort, and it will take time and persistence to assimilate to this new experience. Be consistent, and eventually the stretch receptors within your muscles will come to crave the ball work. *The balls are merely a reflection of the tissue beneath. If the balls feel like stones, the condition of your myofascia may be stone-like.* You'll notice when rolling out your less-tense muscles that the balls may feel supple and yielding, and that again is a reflection of the condition of your tissues.

Eventually, when you have erased your pain, you will feel *pleasant pressure.*

Can I just use tennis balls instead?

Nope. Tennis balls give some pressure, but there are three major differences between tennis balls and the Roll Model Balls:

1. The slippery felt surface of a tennis ball does not provide any grip. The Roll Model Balls are made of a high-grip rubber that literally takes a hold of the many layers of skin, fascia, and muscle while providing penetrating pressure all the way to the bone.

2. Tennis balls are hollow inside and filled with air. They easily flatten with heavy pressure like your body weight. They cannot knead, compress, and trace the body's textures and contours like the dense and durable grip-rubber composition of the Roll Model Balls can.

3. The Roll Model Balls are designed to nurture and give feedback to your body as the rubber yields to layers of muscle and flesh. A tennis ball is designed to be struck with a racquet!

What about harder balls like golf balls, baseballs, or lacrosse balls?

Although sports balls can be beneficial for some people, they are not "one size fits all" balls for a broad range of users. Harder balls like baseballs lack the grip of the Roll Model Balls and are not able to yield at all as they abut the bony surfaces of the body. When a hard ball hits bone with a larger load of pressure and with a mass of soft tissue between the ball and bone, it puts the soft tissue in a very vulnerable state, often resulting in pinching or bruising. These harder balls, lacking a "softer touch," are especially incompatible with larger nerves.

How do I know if I'm in the right spot?

Like riding a bike, it takes time and practice to recognize whether you're in the right spot. Our bodies can be as unknown to us as the depths of the ocean, but with repetition, you will eventually come to know each of the target points within the sequences. Refer often to the images and review your bony landmarks. Last but not least, look for the signs of release to reinforce that you are indeed unraveling your tension.

Indicators that signify release include:

- Feelings of relief, warmth, and relaxation
- A subsiding of tension
- A decrease in pain
- An increase in emotional well-being
- An increase in range of motion
- A decrease in sensations of pain at end range of motion
- An increase in awareness of targeted tissues, or an enhancement of your EmbodyMap (see page 110)

These release signs can appear after the balls are positioned, when they are adjusted, after they are removed, or during all three of these phases.

How often should I use the balls?

As often as you like! Five to twenty minutes a day will definitely have you on your way to remodeling your tissues to make lasting change. But you can get quick relief in as little as two minutes. My friend Kelly Starrett follows this rule:

Roll until you make change or until you've stopped making change.

It is possible to overdo rolling. The balls are small stretch instruments: wherever they go, they create stretch into your tissues. Keeping a ball in one place for too long can overstretch and weaken your tissues' elasticity and reactivity. It is not possible to say what the exact time frame is; it depends on the condition of your tissues and the area you are rolling. Discontinue ball use on an area if it does not make you feel better or if you become bruised from excessive or aggressive use.

What is the difference between the balls?

The different sizes of Roll Model Balls exert different levels of pressure on your body. Here is a basic outline of how much pressure each one imparts into your tissues.

- **Original Yoga Tune Up (YTU) Ball** feels like the pressure of a thumb.
- **PLUS Ball** feels like the pressure of an elbow.
- **ALPHA Ball** feels like the pressure of a fist.
- **Coregeous Ball** feels like the pressure of a broad, flat hand.

Each of these balls is made from a grippy natural rubber that has springy yield so that it can get deep into your tissues, yet roll safely around and over bony prominences. The inflatable Coregeous Ball is the largest. It is the gentlest of the collection and exerts the least stress on your tissues. The rest of the balls are made of solid rubber and supply firmer pressure, as outlined above.

Note: Using the Original YTU, PLUS or ALPHA Balls in pairs and/or cinched in the Snug-Grip Tote reduces the amount of pressure that a single ball exerts.

Which ball is the best for me to use on my _____?

Your size, weight, mass, and tolerance to deep touch differ from those of the person next to you, behind you, or in front of you. All of us come wired with our own tolerance to deep touch. The health condition of your tissues also plays a large role in which ball is going to feel best on your different body parts at different times and for different needs.

If you have a small frame and very little myofascial mass, you may be more sensitive to the balls' pressure, as you have less soft tissue to cushion you from the touch of the balls. You may want to use the Coregeous Ball to familiarize your body with these tools before moving on to the smaller balls. Because of your lesser mass, any of the smaller rubber balls will be able to make its way into the depths of your tissues.

If you are a larger-massed individual, you may find that the smaller balls are absorbed by your tissues and thus don't reach as deeply into certain areas of your body. The larger PLUS or ALPHA Balls may be a better option than the smaller YTU Therapy Balls.

The sequences in chapter 8 suggest which balls to use, but you can also browse the images throughout the book to see how other Roll Models use the different-sized balls in a variety of ways. Trust your instincts and experiment.

Here's an at-a-glance view:

- **Original YTU Balls** can roll almost everywhere but are especially deft at maneuvering into smaller spaces near bones, such as the hands, feet, face, rotator cuff, spine, and pelvic floor.
- **PLUS Balls** satisfy whole-body needs and move well on the thighs, lower legs, outer shoulders, and muscles of the back. They are less helpful for the face.
- **ALPHA Balls** are very satisfying when used on larger areas of the body, like the buttocks and thighs. Using the ALPHA on hands and feet will not give you the point specificity on these finer bones, but these large balls can provide global shear.
- **Coregeous** is best suited to the torso; it is less useful on smaller body parts and limbs.

Is there a special diet you recommend while learning to be a Roll Model?

I am not a nutrition expert, but I do try to follow an anti-inflammatory diet for the most part. I limit caffeine, alcohol, and sugar. I eat a lot of healthy fats, such as avocado, flax, and walnut oil. I also fill my plate with fresh veggies and whatever proteins my body craves. And I consume dark chocolate daily! The most important factor is water. I drink it as soon as I wake up and probably drink 2+ gallons per day.

So my number-one recommendation is to drink plenty of water, as hydration is key for maintaining elasticity in the body's connective tissues. As the Roll Model Balls knead, compress, and move fluids around, fresh oxygenated blood streams in to maintain homeostatic balance in all the cells in the area. Any area that was adhered, locked up, or scarred will also be completely dehydrated, like a dried-out sponge that needs to be rejoined to the aqueous environment surrounding it. Rolling with the Roll Model Method creates friction to release stuckness between your tissues. Fresh fluids rush into these once-stiff areas while their waste products are escorted out. (This is why drinking water frequently is critical!) This friction also increases local heat in the area, which is a clear sign that blood flow is on its way into these dormant and forgotten areas. Free-flowing circulation is the most important part of maintaining healthy tissues.

I recently injured my _____; is it safe to use the balls on it?

Many variables are at play when we try to define "injury," "pain," "safety," and so on. When you are in an acute phase of injury, seek professional help. Pain is scalable and subjective; one person's bruised knee may be another person's unbearable catastrophe requiring crutches. As the author of this book, I am not in your body, so I am unable to know what you feel, your personal pain threshold, or your relationship to pain. If you've been to a professional and are ready to recover, create a conservatively sensitive approach to help yourself. This means developing keen self-listening skills as you roll the balls across tissues that host chronic aches or pains. Do not use the balls directly on inflamed tissues; instead, address the perimeter tissues around the inflamed area or other more remote tissues that are "uptown," "downtown," or "across town" from the injury. Also remember that the rest of your body will compensate to protect the injury, so other structures of the body will definitely need some Roll Model Ball therapy.

My Roll Model Balls are getting a bit soft; should I replace them?

In short, yes and no. Let me explain:

When you first use the balls, they are indeed firmer. Your body is also firmer–that is, riddled with knots–so those tissues are "tighter" and more resistant to massage. The myofascia (muscles and fascias) naturally resists the balls' pressure at first, because the soft tissues of your body were most likely bound up. In this state, they also react to deep pressure by tightening and armoring, so you actually feel more sensation. This sensation is not necessarily associated with the knots, but is caused by general muscle guarding known as the Muscle Spindle Response.

With frequent use, the balls do begin to change in texture; they soften, becoming more pliable and grippy. At the same time, your tissues become more compliant, used to being stretched, mobilized, and maneuvered by the balls. This interplay between ball texture and tissue texture changes with use of the balls *and* your body's familiarity with the types of pressure, traction, and "touch" of the balls within your tissues. The balls get softer, and your tissues become less resistant. The upshot is that you actually *feel the balls less* because the balls are softer, and best of all, SO ARE YOU!

It is not necessary to feel "pain" every time you use the balls. Not feeling pain does not mean that the balls are working less for you. *It doesn't have to hurt to work.*

Balls that have been with you for some time and have softened up by absorbing your tension are also the perfect texture for extra-delicate structures, like your face, as well as extra-bony prominences, such as your wrists, hands, elbows, knees, and ankles.

Should a ball become a bit deformed or oval-shaped and not spring back into a perfect sphere, it can have further "life." Its squishier texture is perfect for use on delicate or bony spots. Its malleability and pliability allow your bones to sink into the rubber and grip hard-to-reach tissues in those areas.

That being said, if a ball completely loses its shape and can't be rolled back into a sphere, it is time to replace that ball for use on some of your larger-mass body areas. The time frame for replacement depends on how often you use the ball and your body mass.

- The Original Yoga Tune Up Therapy Balls have a three- to six-month life, depending on use.
- The PLUS Balls have a six- to twelve-month life, depending on use.
- The ALPHA Balls last the longest and may need to be retired after nine to fifteen months.
- The Coregeous Ball can live on indefinitely but can lose some of its grip over time based on the dirt and oils it collects.

TIP: I never throw "used" balls away unless they become oxidized and completely lose their grip. If they are soft and still have grip, I give them to students who are extra-sensitive to touch. Once these sensitive students get used to the softer balls, I graduate them to their own new, firmer pair.

How do I care for and clean my Roll Model Balls?

1. The solid rubber balls are made of a natural rubber and will oxidize if exposed to moisture or prolonged light, becoming slick and hard over time. To prevent oxidation, store them in a bag or drawer when not in use (but never in a bag with wet clothes or towels).

2. Clean the balls with a damp cloth and natural soap, yoga mat cleaner, or sanitizing wipes. Dry them completely with a towel before storing.

3. If you are storing large quantities of balls for group use, make sure that your storage container provides complete coverage.

How do I modify the ball placement if I feel really uncomfortable while rolling?

You may not "have a ball" the first (or second or third!) time you get down and roll. Feeling your aches, pains, and stuckness can be a bummer no matter how healthy you are. Some areas of your body may tolerate massive pressure, while others may be squeamish. I have shared this work with hundreds of thousands of people and have found a way for almost everyone to engage in rolling.

If rolling is causing you more discomfort than you can tolerate, here is a list of suggested modifications:

1. Change your relationship to gravity; take your balls to the wall (or a bed or sofa).

2. Use a larger ball on that area of your body.

3. Use two balls instead of one.

4. Move the balls uptown, downtown, or across town (that is, above, below, or to the side of the area you are rolling).

5. Stay on the surface with skin-rolling or shear and minimize your depth.

6. Contract/relax until you achieve change or stop making change.

7. When in doubt, use the Coregeous Ball.

Is it safe to use the Therapy Balls during pregnancy?

The various sizes of the Roll Model Balls are perfectly safe to use during pregnancy, especially if you were rolling before becoming pregnant. The general rule during pregnancy is not to jump too aggressively into any new activity, but to build your tolerance slowly and with great awareness. For example, you would not run a marathon without having trained for one. Nor would you start lifting heavy weights if you had not been taught proper form. If you jump into either of these scenarios while pregnant (or not pregnant), you might find yourself injured.

Use common sense, and start slowly. If you've never used the Therapy Balls and are currently pregnant, start with your hands and feet on day one. Then, on day two, progress to your calves and knees, followed by your forearms and elbows. Each time you use the balls, gauge whether you feel better or worse afterward. If you feel worse, you probably went too deep or used the balls for too long. If you feel great, keep adding new body parts.*

The one caution is to avoid using the Coregeous Ball directly on your abdomen during pregnancy if you have never done so before. It's not the best time to experiment with that particular area of your body. Post-delivery, the Coregeous Ball abdominal techniques will be a useful part of your rehab. By all means, you can use the Coregeous on your chest and sternum during pregnancy to help you master the dynamic breathing mechanics outlined in this book (see chapter 7). As your belly grows, you can do this same sternum rollout against a wall.

* For in-depth prenatal and postnatal instruction, see my webinar "Healthy Pregnancy, Healthy Baby: Dispelling Myths of Prenatal Exercise, Diet and Self-Care" at www.creativelive.com/courses/healthy-pregnancy-healthy-baby-jill-miller

Is it safe for kids to use the balls?

I get asked this question all the time, especially by parents whose kids play sports. Typically, their kids have already used the balls, as they've seen Mom or Dad roll and just imitate what they see. I also have heard from a number of folks around the globe who share the balls with kids in their classrooms or PE classes (see page 404), or for complementary therapies. I believe we are creating a "roll-volution" where we can help our children become more body smart than our generation. If we lead by example and empower ourselves with self-care healthcare, then we can help future generations prevent injuries and musculoskeletal disease.

Many activities that appeal to children carry a much higher risk of injury than rolling around on rubber balls, but that being said, here are some guidelines:

1. Always consult the child's physician first.

2. Follow all of the guidelines and modifications as you would for yourself.

3. Pay close attention to good pain and bad pain, as outlined in chapter 2.

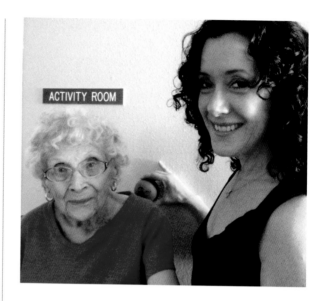

// *My student Clemi is 102! She started yoga at 99. She just walked into my seniors yoga class one day and said she needed to exercise. She is still going strong and sassy! She especially likes rolling out her shoulders because she says it just feels so good! At 102, I believe that is the only reason you need!* //

–Cathy Favelle,
Wautoma, Wisconsin

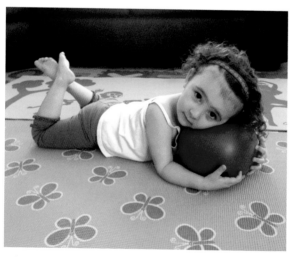

Wise beyond her three years, Twyla is a budding Roll Model. Her mom, Amy Deguio, often finds her resting her ribs and abdomen on the ball and practicing her breathing, just like her mommy.

Roll Model Lingo

Glossary of Terms

Note that this list of terms is by no means exhaustive. I have crafted lean and limited definitions of these terms, and I am defining them in the context of this book.

Adhesion–An area of the body loaded with an excess of collagen that limits tissue motion and fluid perfusion. Adhesions are often the remnants of scars. Massage therapy expert Sandy Fritz adds that they are "inappropriate connective tissue connections."*

Aponeurosis–A broad, flat tendon that connects muscle to muscle or connects a muscle to itself–for example, the central tendon of the diaphragm or the thoracolumbar fascia of the lower back.

Autonomic–The part of the nervous system that acts automatically of its own accord. It is involuntary.

Body blind spot–An area of the body lacking in body sense. These areas are typically overused, underused, misused, or abused and are often the catalysts for pain and injury.

Compress–To load a ball against your body in a static/non-motion-based manner.

Connective tissues–All tissues that are formed from the mesoderm of an embryo. These include blood, lymph, fascia, tendon, ligament, cartilage, and periosteum.

Contract/relax–A quick method of removing internal muscle bracing while using a ball. The muscle in contact with the ball is deliberately tightened and held for a length of time, then consciously released.

CrossFiber–To manipulate a ball perpendicularly or obliquely to the line of pull of a myofascial structure. This is akin to pulling a violin bow across the strings or crossing them at an angle. See also *myofascia*.

Deep fascia–Fascia that has a definitive crimp-like appearance and is highly organized in its arrangement. It can be found surrounding muscles or as a thickened, broad aponeurotic tendon layer. See also *aponeurosis, fascia*.

EmbodyMap–Your constant positional sense of your relationship to your body in stillness or in motion. Your keen perception of your inner proprioceptive landscape.

Enteric–A branch of the nervous system that governs gastrointestinal processes.

Extracellular matrix–The environment between and surrounding the body's cells that permits cells to "breathe," replicate, move, and die.

Fascia–The fibrous and gelatinous bodywide web that forms the body's living seams, protection, and repair system. It is the soft-tissue scaffolding that gives the body its form and shape. It links muscular proteins and other connective-tissue structures like bones, ligaments, and tendons to one another.

Global shear–A technique that uses larger balls to maximize the motion of fascial slide and glide from superficial to deep. Shear quickly warms up the body and heightens proprioception.

Ground substance–(1) The amorphous, gel-like, noncellular component of the extracellular matrix in which the fibers and cells of connective tissue are embedded. (2) The clear, fluid portion within a cell's membrane. Both the ground substance within cells and the ground substance of the extracellular matrix are affected by loads and

---

* Sandy Fritz, *Sports & Exercise Massage: Comprehensive Care for Athletics, Fitness and Rehabilitation* (Mosby, 2013).

pressures while providing suspension and support to microscopic structures of the body. See also *extracellular matrix.*

Hyaluronic acid–A lubricating fluid produced by fascial tissues throughout the body. This fluid permits slide & glide among the multiple layers of soft tissue.

Line of pull–The direction of motion designated by the organization of muscle fibers and fascia relative to their muscle origin and muscle insertion attachment sites. For example, the line of pull of the quadriceps is from the upper tibia (top of the shin) to the ilium (uppermost pelvic bone). See also *muscle origin, muscle insertion.*

Loose fascia–Refers to the fascias that cannot be categorized as either superficial or deep. Loose fascia is found as an intervening connecting layer between layers of deep fascia and as a membranous layer between superficial and deep fascias.

Mesoderm–The middle of the three primary layers from which an embryo develops. The mesoderm spawns many bodily tissues and structures, including all connective tissues.

Muscle bracing–The exact opposite of the effect you want to create while rolling. Muscle bracing occurs when the muscle spindles sense that too much stretch is happening. Instead of allowing the stretch to occur, the muscle contracts to protect itself and the underlying structures and locks itself into a hardened, tensed state. Bracing can happen when a tool is perceived as too hard, a stroke against the body is too fast, or the body is in a state of global tension. See also *muscle spindles.*

Muscle insertion–The portion of a muscle that moves more during a contraction (often more distal, or farther from the midline, the body's axis).

Muscle origin–The portion of a muscle that moves less during a contraction (often more proximal, or closer to the midline, the body's axis).

Muscle spindles–Stretch receptors (mechanoreceptors) within myofascial structures. They are located within the perimysial sheath of muscle fascicles. See also *myofascia.*

Myofascia–Refers to the actual familiar-named muscle structures with their associated interpenetrating fascias.

Parasympathetic–The branch of the autonomic nervous system that creates down-regulatory, rest, digest, and repair responses. See also *autonomic.*

Perfusion–The body's process of transferring fluids, nutrients, and waste into and out of tissues and blood vessels.

Periosteum–The dense connective-tissue membrane surrounding bones.

Peripheral nervous system–Refers to the nerves not directly within the skull or spinal bones. The nerves that branch out from the central nervous system.

Petting-zoo soft–My cutesy way of describing the ultimate state of pliable perfection in tissues warmed, rolled, and cared for after a Roll Model Therapy Ball session; the ideal result of erasing pain and rubbing out knots, kinks, and adhesions. For example: *Her upper trapezius was petting-zoo soft after three minutes of rolling!*

Pin/spin & mobilize–To compress and twist a ball against the body to gather soft tissue and create massive shear, and then mobilize the body part in contact with the ball or a body part directly connected to the area in contact with the ball.

Proprioception–The body's sense of itself; its inner GPS system.

Resting tone–Refers to the level of resistance within a muscle while it is passive and "at rest."

Septa–A connective-tissue partition. A deep fascia "dividing line," "fence," or "soft-tissue curtain" between different myofascial structures. See also *myofascia.*

Shear–A mechanical action or stress that causes motion and slide among contiguous body parts in a direction parallel to their plane of contact. Shear involves using a ball to create a force that maneuvers one tissue layer laterally across the layer beneath it. Shear force mobilizes your tissues so that they slide and transition some distance away from their starting point before they recoil and return to their original position, and provides immediate heat to the area. See also *skin-roll*.

Skin-roll–To use the grip and tackiness of the Roll Model Balls to maneuver the skin and underlying fascias. Skin-rolling enhances slide & glide among fascial layers from superficial to deep. It can be performed by:

1) Pinning a ball against the skin, latching it to a fixed point like Velcro, catching traction, and moving the ball while it remains stuck to the skin.

2) Lying atop the ball and moving the body over the ball to create rippling shear as the ball grips the skin while the body maneuvers over it.

See also *shear, global shear.*

Slide & glide–The ability for motion and movement to occur among fascias and the structures they interconnect.

Somatic–The part of the peripheral nervous system that transfers the motor and sensory nervous system from the central nervous system (brain and spinal cord) to the periphery and back. See also *peripheral nervous system.*

Strip–To use a ball to maneuver along the line of pull of a muscle, tracking through origin to insertion or vice versa. See also *line of pull.*

Superficial fascia–Fascia that has an alveolar collagen/elastin structure and can contain adipose (fat) cells. Superficial fascia is usually found directly beneath the skin. Superficial fascia often defines a person's physical shape and has a spongy, springy texture. When your aunt pinches your cheeks, she's going after superficial fascia.

Sympathetic–The portion of the central nervous system devoted to arousal, fighting, and fleeing.

Tendon–A connective tissue that joins muscle to periosteum. "Flat" tendons are known as *aponeuroses*. See also *periosteum.*

Trigger point–A highly sensitive and hyperirritable area within a muscle that often refers pain to other areas. Commonly referred to as a *knot.*

Viscoelasticity–The property of fascia that permits motion due to its inherent fluidity and plasticity. Fascia is gelatinous, viscous, and fibrous. These elements permit gradual change in the shape of fascia over time.

Anatomy lingo can be both professorial and personable. If you instruct others to roll, practice using both to become a ball "cue-master" (see page 418).

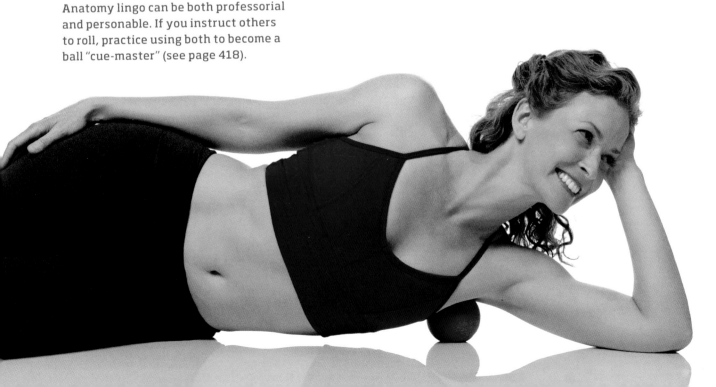

Cue Menu for Ball Techniques

Because these are "hands-off" treatments, coaches, teachers, and trainers must develop keen cueing to help students and clients find their targets safely and effectively. As you guide your students through Roll Model moves, develop active verb cues that come from your own somatic language experience. Craft unique and vivid cues that bring their bodies to life! The more you savor your own experiences and communicate them to your students, the more authentic you will be in teaching the sequences. The following are some action-filled verb cues that you can use instead of the technical "technique terms."

BALL PLOW

Clear off the bone
Dig
Dissect
Fluff
Partition
Pile
Ripple
Rubber claw
Scrape
Seam rip
Unfold

BALL STACK

Clamp and partition
Latch and bite
Pinch and pluck
Python
Rubber suture
Squash and disassemble
Vise grip

CONTRACT/RELAX

Arnold Schwarzenegger/puppy-dog soft
Pump/slack
Squeeze/disengage

Stiffen/soften
Tense/release
Tighten/let go

CROSSFIBER

Asterisk
Cut
Detour
Grill
Hashtag
Rake
Rock
Scootch
Score
Scrape
Scratch
Slice
Tease

PIN/SPIN & MOBILIZE

Bolt/drill and bend
Dent/pickle and fan
Lock/crinkle and maneuver
Mark/whirlpool and scrape
Poke/swivel and track
Stick/twist and pivot
Tuck/gather and navigate

PIN & STRETCH

Crease and fold
Dot and spindle
Hold and bend
Place and stir
Squash and close
Tack and pivot

SKIN-ROLLING/ SHEAR

Clamp
Crimp
Crinkle
Gather
Grind
Pickle
Pinch
Prune
Scrunch
Skid
Slurry
Turbulate

STRIPPING

Brush
Comb
Glide
Line
Navigate
Noodle
Slide
Slit
Steer
Trail

SUSTAINED COMPRESSION

Burrow
Cradle
Dent
Fix
Mark
Nudge
Place
Plunk
Pock
Rivet
Squish
Staple
Tuck

Recommended Reading and Viewing

Books

Alignment Matters: The First Five Years of Katy Says, by Katy Bowman (Propriometrics Press, 2013)

Anatomy of Hatha Yoga: A Manual for Students, Teachers, and Practitioners, Revised Edition, by H. David Coulter (Body and Breath, 2010)

Anatomy Trains: Myofascial Meridians for Manual and Movement Therapists, 3rd Edition, by Thomas Myers (Churchill Livingstone, 2014)

Becoming a Supple Leopard: The Ultimate Guide to Resolving Pain, Preventing Injury, and Optimizing Athletic Performance, by Dr. Kelly Starrett with Glen Cordoza (Victory Belt, 2013)

The Body Bears the Burden: Trauma, Dissociation, and Disease, 3rd Edition, by Robert Scaer (Routledge, 2014)

Cells, Gels and the Engines of Life, by Gerald H. Pollack (Ebner & Sons, 2001)

Fascia: Clinical Applications for Health and Human Performance, by Mark Lindsay (Cengage Learning, 2008)

Fascia: The Tensional Network of the Human Body, by Robert Schleip, Thomas W. Findley, Leon Chaitow, and Peter A. Huijing (Elsevier, 2012)

Fascia in Sport and Movement, by Robert Schleip (Handspring Publishing, 2014)

Free+Style: Maximize Sport and Life Performance with Four Basic Movements, by Carl Paoli and Anthony Sherbondy (Victory Belt, 2014)

Freedom from Pain, by Peter A. Levine and Maggie Phillips (Sounds True, 2012)

Groundworks: Narratives of Embodiment, edited by Don Hanlon Johnson (North Atlantic Books, 1997)

A Handbook for Yogasana Teachers: The Incorporation of Neuroscience, Physiology, and Anatomy into the Practice, by Mel Robin (Wheatmark, 2009)

The History of Massage: An Illustrated Survey from Around the World, by Robert Noah Calvert (Healing Arts Press, 2002)

Job's Body, by Deane Juhan (Barrytown/Station Hill Press, Inc., 2003)

The Key Muscles of Yoga, by Ray Long (Bandha Yoga, 2009)

Kinesiology: The Skeletal System and Muscle Function, 2nd Edition, by Joseph E. Muscolino (Mosby, 2010)

The MELT Method, by Sue Hitzmann (HarperOne, 2013)

Move Your DNA: Restore Your Health through Natural Movement, by Katy Bowman (Propriometrics Press, 2014)

The Muscle and Bone Palpation Manual with Trigger Points, Referral Patterns and Stretching, 2nd Edition, by Joseph E. Muscolino (Mosby, 2014)

The Muscular System Manual: The Skeletal Muscles of the Human Body, 3rd Edition, by Joseph E. Muscolino (Mosby, 2009)

Power, Speed, Endurance: A Skill-Based Approach to Training, by Brian MacKenzie (Victory Belt, 2012)

Pride and a Daily Marathon, by Jonathan Cole (Bradford Books, 1995)

Ready to Run: Unlocking Your Potential to Run Naturally, by Dr. Kelly Starrett with T.J. Murphy (Victory Belt, 2014)

Sports & Exercise Massage: Comprehensive Care for Athletics, Fitness, and Rehabilitation, 2nd Edition, by Sandy Fritz (Mosby, 2013)

Trail Guide to the Body, 4th Edition, by Andrew Biel (Books of Discovery, 2010)

Waking the Tiger: Healing Trauma, by Peter A. Levine and Ann Frederick (North Atlantic Books, 1997)

Why Fascia Matters, by Brooke Thomas (ebook; available at www.liberatedbody.com/product/why-fascia-matters/)

Yoga Body: The Origins of Modern Posture Practice, by Mark Singleton (Oxford University Press, 2010)

Websites

www.yogatuneup.com: Jill Miller's website.

www.blog.gaiam.com/blog/author/jillmiller: Jill Miller's blog.

nutritiousmovement.com/blog: Katy Bowman is a human biomechanics expert.

www.rogercoleyoga.com: Roger Cole is a sleep science and relaxation response expert.

erikdalton.com: Erik Dalton has produced excellent massage resources and offers many free videos.

www.gilhedley.com: Gil Hedley leads compassionate dissection workshops.

www.meltmethod.com: Sue Hitzmann teaches about fascia wellness.

www.drlepp.com: Dr. David Lepp is my favorite chiropractor in the San Francisco Bay Area.

powerspeedendurance.com: Brian MacKenzie and his team outline proper running mechanics.

www.anatomytrains.com: Thomas Myers is a leader in the fascia field.

www.ted.com/talks/vs_ramachandran_the_neurons_that_shaped_civilization.html: V.S. Ramachandran discusses mirror neurons.

matthewremski.com/wordpress/multimedia/wawadia/: Matthew Remski's brilliant series of articles entitled "What Are We Actually Doing in Asana?" takes a deep look at yoga-related injuries.

www.mobilitywod.com: Dr. Kelly Starrett has an astonishing blog loaded with videos about movement and mobility.

www.liberatedbody.com: Brooke Thomas has a fascia facts and functional movement blog.

www.chiropracticbodywork.com: Dr. Christopher Tosh is my favorite Los Angeles-based chiropractor and Active Release Therapy specialist.

www.activerelease.com: Information about the Active Release Technique.

fasciaresearchsociety.org: The website for the Fascia Research Congress.

www.usabp.org: The website for the United States Association for Body Psychotherapy.

Videos

Coregeous® DVD–Jill Miller; www.yogatuneup.com

On-Demand Pain Relief Massage Therapy Kit: 11 Guided Routines on 2 DVDs–Jill Miller; www.yogatuneup.com

Treat While You Train DVD–Jill Miller, Kelly Starrett, Tune Up Fitness Worldwide; www.yogatuneup.com

Quickfix Rx: KneeHab DVD–Jill Miller; www.yogatuneup.com

Healthy Pregnancy, Healthy Baby: Dispelling Myths of Prenatal Exercise, Diet and Self-Care webinar–Jill Miller, Kelly Starrett, Juliet Starrett, Katy Bowman, Esther Gokhale, Sarah Fragoso, Eden Fromberg; www.creativelive.com/courses/healthy-pregnancy-healthy-baby-jill-miller

Yoga Link / Core Integration DVD–Jill Miller; www.pranamaya.com/products/dvds/miller-core.html

Living fascia videos by J.C. Guimberteau; endovivo.com/en

Gil Hedley's YouTube channel is rich with anatomy content; www.youtube.com/user/somanaut

❚❚I am a big promoter of the Coregeous *DVD. I started practicing it three times a week with the Therapy Ball segment, and it cured my rotator cuff problem and in turn also cured my golfer's elbow in my right arm. I was not expecting these benefits from the routine! I am a longtime swimmer and just got used to the constant twang in my right shoulder and a cortisone shot every now and then. No more!❚❚*

–Jim Hinton, Swim Coach, Asheville, North Carolina

Extra-Special Subject: A Ruff Roller

Krystin Zeiger, 34, and Chloe (the lucky mutt), 6
Yoga Instructor
Redwood City, California (formerly Houston, Texas)

Hi Jill,

I really appreciate your interest in including Chloe in your book and would love to share her story with you!

CHLOE'S ANXIETY:

Chloe was rescued from a puppy mill February 2008 at just a few weeks old. When I adopted her that September from a shelter, I was given some heartbreaking info about her background. She had been in the same iron cage for six months, had never seen grass, never been on a leash, and rarely was allowed to spend time with other dogs "because of her temperament and hyperactivity." So she was moved to the back only to be "shown" during free adoption weekends.

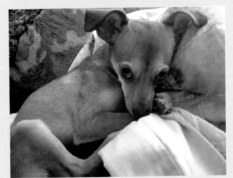

Chloe in her new home, just an hour after she was adopted.

After I was "warned," they brought "Ramsey" (for "rambunctious") to me. Yes, she was hyper, peed all over me, but then curled up in my lap with her big blue eyes staring up at me, and I was sold. When I brought her home, she was a completely different puppy: curious, affectionate, and desperate to love and be loved!

The vet determined she was underweight, she had fleas, and her kneecaps were prone to popping out (bilateral patellar luxation). Over the next two weeks, she was housetrained, gained a few ounces, and had become the most loving, well-behaved puppy I'd ever had. Then Hurricane Ike hit, along with a tornado that demolished several neighbors' homes and took off part of my second-story walls and some of the roofing.

Chloe seemed okay in those few weeks during the aftermath, but when I returned to work I began to notice her anxiety. I would come home and find her shaking and panting under my bed. She was much worse when it rained, even if it was for a few minutes. Then she stopped eating. The vet suggested putting her on Xanax! I was hesitant, but her panic episodes kept happening, so I started giving her the meds, which gave a little relief. After a few days and doses, it didn't seem to do much other than make her walk into walls. I decided it was time for a new approach.

I began using techniques I'd learned volunteering at a couple of women's shelters and crisis centers. One that really seemed to work was placing ice or a cold compress somewhere near or on her body. It seemed to calm her breathing and heart rate and kept her grounded and present. Once the panic episodes started to shorten and occur less frequently, I gradually introduced her to rain. I held her the first few times, then put her on a leash. It took about a month before the panic seemed to dissipate altogether.

All was good until I took Chloe to my parents' lake house for July Fourth 2012. The second she heard that first firework, she was back at square one. Nothing helped. Her anxiety was much worse than it'd ever been and escalated to anxiety with any kind of loud, sudden sound. The vet doubled her Xanax dose and added Tramadol, a narcotic for severe pain. I thought, seriously?! Hell no!

TUNE UP THERAPY:

I spent most of 2013 living out of a suitcase in a terminal, on an airplane, or in a hotel. Trainings, teaching, clients in NY, NM, CA, HI, TX, blah! It was the first time Chloe was away from me for longer than a weekend. And then

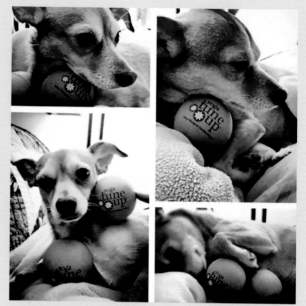

Chloe, the anxious mutt, rubs herself on her mama's Roll Model Balls. She never chews, only rolls and rubs.

came the light at the end of the tunnel . . . Yoga Tune Up Training. You may recall that during training, I had multiple bilateral kidney stones. I was actually scheduled to have my stones removed through high-intensity shock wave therapy (lithotripsy) at that time, but put it on hold because . . . let's just say I had a gut feeling. And lo and behold, I left the training stone free! I had a new set of balls, but no stones. ;) Jill Miller, you changed not only my life, but those close to me, my clients, and of course Chloe!

Along with the anxiety, Chloe's bilateral patellar luxation was getting much worse, so bad that the vet was suggesting surgery. When I spoke to her, I was given the "wait and see" talk. Those words tend to fall short in my spoken or written vernacular, much less received. I tried to translate my rehabilitation through Yoga Tune Up Training into Chloe terms. I returned to Houston on July 2, knowing that in two days Chloe's worst enemy would cause some serious stress. After greeting her for the first time in over a month, I opened my suitcase, and the first thing she pulled out were my toted Therapy Balls. She was immediately intrigued and started pushing them around with her nose. I got on the floor, placed them under my low back, and let out a long plane ride sigh of relief. Chloe sat and stared with kind of a weird fascination-I think what she picked up on the most was how calm I was. As I was lying there in a mini corpse pose, I heard these little paw sounds scratching but remained still and quiet. Fifteen minutes or so later, I slowly peeled off the floor and circled my gaze around the room to find no Chloe and a missing Therapy Ball. I quietly walked downstairs and found her sleeping with the ball wrapped between her paws, nested against her chest.

"PAWPRIOCEPTION":

We got though the fireworks that July Fourth with little stress. During moments of intense noise, either my husband or I would do a gentle ball massage on Chloe's neck.

Now, six months later, she has two sets, the ALPHA and has recently been stealing my Pluses that she sleeps with. The past few weeks we've been working on real downward dog. I place one ball a couple feet from where she's sitting, and as she goes to reach with one paw she extends the opposite on the mat to balance. Chloe's got some serious "pawprioception"! I follow her cues, study her movement, and can get a sense of where she wants the ball. Until she has the ability to miraculously grow opposable thumbs, of course I have to assist.

Chloe is incredibly smart and has developed some amazing body awareness fairly quickly. I can tell she's trying to move the balls closer to the muscles surrounding her knees and will whine when I don't help with an adjustment. A couple weeks ago she started sleeping with the Alpha resting under one thigh while extending the opposite leg, which looks kind of like a modified Leg Stretch #3. And to get that nice lateral stretch, she extends both arms in the air, lets out a sigh, and drops them to the opposite side. You can see her breath slowly rise and fall for a minute or two, and then she positions her body and ball to work the other side. I believe she's earned the right to say/bark/think, "I am a student of my body."

To make a very long story short, the Roll Model Therapy Balls have magic in them! My original intentions for Chloe were to eliminate anxiety and medication. Every day she surprises me. She has very little, if any, anxiety, has more energy during the day, sleeps like a rock, is much kinder to her sister, and is just all around a happier, healthier dog. She's living proof that your creation has and will continue to evolve!

Thank you, Jill, for everything you do, share, and teach. The world of movement (and the world in general) is blessed to have you in it!

Love and Light,
Krystin

P.S. The night I got home from a recent visit to the hospital, the first thing nurse Chloe did was nuzzle her Roll Model Ball under my neck.

P.P.S. Chloe's current drug protocol: Glyco-Flex for joint support. She also recently kicked her 0.25 milligrams of Xanax during plane rides.

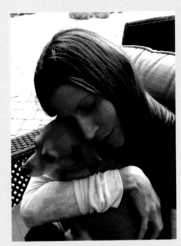

Chloe and Krystin.

Acknowledgments

Thank you to my teachers, who showed me the way by asking me to find my own way: Glenn Black, Lynne Blom, Tim O'Slynne, David Downs, Gil Hedley, and Ellen Heed.

Thank you to my "first student," Lillee Chandra. It was during a session with you that I truly recognized the importance of what I was teaching. Thank you, Maura Barclay-Creighton, for insisting that you should teach this work because it healed you and for encouraging me to craft a teacher training program. And thank you Sarah Court and Trina Altman for your ROLL in getting this work into the world. You have all touched this book far more than you'll ever know.

Thank you, Lashaun Dale, for your insight and understanding of the importance of this work.

Thank you to Equinox Fitness Clubs and Pure Yoga for your invaluable support: Lisa Wheeler, Carol Espel, Keith Irace, Delf Enriquez, Stephanie Vitorino, Amy Dixon, Tandy Gutierrez, Laina Jacobs, and Kay Kay Clivio.

Thank you, Jessica Smith and Phil Swain, for fifteen years of support at YogaWorks.

Thank you, Sherry Yard, for inspiring an organizing principle of my training manual and feeding my sweet tooth.

Thank you to 2 Market Media team for your insights: Hank Norman, Steve Carlis, Terri Trespicio, and Jani Moon.

Thank you, Kim Haun, for always supporting our video endeavors and bringing your brilliant eye.

Thank you, Tom Danon and Nathan Ruyle, for your editorial perseverance.

Thank you to our Roll Model trailer video production team: Vance Jacobs, Eddie Filian, Colin Sims, and David Ventura; and talent: Jessica Hooper, Nicole Quibodeaux, Jeff Rancillo (and Sol City CrossFit), Delf Enriquez, and the Schiller family.

Thank you Tom Ivicevic and Carol Scott for being so darn cool and supportive.

Thank you Maria Gillespie, Harijot Khalsa, Brooke Siler and Elena Brower for sparking small ideas that I've grown into big tangible things.

Thank you to our graphic designers, Liz Ross and Heidi Broecking, for helping make us look so good.

Thank you to the body doctors who frequently change my mind and help me better my body: David Lepp, Sean Hampton, Dawn McCrory, and Chris Tosh.

Thank you to my publishing team at Victory Belt: Erich Krauss, Glen Cordoza, Michele Farrington, Susan Lloyd, and Jenny Castaneda. To the design team who brought my vision to life: Holly Jennings, Ismael Pinteño, Sean Farrington, Lance Freimuth, and the rest of your gifted team. And to Pam Mourouzis, whose edits were impeccable.

Thank you to all the Roll Models for their stories: Sharon Alkerstedt, Carlton Bennett, Lee Callans, Diane "V" Capaldi, Sarah Court, Tiffany Creswell-Yeager, Lisa Highfield, Karen Hypes, Jennifer Jennings, Eric Johnson, Amanda Joyce, Karen Kroll, Todd Lavictoire, Jennifer Lovely, Helen MacAvoy, Rebecca Moss, Carolyn Philips, Greg Reid, Emily Sonnenberg, Joanne Spence, Kelly Starrett, Lori Weider, Elizabeth Wipff, Krystin Zeiger, and Chloe.

Thank you to the operations team at Tune Up Fitness Worldwide for being my backbone: Robert Faust, Annie Brown, Nicole Quibodeaux, and Alexandra Ellis.

Thank you to my parents.

Thank you to Brian MacKenzie, Kelly Starrett, and Carl Paoli, the Victory Belt authors who paved the movement road before me.

Thank you to Tony Gardner, Carol Leggett, and Lawrence Ineno for "first stage" book support.

Thank you, Keith Wittenstein, for the best introduction ever.

Thank you to the whole crew at San Francisco CrossFit and to #Blondtrepreneur Juliet Starrett.

Thank you, Kelly Starrett, brother from another mother...you get your own line here.

Thank you, Katy Bowman, sister from another mother; I love your body brains.

Thank you for diving into research, Dr. Steven Capobianco and Robyn Capobianco.

Thank you to Rasmani Orth and the Kripalu Institute for welcoming my coursework.

Thank you for your spectacular friendship, Max "maxintosh" Miller, Carol Beitcher, and Chip Rosenbloom.

A warm thank you to Dr. Robert Schleip for organizing the "fascianistas" of the world and for sharing pages of your new book with me. You are a visionary.

Thank you, Manduka, for supplying me with the most beautiful yoga mats and blocks on the market.

Thank you to the hundreds of Yoga Tune Up Trainers and Teachers worldwide. You are improving lives every day and leading by example. You are all Roll Models.

Thank you to my readers, Dr. Laurie Bruckner, Sarah Court, Beth McNamara, Christopher Walling, and Robert Faust, for peering into the pages and giving me brilliant edits and guidance.

Special thanks to Sarah Court for collecting and composing many of the Roll Model stories in this book. Your eyes, ears, edits, and writing mastery are exceptional. You have the uncanny talent of being a translator for my own brain. You keep me on track and always have my back with your feedback. Your integrity, commitment, and grammar skills dazzle me. I love you.

Extra-special thanks to integrated anatomy pioneer and somanaut Gil Hedley for your anatomy mentorship and for allowing me to share your impeccably photographed images of fascia as the basis for the fascia illustrations in this book.

And thank you, Robert Faust, for all you do for me, us, and our business.

Photos of: Dawn Adams, Annelie Alexander, Trina Altman, Maura Barclay-Creighton, Laurel Beversdorf, Jennifer Black, Kevin W. Boyle, Sandy Byrne, Lillee Chandra, Nancy Cochren, Drew Corrigan, Sarah Court, Adam Dugas, Taylor Dunham, Daniel B. Edwards, Alexandra Ellis, Alyssa Farrell, Cathy Favelle, Oliana Gegprifti, Renee Holden, Alex Iglecia, Bridget Ingham, Kayla Irvys, Louis Jackson, Lynda Jaworski, Dagmar Khan, Ariel Kiley, David Kim, Sarah Kusch, Melissa Labatut, Todd Lavictoire, Matt Leger, Stephanie Leger, Heather Lindsay, Terry Littlefield, Brian MacKenzie, Mimi Martel, Anthony Martinez, Kristin Marvin, Dr. Stuart McGill, Yasmen Mehta, Max Miller, Matt Nadler, Blair Ofner, Alex and Kevin Quibodeaux, Holli Rabishaw, Regina Santos, Kimberly Shultz, Jennifer Slot, Matt Sharpe, Luke Sniewski, Elissa Strutton, Brooke Thomas, Amanda Tripp, Dinneen Viggiano, Marion Vu, Jennifer Wesanko, Maricarmen Wilson (inspiredshakti.com), Elizabeth Wipff, Keith Wittenstein, Nikki Wong

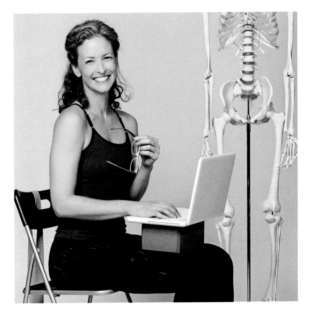

Sarah Court

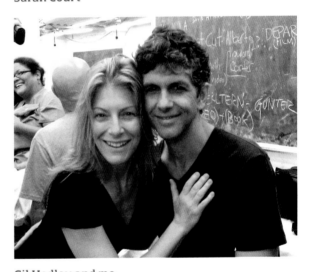

Gil Hedley and me

Cover design and technique icons: Heidi Broecking

Cover photo: Bradford Rogne

Cover model: Sarah Kusch

Book sequence photography: Glen Cordoza

Additional interior photography: Aliya Alewine, Stacy Berg, Erica Camile, Gina Conte, Shawn De Salvo, Amy Deguio, Taylor Dunham, Alexandra Ellis, Giancarla Griffith-Boyle, Matt Huber, Samantha Jacoby, Karen Kirkland, Anette Kraemer-Botosic, Mark Leibowitz, Heather Lindsay, Gillian Mandich, Kate Morgan, Sabrina Polizzi, Michael Sanville, Todd Vitti

Book design by: Yordan and Boryana Terziev

Index

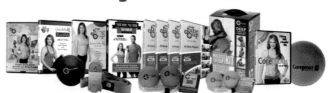